FEMTOSECOND LASER-ASSISTED CATARACT SURGERY

FACTS AND RESULTS

FEMTOSECOND LASER-ASSISTED CATARACT SURGERY

FACTS AND RESULTS

Edited by
Zoltán Z. Nagy, MD, PhD, DSc
Professor of Ophthalmology
Department of Ophthalmology
Semmelweis University
Budapest, Hungary

SLACK
INCORPORATED

***The Classic Papers in Section II were previously published as articles in the* Journal of Refractive Surgery.**

www.Healio.com/books

ISBN: 978-1-61711-996-5

The procedures and practices described in this publication should be implemented in a manner consistent with the professional standards set for the circumstances that apply in each specific situation. Every effort has been made to confirm the accuracy of the information presented and to correctly relate generally accepted practices. The authors, editors, and publisher cannot accept responsibility for errors or exclusions or for the outcome of the material presented herein. There is no expressed or implied warranty of this book or information imparted by it. Care has been taken to ensure that drug selection and dosages are in accordance with currently accepted/recommended practice. Off-label uses of drugs may be discussed. Due to continuing research, changes in government policy and regulations, and various effects of drug reactions and interactions, it is recommended that the reader carefully review all materials and literature provided for each drug, especially those that are new or not frequently used. Some drugs or devices in this publication have clearance for use in a restricted research setting by the Food and Drug and Administration or FDA. Each professional should determine the FDA status of any drug or device prior to use in their practice.

Any review or mention of specific companies or products is not intended as an endorsement by the author or publisher.

SLACK Incorporated uses a review process to evaluate submitted material. Prior to publication, educators or clinicians provide important feedback on the content that we publish. We welcome feedback on this work.

Published by: SLACK Incorporated, 6900 Grove Road, Thorofare, NJ 08086 USA
Telephone: 856-848-1000, Fax: 856-848-6091, www.Healio.com/books

Contact SLACK Incorporated for more information about other books in this field or about the availability of our books from distributors outside the United States.

Library of Congress Cataloging-in-Publication Data

Nagy, Zoltan Z. (Zoltan Zsolt), 1961- author.
Femtosecond laser-assisted cataract surgery : facts and results / Zoltan Z. Nagy.
p. ; cm.
Includes bibliographical references and index.
ISBN 978-1-61711-996-5 (alk. paper)
I. Title.
[DNLM: 1. Cataract Extraction--methods. 2. Laser Therapy. WW 260]
RE451
617.7'42059--dc23
2014009011

Printed in the United States of America.

Last digit is print number: 10 9 8 7 6 5 4 3 2 1

Dedication

To my family—
to Ildikó, my wife, and to my daughters, Daniella and Lili.

Contents

Acknowledgments

I would like to acknowledge all my co-authors, who helped from the first femtolaser cataract surgery through the later years. I am especially thankful to Professor Tibor Juhasz, Ron Kurtz, Eric Weinberg, Trudy Larkins, and to many others who had a strong belief that femtolaser technology would change anterior segment surgery of the eye.

About the Editor

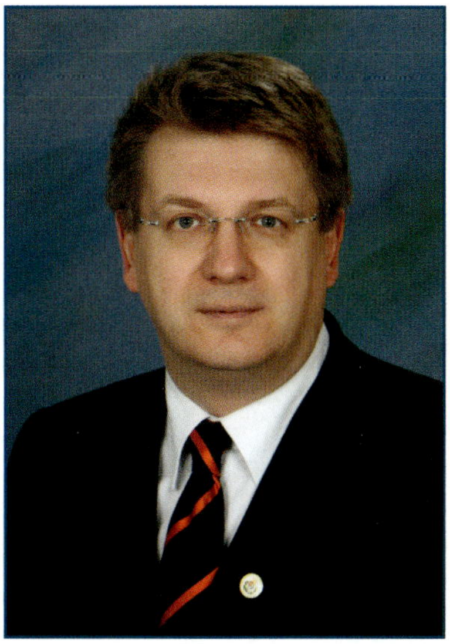

Zoltán Z. Nagy, MD, PhD, DSc is a Professor of Ophthalmology in the Department of Ophthalmology at Semmelweis University, Budapest, Hungary. He received his MD in 1986 at the Szent-Györgyi Albert Medical University, Szeged, Hungary. In the same year, he started his residency program in ophthalmology. After specialization in general ophthalmology, he received a scholarship in the Department of Ophthalmology in Erlangen at the Friedrich Alexander Universität Erlangen-Nürnberg with Professor Gottfried Otto Naumann. In Erlangen he studied the role of secondary ultraviolet exposure in eyes that had had refractive surgery before. He published an article in *Ophthalmology* (1997) on the harmful role of ultraviolet exposure in eyes with previous photorefractive keratectomy during the avascular corneal healing. Afterward he did a fellowship at Moorfields Eye Hospital in London, England.

Dr. Nagy is a dedicated anterior segment surgeon. In 2008, he performed the first femtosecond laser cataract surgery in a human eye. His scientific contribution was awarded with the Waring Prize in 2010 in New York. In 2012, he received the Casebeer Prize from the International Society of Refractive Surgery, among numerous other awards. He and his co-workers published more than 20 peer-reviewed articles in the field of femtolaser-assisted cataract surgery. He receives invitations for live surgery events as a surgeon and presenter during international congresses. Presently he serves as Dean of the Faculty of Health Sciences at Semmelweis University.

Contributing Authors

Ahmed A. Abdou, MD, PhD (Classic Paper 12)
Vissum Corporation
Alicante, Spain
Ophthalmology Department
Assiut University Hospital
Egypt

Jorge L. Alió, MD, PhD (Classic Papers 2, 7, 12)
Department of Ophthalmology
Universidad Miguel Hernández
Vissum Corporation
Alicante, Spain

Roberto Bellucci, MD (Foreword)
Director of Hospital Ophthalmology
Hospital and University of Verona
Verona, Italy

Zoltán I. Bocskai (Original Chapter 5)
Department of Structural Mechanics
Budapest University of Technology and Economics
Budapest, Hungary

Imre Bojtár, PhD, CSc (Original Chapter 5)
Department of Structural Mechanics
Budapest University of Technology and Economics
Budapest, Hungary

Eric Donnenfeld, MD (Foreword; Classic Papers 2, 9)
Clinical Professor of Ophthalmology
New York University
New York, New York
Trustee
Dartmouth Medical School
Hanover, New Hampshire

Árpád Dunai, MD (Original Chapter 8)
Department of Ophthalmology
Semmelweis University
Budapest, Hungary

Mónika Ecsedy, MD, PhD (Original Chapter 9; Classic Paper 10)
Department of Ophthalmology
Semmelweis University
Budapest, Hungary

Roberto Fernández-Buenaga, MD (Classic Paper 12)
Vissum Corporation
Alicante, Spain

Tamás Filkorn, MD (Original Chapters 6, 7; Classic Papers 1, 2, 8, 10, 11, 12, 13, 14, 15)
Department of Ophthalmology
Semmelweis University
Budapest, Hungary

Róbert Gergely, MD (Classic Papers 13, 15)
Department of Ophthalmology
Semmelweis University
Budapest, Hungary

Andrea Gyenes, MD (Original Chapter 13; Classic Paper 15)
Department of Ophthalmology
Semmelweis University
Budapest, Hungary

Éva Horváth, MD (Original Chapter 6; Classic Paper 8)
Department of Ophthalmology
Semmelweis University
Budapest, Hungary

Jaime Javaloy, MD, PhD (Classic Paper 12)
Vissum Corporation
Alicante, Spain
Division of Ophthalmology
Universidad Miguel Hernández
Alicante, Spain

Éva Juhász, MD (Original Chapter 13; Classic Paper 14)
Department of Ophthalmology
Semmelweis University
Budapest, Hungary

Tibor Juhasz, PhD, DSc (Original Chapter 1; Classic Paper 2)
Department of Ophthalmology
Semmelweis University
Budapest, Hungary
Department of Ophthalmology
University of California–Irvine
Irvine, California

Zoltán Kiss, PhD (Original Chapter 5)
Department of Polymer Engineering
Budapest University of Technology and Economics
Budapest, Hungary

Michael C. Knorz, MD (Original Chapters 6, 7, 8; Classic Papers 2, 3, 4, 5, 6, 7, 8, 9, 11, 13, 14)
Medical Faculty
Mannheim of Heidelberg University
FreeVis LASIK Center
Medical University of Mannheim
Mannheim, Germany

Illés Kovács, MD, PhD (Original Chapters 6, 7, 9, 11; Classic Papers 3, 4, 7, 8, 9, 10, 11, 15)
Department of Ophthalmology
Semmelweis University
Budapest, Hungary

Kinga Kránitz, MD (Original Chapters 4, 6, 8, 11, 13; Classic Papers 2, 3, 4, 5, 6, 7, 9, 13, 15)
Department of Ophthalmology
Semmelweis University
Budapest, Hungary

Ronald R. Krueger, MD, MSE (Foreword)
Professor of Ophthalmology
Lerner College of Medicine of Case Western Reserve University
Medical Director
Department of Refractive Surgery
Cole Eye Institute
Cleveland, Ohio

Kata Miháltz, MD, PhD (Original Chapter 7; Classic Papers 3, 4, 5, 6, 7, 10, 11)
Department of Ophthalmology
Semmelweis University
Budapest, Hungary

Rudy M. Nuijts, MD, PhD (Classic Paper 9)
University Eye Clinic Maastricht
Maastricht University Medical Centre
Maastricht, The Netherlands

Gábor László Sándor, MD (Original Chapter 5; Classic Papers 5, 9, 14)
Department of Ophthalmology
Semmelweis University
Budapest, Hungary

Melvin Sarayba, MD (Classic Paper 1)
LenSx Lasers Inc
Aliso Viejo, California

Gabor Mark Somfai, MD, PhD (Original Chapter 9)
Department of Ophthalmology
Semmelweis University
Budapest, Hungary

Felipe Soria, MD (Classic Paper 12)
Vissum Corporation
Alicante, Spain

Andrea Szigeti, MD (Classic Papers 6, 14)
Department of Ophthalmology
Semmelweis University
Budapest, Hungary

Ágnes I. Takács, MD (Original Chapters 5, 6, 7, 13; Classic Papers 1, 2, 3, 4, 5, 6, 7, 8, 10, 11, 13, 14, 15)
Department of Ophthalmology
Semmelweis University
Budapest, Hungary

Preface

For the past five decades, ophthalmology has had a pioneering role in laser application. Recently, femtolaser technology has conquered ophthalmic surgery; femtosecond lasers were first used in corneal application and then in critical steps of cataract surgery. Lasers do not replace good surgeons but help good surgeons provide consistent results for both patients and ophthalmologists. At present, central continuous curvilinear capsulorrhexis, fragmentation/liquefaction, and corneal wound and arcuate corneal incisions are the most prominent features of the femtolaser method. Peer-reviewed results are needed to establish the exact role of femtolasers in cataract surgery. Consistent surgical results are needed to fully benefit from premium lenses that correct for presbyopia and corneal astigmatism and correct for higher-order aberrations in eyes having had refractive surgery before.

I consider myself a lucky man. When I first heard about the possible application of femtolasers in cataract surgery, I felt the same excitement as when I started to perform refractive surgery in the early 1990s. When I saw the first excimer laser treatment, I immediately felt that it would change my life. I performed all kinds of refractive and cataract surgeries. Later, during an American Academy of Ophthalmology meeting in New Orleans, I met Professor Juhasz and first learned about the possibilities of femtolaser cataract surgery. Once again I felt optimistic and excited, and in August 2008, we performed the first capsulorrhexis in a human eye with the femtosecond laser. And it worked immediately.

Of course, it was a long journey before we could demonstrate the method during a live surgery transmitted from Budapest to the Vienna European Society of Cataract & Refractive Surgeons (ESCRS) meeting. My responsibility was huge; according to estimates, more than 3000 ophthalmologists witnessed the first femtolaser-assisted cataract surgery. A responsible and very helpful team was behind me; everyone knew his or her task. Everything went according to plan, the method received FDA and CE approval, and the first machine was launched during the Vienna ESCRS meeting.

By now, more than 150,000 surgeries have been performed worldwide; different platforms offer newer methods and possible applications for surgeons and patients. During local and international meetings, femtolaser cataract surgery is often discussed; symposia, courses, and free papers are dedicated to the method.

This book summarizes the 5-year results of our team, focusing on the most important results. Besides clinical results with cataract and corneal applications, basic research regarding the strength of the anterior capsule is also presented. The most important publications of our team are also included in the book.

Hopefully surgeons will benefit from the book and the method. As femtolaser data collection and evaluation continue, I conclude with the words of Charles Kelman: "Doctors debate and patients decide."

—Zoltán Z. Nagy MD, PhD, DSc

Foreword

While reading this excellent book by Prof. Nagy, it seems impossible that only three decades ago cataract surgery meant intracapsular cryoextraction for most ophthalmic surgeons. At that time, nobody could imagine all the developments both in the technique and in the implants that took place in just a few years. The advent of intraocular lens (IOL) implantation prompted surgeons toward extracapsular extraction, phacoemulsification led to foldable IOLs, which in turn originated the microincision cataract surgery evolution. This evolution could not have happened without the sacrifice and the visionary ideas of a few doctors really interested in innovation. Innovators are those unsatisfied with current technology who are able to invent and walk along never-conceived paths. History tells us that they are usually laughed at and then fought with before their ideas are accepted and they are recognized as masters. Luckily, we are living in different times now, times of incredibly rapid change that do not consider innovation and opportunity a danger.

The application of femtosecond laser technology to cataract surgery is the latest innovation in the most frequently performed surgery in the world, and it appears to be a revolution rather than an evolution. The ability to perform intraocular surgery in a closed eye dates back more than 30 years ago to the first laser applications to the retina and to the posterior capsule, but only with the advent of devices that could measure the inner eye was a real cyber knife developed for ophthalmology. With femtosecond laser application to cataract surgery, we can program the laser part of the surgery at the computer, and the laser will perform every maneuver without mistakes. The expert surgeon will appreciate the increased precision, especially of the capsulotomy; the novice surgeon will experience a quick and safe way to surgery.

Prof. Nagy's working group in Budapest, Hungary, is recognized and appreciated for introducing the femtosecond laser in cataract surgery. The first procedure was performed in Budapest in 2008, and since then a lot of work has been done and a number of papers published in the international literature. As femtolaser cataract surgery is spreading all around the globe, we still look at Budapest to discover ideas, applications, and results. Femtolaser cataract surgery is still in its infancy, and the growing interest of surgeons and technicians will probably lead to a brilliant future in the final interest of our patients.

The latest advancements of Prof. Nagy's team are reported in the first part of this book, a true "femto-manual" that every ophthalmic surgeon should read. There we can find the dreams and the reality of daily work carried out for many years. The second part is a collection of papers previously published by Prof. Nagy and co-workers in the international literature still endowed with the freshness and excitement of novelty. Having them together in a single book will help those interested in original, peer-reviewed papers for scientific purposes.

As the improved visual and refractive results obtained with the femtolaser in comparison with phacoemulsification alone are receiving wider confirmation, we already know that the precision and repeatability of the capsulotomy removes one of the most important factors affecting the outcome. As a consequence, we will increase our knowledge of IOL- and patient-related factors, and the very study of new IOL material and design will be shorter and more precise. In this respect, femtolaser cataract surgery will have a positive impact on the entirety of implant surgery. We as surgeons will also be affected. Progressive automation will affect our ability to perform old maneuvers, and it might be difficult to teach and to learn capsulorrhexis in the future. Other concepts and solutions will be implemented and developed. We can't stop evolution. We all want to read many books as innovative and as exciting as this one.

—Roberto Bellucci, MD
Director of Hospital Ophthalmology
Hospital and University of Verona
Verona, Italy

Foreword

We are now witnessing the natural progression of cataract surgery from intracapsular, to extracapsular, to phacoemulsification, and now to the femtosecond laser. With any new disruptive technology there are pioneers who provide the leadership and direction to take an innovative idea and create the transformation that will change the future of our specialty. Dr. Zoltán Nagy is the undisputed innovator most responsible for the clinical development of femtosecond laser-assisted cataract surgery. Not only was Dr. Nagy the first to perform the full spectrum of femtosecond laser cataract surgery, he is also the leading author in the peer-reviewed literature. Dr. Nagy constantly asks and answers the question of how can we improve our surgical techniques to the betterment of our patients. He is a superb surgeon with many techniques to his credit, but most remarkably, he possesses the rarest of all personal attributes. He is an original thinker. Dr. Nagy is bold, creative, logical, and innovative, and his patient care is firmly and well grounded on the fundamental principle that no matter what we do, our patients come first.

The future of cataract surgery will lie in our ability to correct the limitations we currently have and produce a more optimized cataract extraction procedure. That future will begin with the increased utilization of the femtosecond laser. Femtosecond laser cataract surgery has already been established as superior to conventional phacoemulsification in several parameters and the potential for improvements is limitless. Aspects of the cataract procedure will be performed with the femtosecond laser that are simply impossible with conventional phacoemulsification. The ability to produce true self-sealing cataract incisions with reverse side cuts should reduce the incidence of endophthalmitis. Atraumatic capsulotomies and lens disruption can be performed in cases of trauma with zonular dehiscence through vitreous in the anterior chamber. Refractive incisions are now computer controlled and do not rely on surgeon skill or experience. The use of a femtosecond laser system will provide faster, safer, easier, customizable, adjustable, and fully repeatable astigmatic incisions. Removing the inconsistencies in the astigmatic procedure will improve our understanding and accuracy of astigmatic incisions and should provide improved refractive results and patient satisfaction. The ability to perform intrastromal ablations for astigmatism management cannot be achieved with manual incisions. The optimal placement of the capsulorrhexis on the center of the capsular bag, over the pupil, or centered on the visual axis will be possible with image guided laser surgery. Finally, intraocular lens design will be revolutionized by the ability to create regular, reproducible capsulotomies and lens disruption.

Femtosecond Laser-Assisted Cataract Surgery: Facts and Results represents the best of Dr. Nagy and his colleagues' unique and original approach to femtosecond laser-assisted cataract surgery. The book is a comprehensive analysis of the benefits and pitfalls of this extraordinary technology designed to make all of us better surgeons. It summarizes all of the best and most useful and practical pearls that have been developed. Dr. Nagy has brought together an internationally recognized group of authors and written a definitive book on femtosecond laser-assisted cataract surgery. This book will be widely read by anterior segment surgeons who wish to add to their surgical armamentarium and will be an important contribution to ophthalmology.

—*Eric Donnenfeld, MD*
Clinical Professor of Ophthalmology
New York University
New York, New York
Trustee
Dartmouth Medical School
Hanover, New Hampshire

Foreword

As the editor of a book on laser-assisted cataract surgery myself,[1] I can tell you that there is a fine line between "hype" and "fact" with laser-assisted cataract surgery. The clear "fact" is the superior precision involved in the laser's incision and excision of ocular tissues. However, with all the commercial investment involved in getting a system, how can one avoid the promotional "hype," and be objective about its true clinical relevance?

Of all the individuals who might be qualified to discriminate between "hype" and "fact," Zoltán Nagy offers the greatest confidence of objectivity in this book, and he does so for several reasons: 1) He is a university Professor of Ophthalmology, who is dedicated not only to patient care, but to the scientific method and education. 2) He has the greatest clinical experience with laser-assisted cataract surgery, as he performed the first procedure in 2008, and has been the first to be clinically involved in all the upgrades and technology modifications of the first commercial system since that time. 3) He is the most prolific author, having published more than 20 peer-reviewed manuscripts on this technology, including the very first publication in 2009,[2] which is Classic Paper 1 of this book. 4) He is an honest educator, who communicates with personal integrity and objectivity, so when he reports on his experience, you can believe it to be true and not "hype."

Up until now, you could listen to or even read about Zoltán's experience in the many lectures he has given and articles he has published. This book now puts all that experience into one source document, and it does so in a way that is very different from other books on the subject. While most books, like my own,[1] compile the experience of many authors, this book is unique in that it highlights, with the help of others, the experience of a single, most experienced author. All, except the first, of its 28 chapters, are authored by Dr. Nagy, with more than half being his published, peer-reviewed manuscripts from the *Journal of Refractive Surgery*. This 5-year experience by one of the primary leaders of laser-assisted cataract surgery, as a controversial and disruptive technology, is an invaluable resource to the many cataract surgeons who are yet unfamiliar with this technology. It is perhaps the most practical resource available to date. Personally, as president of the International Society of Refractive Surgery, I am proud of Zoltán's accomplishments, and impressed at the scope of his contribution in helping to make laser-assisted cataract surgery a part of refractive surgery. I look forward to his continued contribution in the future, as refractive laser-assisted cataract surgery moves more and more into mainstream ophthalmology.

—*Ronald R. Krueger, MD, MSE*
Professor of Ophthalmology
Lerner College of Medicine of Case Western Reserve University
Medical Director
Department of Refractive Surgery
Cole Eye Institute
Cleveland, Ohio

References

1. Krueger RR, Talamo JH, Lindstrom RL. *Textbook of Refractive Laser Assisted Cataract Surgery (ReLACS)*. New York, NY: Springer; 2013.
2. Nagy Z, Takacs A, Filkorn T, Sarayba M. Initial clinical evaluation of an intraocular femtosecond laser in cataract surgery. *J Refract Surg*. 2009;25(12):1053-1060.

Introduction

I performed the first femtosecond laser-assisted cataract surgery in a human eye in August 2008. I knew that it might be a historical date in cataract surgery in the future. Of course, the first capsulotomy, lens fragmentation, corneal wound creation, and arcuate keratotomy seemed easy at first glance, but there was much developmental work required by the team behind me until we were able to present the first clinical results during a San Francisco meeting.

After the first femtolaser cataract surgeries, I realized that although this technology is not principally different from traditional phacoemulsification, it needs another approach. There is a learning curve and surgeons should accept it before starting the procedure.

Femtolaser technology offers an alternative approach toward the first clinical steps of lens surgery, offering higher predictability and safety during capsulotomy, fragmentation, and wound creation. It may provide a sound basis for further developments both in cataract and corneal surgery. If newer lenses appear, the surgical technology might be able to achieve all the results that the new lenses might promise. This is surely not a technology to replace good surgeons but one to help good surgeons.

With this book I tried to summarize all of our experiences from the starting point until now. Along with my co-authors, I write for those just starting femtolaser-assisted cataract surgery and also for those who are already advanced and skilled femtolaser users.

Personal thoughts and advice are important when starting with a new technology; in this book I try to share mine with the reader.

I am very thankful to my family, teachers, colleagues, co-workers, and surgeons who actively helped and may help further in the mission of improving vision and cataract surgery by using femtolaser technology.

—Zoltán Z. Nagy MD, PhD, DSc

SECTION I

Original Chapters

Competing Femtosecond Laser Technologies for Cataract Surgery

Tibor Juhasz, PhD, DSc

Abstract

Rapid development of competing femtosecond laser technologies for cataract surgery has occurred during the past several years. These technologies differ in their appearance, software, and patient interface, but they all have the same basic characteristics. They all apply some type of 3-dimensional optical imaging modalities to determine the exact locations of the surgery targets, and they all use femtosecond laser pulses to perform the surgical incisions. Because of their confined tissue effects and minimized collateral tissue damage, femtosecond lasers, which became practical technically in the early 1990s, soon became considered for high-precision ocular surgery. Corneal femtosecond laser surgery was the first application attempted with this technology in the late 1990s due to relatively easy laser beam delivery, referenced from a contact lens placed on the ocular surface. Over the past decade, these devices have become the dominant tool for LASIK flap cutting in many countries. The addition of a high-precision imaging technique enabled accurate targeting of tissue beyond the cornea, such as the crystalline lens, allowing the development of femtosecond laser cataract surgery. In this chapter, basic principles and operational characteristics of femtosecond laser technology for cataract surgery are generally described. Similarities and differences between the competing technologies are also discussed.

Newly developed laser technologies, such as femtosecond lasers, have gained early applications in ophthalmic surgery. Femtosecond lasers utilize photodisruption to mediate their surgical effects. Photodisrution is a complex, nonlinear process based on ionization in transparent tissue. As in inorganic materials, tissue photodisruption begins with laser-induced optical breakdown, when a strongly focused, short-duration laser pulse generates a high-intensity electric field, leading to the formation of a mixture of free electrons and ions that constitutes the plasma state.[1] The optically generated hot plasma expands with supersonic velocity displacing surrounding tissue.[1-5] As the plasma expansion slows, the supersonic displacement front propagates through the tissue as a shock wave. The shock wave loses energy and velocity as it propagates, relaxing to an ordinary acoustic wave that dissipates harmlessly.[6] Adiabatic expansion of the plasma occurs on a time scale that is short in comparison to the local thermal diffusion time constant, thereby confining thermal damage. The cooling plasma vaporizes a small volume of tissue, eventually forming a cavitation bubble. The cavitation bubble consists mainly of CO_2, N_2, and H_2O, which can diffuse out from the tissue via normal mechanisms.[7]

Photodisruption with the nanosecond-pulsed neodymium:yttrium-aluminum-garnet (Nd:YAG) laser was already well established clinically in the early 1980s for procedures such as posterior capsulotomy and internal sclerostomy.[8] These procedures were associated with relatively large collateral tissue damage zones due to the high-energy threshold associated with the nanosecond pulse durations. Laser–tissue interaction studies have shown that the photodisruption threshold (and therefore the amount of laser energy deposited in the tissue) can be markedly decreased when the pulse duration is shortened to the hundred femtosecond range.[9] The decreased laser pulse energy results in smaller shock waves and cavitation bubbles. Incisions are created by scanning the focal spot of the laser pulse so that the cavitation bubbles are coalescing, thus creating a cleavage in the tissue. The markedly reduced cavitation bubble size of the femtosecond laser photodisruption provides more precise incisions

Nagy ZZ, ed. *Femtosecond Laser-Assisted Cataract Surgery: Facts and Results* (pp 3-10).

while the most important consequence of the reduced shock wave range is minimized collateral damage in the tissue adjacent to the incisions. Additionally, the development of compact diode-pumped femtosecond laser technologies, such as Nd:glass and ytterbium based laser crystals has further enabled commercial developments of femtosecond laser technologies for ophthalmic surgery.[10]

Operating Principles of Ophthalmic Femtosecond Lasers

Cataract surgery with intraocular lens (IOL) implantation is the most common ophthalmic surgical procedure worldwide. It is also the most common surgery that corrects refractive error, performed over five times more frequently than corneal refractive surgery.[11] Phacoemulsification is the dominant form of cataract surgery in developed countries, accounting for more than 90% of procedures.[12,13] While there has been a number of recent developments in IOL technology, the basic phacoemulsification procedure has remained largely unchanged over the past 20 years, involving a series of individual steps including corneal incision creation, capsulorrhexis, and phacofragmentation.

Although highly successful, each of these manual steps presents an opportunity for improvement in both safety and effectiveness. For example, manual capsulorrhexis results in capsular tears in approximately 1% of cases, and its limited diameter predictability can affect IOL centration, postoperative anterior chamber depth, and posterior capsular opacification rates.[14-18] Separately, the surgical challenges posed by nuclear chopping techniques have hindered widespread adoption, despite evidence that they reduce ultrasound requirements relative to traditional phacoemulsification.[18]

The precision of femtosecond lasers can potentially be directed toward the various steps in cataract surgery.[9,19-22] To understand the operating principles of cataract femtosecond lasers, however, it is important to briefly review the characteristics of corneal-only femtosecond lasers, which were developed prior to the cataract lasers.

Operating Principles of Corneal Femtosecond Lasers

The cornea presents an attractive initial target for femtosecond laser surgical applications because it is easily accessible and lacks blood vessels. Only 500- to 600-μm thick centrally, the cornea allows delivery of femtosecond pulses with negligible nonlinear effects. The cornea is highly transparent in the near infrared region, up to 1.2-μm wavelength, allowing the use of the near infrared femtosecond lasers without any restrictions.

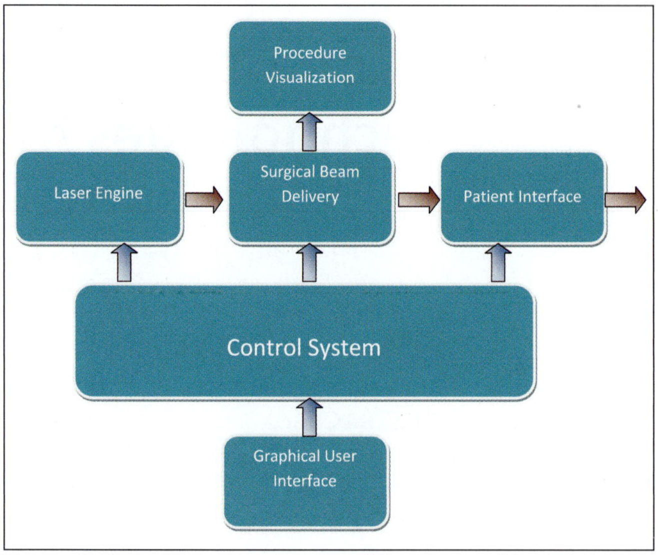

Figure 1. The schematics of a corneal femtosecond laser.

A block diagram of a corneal femtosecond laser is shown in Figure 1. The most important building blocks are the laser source (or engine), the delivery system, the patient interface, and the control system.

Since high-precision cutting of the cornea requires generation of cavitation bubbles that are less than 10 μm in diameter, the use of low-energy laser pulses is necessary. This requirement puts a strong limitation on the pulse duration of the laser. Earlier investigations on the photodisruptive damage threshold on the surface of corneal tissue indicated that a considerable decrease of the damage threshold can be obtained as the pulse duration decreased from the nanosecond range to the hundred femtosecond pulse duration range.[10] Accordingly, the pulse duration of commercially available femtosecond lasers ranges from 200 to 800 fs.

To minimize collateral tissue effects, the per pulse energy of the corneal femtosecond lasers is best set as close as possible to the photodisruption breakdown threshold. While the first commercial lasers were introduced with pulse energies from 1 to 3 μJ, more recent corneal systems operate in the sub-μJ energy range.

Because creation of a corneal flap requires several million laser pulses and very short procedure times are desired, the repetition rate of corneal femtosecond lasers must be very high. In fact, repetition rate has been the key technology driver during the development of corneal femtosecond lasers. While the first femtosecond laser had a repetition rate of 15 KHz at introduction (IntraLase Inc, Irvine, California), all systems now are marketed with much higher repetition rates, from 150 kHz up to the megahertz range (Ziemer AG, Port, Switzerland). While repetition rate is an important parameter, the procedure time is not inversely proportional with this value. Because lasers with higher repetition rates also utilize lower energy pulses that are placed closer to each other, more total pulses are required than lower repetition lasers, somewhat limiting the potential reduction in procedure time. While the procedure time for the first IntraLase laser was approximately 1 minute, most currently marketed lasers create flaps in approximately 10 to 20 seconds.

Although the femtosecond laser source is the technologically most advanced building block of a corneal laser system, the beam delivery device is equally important and expensive. The most important property of the beam delivery device is the numerical aperture of the focusing objective that determines the spot size of the system. Achieving smaller spot size allows the system to use smaller laser pulse energies and provides higher flap depth precision. Therefore, the designers of all commercially available corneal femtosecond laser systems try to achieve the smallest possible spot size allowed by the geometry of the human head. It is difficult to compare spot sizes of the different corneal lasers, since numerous definitions of the spot size are used in the literature, but most companies are quoting their system's spot size in the 2- to 3-μm diameter range. One of the most challenging difficulties of the beam delivery system design is achieving a homogeneous and distortion-free spot size in the entire cylinder shaped scanning volume with usual dimensions of 10 mm in diameter and 1 mm in height. The beam is scanned within this volume using a 3-dimensional scanning system. Depth scanning (usually referred to as Z directional scanning) is achieved by a moving lens, and lateral scanning (X-Y scanning) is achieved by angular movement of small mirrors attached to fast scanning motors.

The spatially confined surgical effect of the femtosecond laser, together with the fine spatial control of the focal spot with respect to the corneal surface, allows the execution of highly precise cuts in the cornea. To accomplish this, all corneal procedures also utilize a suction ring and a contact lens (flat or curved) located at the tip of the laser delivery system. The suction ring fixates the eye, allowing the corneal anterior surface to temporarily assume the curvature of the contact glass (Fig 2). The depth of the cut is calibrated relative to the lower surface of the contact glass, which provides a reference surface for the calibration of the laser, achieving depth precision of less than 10 μm.[23] A flap is created by scanning a spiral or raster pattern of laser pulses at the desired depth to create a resection plane parallel to the applanated corneal surface. An arc is then scanned with progressive movement closer to the surface to create a hinged side-cut. Following creation of the flap, the suction ring is released and the applanating contact lens removed. The flap is then elevated to facilitate excimer laser treatment.

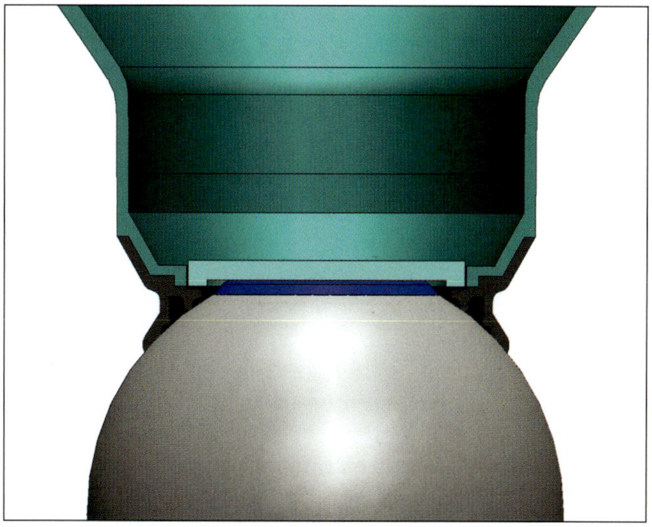

Figure 2. The flat applanating patient interface.

Clinical studies indicate that reproducible 100-μm thick corneal flaps can be created for LASIK surgery.[23] The accuracy and reproducibility of femtosecond laser flaps generally surpass those created with traditional mechanical microkeratomes, thereby enabling more consistent outcomes and safety.[23,24]

Since 2001, several corneal femtosecond laser systems have been introduced, primarily for LASIK flap creation.[24] Although there are several new devices available on the market today, the majority of the flap cutting procedures is still performed by different generations of the IntraLase device (Abbott Medical Optics, Santa Ana, California).

While flap creation is the most common application of the corneal femtosecond lasers, several stand-alone refractive procedures that use only the femtosecond laser are under clinical investigations. These include removal of laser-cut lenticules,[25] as well as the combination of direct volumetric tissue destruction and corneal biomechanical changes induced by selective femtosecond laser treatment.[26]

In addition to refractive corneal procedures, corneal femtosecond laser technology has also been evaluated for various corneal transplantation procedures. Faster visual rehabilitation and improved refractive outcomes have been reported when femtosecond laser cuts were used to create self-sealing corneal cuts in full-thickness corneal transplantation surgery.[27]

Operating Principles of Cataract Femtosecond Lasers

Among the several important differences between corneal and cataract laser surgical systems, the most important is the difference in the targeted tissue. By definition, corneal lasers target only corneal tissue, while cataract lasers have three tissue targets: the crystalline lens, the anterior lens capsule, and the cornea. This obviously drives major differences in technical requirements, since corneal systems deliver laser energy only to approximately 150-µm depth, while cataract systems are required to cut tissue located as deep as 9 mm from the corneal surface. Since laser energy needs to be delivered considerably deeper into the eye, losses that occur during beam propagation must be compensated by the laser source. Due to limitations in the focusing cone angle when the crystalline lens or the lens capsule is targeted, the achievable laser spot size is also larger in the lens than in the cornea, further contributing to the need for larger laser energy for incisions in the crystalline lens. Although reduction in the required laser energy may occur as delivery system technology improves, currently the use of pulse energies in the 5-µJ range is required in the lens.[28]

While corneal cuts can be performed with the same spot size the system produces in the lens, a smaller spot size in the corneal cuts allows the use of smaller laser pulse energies, which is advantageous as we know from the corneal laser experience. Therefore, the development of a delivery system that can deliver a variable focusing cone angle may be desirable, though this introduces considerable additional complexity for the surgical beam delivery system.

Since the anterior chamber depth and the lens thickness vary from patient to patient, there is a clear necessity for an accurate ranging device that locates the exact position of the surgical target. To date, all femtosecond laser cataract surgery systems have based this ranging device on some form of optical imaging. Three companies (Alcon LenSx Inc, Aliso Viejo, California; OptiMedica Corp, Santa Clara, California; and Bausch + Lomb–Technolas Perfect Vision AG, Munich, Germany) use optical coherence tomography (OCT) technology, while one company (LensAR Inc, Winter Park, Florida) uses a Scheimpflug imaging–based device to locate the targeted tissue. After obtaining the image of the anterior segment of the eye, some level of image processing is necessary in order to locate and visualize the targeted tissue. Thus, the block diagram of a cataract surgical laser, shown in Figure 3, is more complex than that of the corneal laser with the addition of a high-precision 3-dimensional imaging system coupled to the beam delivery device and an image-processing and visualization unit that provides information to the user and feeds back to the control system. While accurate cross-calibration in between the imaging and the beam-scanning devices is important, the requirement for resolution of the 3-dimensional imaging device is determined by the surgical beam delivery device. Since higher accuracy than the depth of focus of the surgical beam focusing objective is not needed, the requirement for depth resolution is approximately 10 µm.

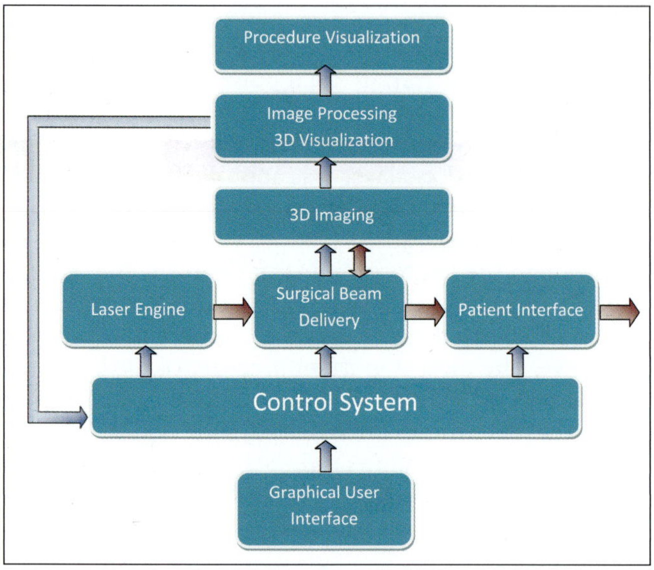

Figure 3. The schematics of a cataract femtosecond laser.

The markedly increased beam delivery range and the addition of the 3-dimensional imaging device increase the complexity of the cataract laser beam delivery system. Clearly, the most complex building block of the cataract laser is the beam delivery device.

The higher per pulse energy requirement increases the average power of the laser source to several times higher than that of a corneal laser engine. Since the maximum average power generated by the specific laser material is limited by available pump power and the thermal characteristics of the laser material, cataract lasers operate at lower repetition rates than corneal systems. To date, repetition rates from 50 kHz up to 100 KHz have been reported for cataract surgery laser systems.

It is important to note, however, that the repetition rate of a cataract system is not such a key driver as it is for a corneal system. In the crystalline lens, faster procedure time can be achieved by using slightly higher laser-pulse energies and placing the spot and layer separation during scanning somewhat further apart. Using larger energy in the cornea may be disadvantageous because it may cause tissue inflammation.[23] However, the lens material is removed during the cataract procedure; therefore, the use of higher energies does not have clinical consequences.

Because procedure times for cataract surgery are somewhat longer than that for corneal flap cutting, and because cataract patients are generally older, any increase in intraocular pressure should be minimized during the laser procedure. Additionally, posterior corneal wrinkles created by applanation of the cornea may reduce the quality of the laser beam delivered to the crystalline lens, resulting in decreased cutting performance. These requirements preclude the use of a flat applanating

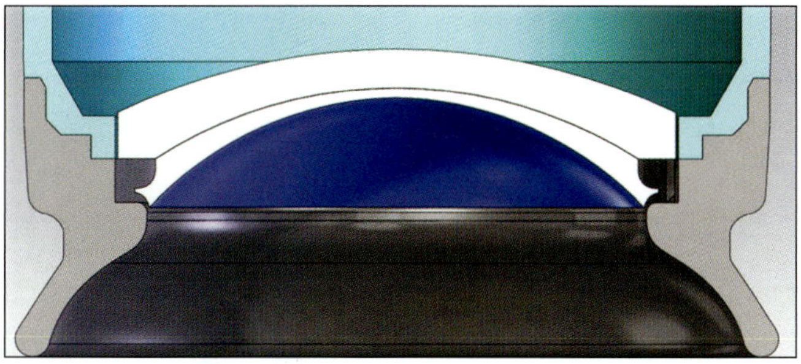

Figure 4. The SoftFit curved patient interface.

patient interface. In fact, the patient interfaces used by competing cataract laser technologies markedly differ. For example, Alcon LenSx introduced a dual curvature soft hydrogel patient interface (SoftFit) that is easy to dock and fully avoids the creation of any wrinkles on the posterior corneal surface (Fig 4). Similarly, the Victus laser applies a curved glass patient interface controlled by intelligent pressure sensors that touch the eye only at the apex, and the gap in between the cornea and the glass is filled with a liquid layer.

Two of the competing companies (OptiMedica and LensAR) have developed a Liquid Optics patient interface (Fig 5). The Liquid Optics patient interface fills the gap between the eye and the delivery optics with a liquid, leaving the cornea close to its native shape, thus also avoiding any posterior corneal wrinkles.

Once the eye is docked to the beam delivery device and the globe is stabilized by applying suction to the patient interface, the position of the corneal surface and the posterior and anterior lens capsule is determined using the 3-dimensional imaging device. After completion of the 3-dimensional image scanning, intelligent image recognition software is used to determine the position of the corneal surfaces and anterior and posterior lens capsule. Automated alignment of the surgical incisions is then performed by the software. Video camera and cross-sectional images of the eye are then displayed with the visualization of the planned surgical incisions. During the final step of procedure alignment, the user approves the position of the incisions or has the power to change their locations using the graphical user interface.

Once the positions of the incisions are accepted by the surgeon, the laser procedure is initiated by pressing a footswitch. Capsulorrhexis, lens fragmentation, and corneal incisions are performed by the scanning system while the user observes the procedures through a video microscope. A flow diagram of the femtosecond laser cataract surgery is shown in Figure 6.

Safety margins to prevent damage to the lens capsule are implemented for incisions performed inside the crystalline lens. Unlike the large shock and acoustic waves generated by ultrasonic phacoemulsification

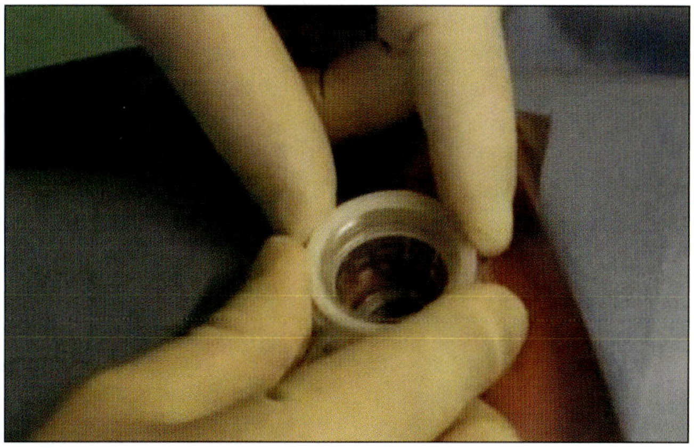

Figure 5. The Liquid Optics patient interface.

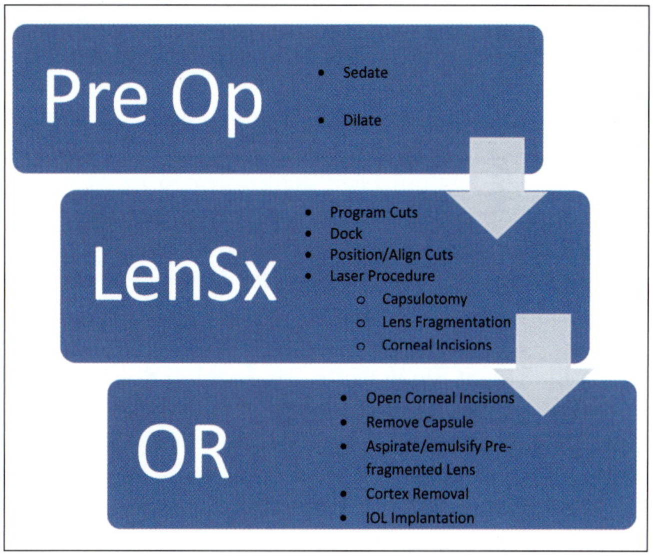

Figure 6. Flow diagram of femtosecond laser cataract surgery.

devices that can be associated with capsular and endothelial cell damage,[29-32] those generated by femtosecond photodisruption dissipate within approximately 30 μm of the targeted lens tissue.[33] The laser wavelength is not absorbed by the cornea, while the maximum retinal fluence is approximately five times less than the multiple shot damage threshold determined by Schumacher et al.[34] These findings are consistent with the safety record established by femtosecond laser corneal surgery systems over several million procedures during the past decade.

Combined Corneal and Cataract Femtosecond Lasers

Ophthalmologists are overwhelmed with highly complex and expensive technology, for diagnostics as well as for surgery. History indicates that patients are eventually accepting of higher prices for new technology, especially if it provides better medicine. It is, however, questionable if an average ophthalmic practice can really afford two femtosecond laser devices—one for the cornea and one for cataract surgery. Thus, it is important to determine the feasibility of a combined femtosecond laser platform for both corneal and cataract surgery.

As we have seen, the requirements for corneal and cataract lasers are markedly different; therefore, merging the two technologies requires some unique engineering solutions. For example, corneal flap cutting requires a hard applanating patient interface and high repetition rate laser, while cataract surgery requires a patient interface that leaves the cornea intact and a lower repetition rate laser. In fact, both the LenSx laser and Victus laser use a patient interface that can easily be modified to a hard applanating interface. Both companies have already demonstrated corneal flap cutting with their lasers and obtained Food and Drug Administration clearances. It is expected that these procedures will be commercially available in the near future.

Cutting a corneal flap with a Liquid Optics patient interface, however, may be technically more challenging, and in fact, it has not been demonstrated to date with this technology. Therefore, it is expected that technologies using the Liquid Optics patient interface may require some further development for corneal flap cutting.

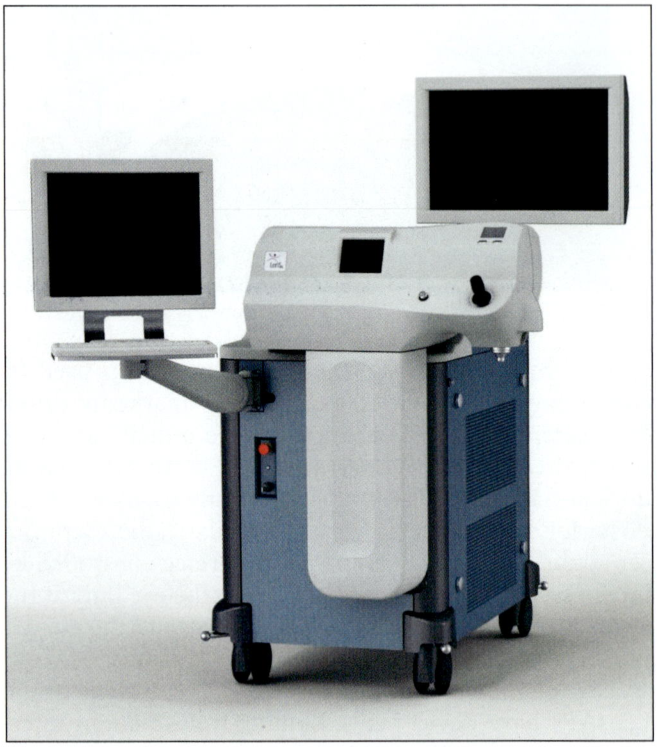

Figure 7. The LenSx laser system by Alcon LenSx Inc.

Brief Description of the Commercially Available Cataract Femtosecond Lasers

To date there are four commercially available cataract femtosecond lasers on the market. The first laser was introduced at the American Society of Cataract and Refractive Surgery meeting in 2011 by Alcon LenSx. The first commercial units were shipped immediately after the meeting. Competitors followed Alcon LenSx approximately 1 to 1.5 years later with the commercial introduction of their lasers.

The LenSx laser from Alcon LenSx is shown in Figure 7. The laser has a small footprint (approximately 2' x 3') and it has a movable gantry to deliver the laser beam to the patient's eye. The range of the gantry motion is designed so that this laser can work with all commercially available patient gurneys. Its SoftFit patient interface is designed to avoid posterior corneal wrinkles to ensure perfect beam quality and spot size for the lens procedures. Docking of the laser system with the SoftFit patient interface is quick and easy, allowing fast completion of the laser cataract procedures. Additionally, Alcon LenSx also optimized OCT scanning patterns to minimize procedure times. In fact, the total procedure time including docking, OCT scanning, capsulotomy, lens fragmentation, and corneal procedures is approximately 2 minutes with this laser. The use of rolling patient beds together with the short laser procedure time allows the user to optimize patient flow with this technology. Thus, despite the additional steps associated with use of the laser, the efficiency of the surgeon is practically unchanged. To date Alcon LenSx has the largest installed base among all the competitors in the field and by far the highest procedure numbers completed. Additionally to the cataract procedures, due to the variable cone angle of the beam delivery device, excellent quality corneal flap cutting was also demonstrated with the LenSx laser.

The Catalys laser system manufactured by OptiMedica is shown in Figure 8. This laser features a solid gantry and a patient bed that is not detachable from the laser. In contrast to the LenSx laser, docking of the patient is established by moving the patient bed, not the beam delivery gantry. It has a noncontact Liquid Optics patient interface applying liquid in between the laser delivery optics and the cornea. This system applies a 3-dimensional OCT scanning pattern to locate the lens capsule and corneal surfaces. Docking with the Liquid Optics interface is more complex; therefore, the total procedure time with the Catalys is approximately 4 minutes. The use of the attached patient bed may require some logistics to move older patients under the laser. Although this technology was introduced somewhat later than the LenSx system, the number of installations is rapidly growing.

The LensAR laser (LensAR Inc), shown in Figure 9, is a small footprint machine designed to use an external movable patient bed, allowing easy patient transfer and well-optimized patient flow. In contrast to all other systems it uses a Scheimpflug imaging device to locate the

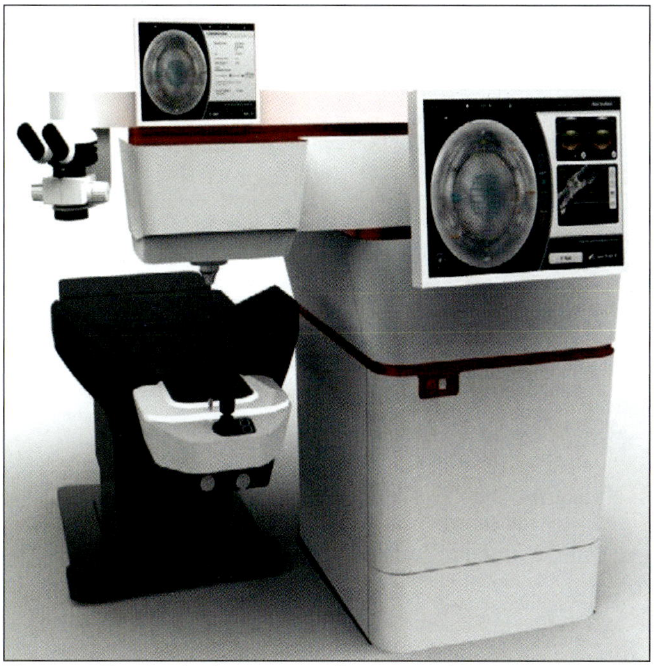

Figure 8. The Catalys laser system by OptiMedica Corp.

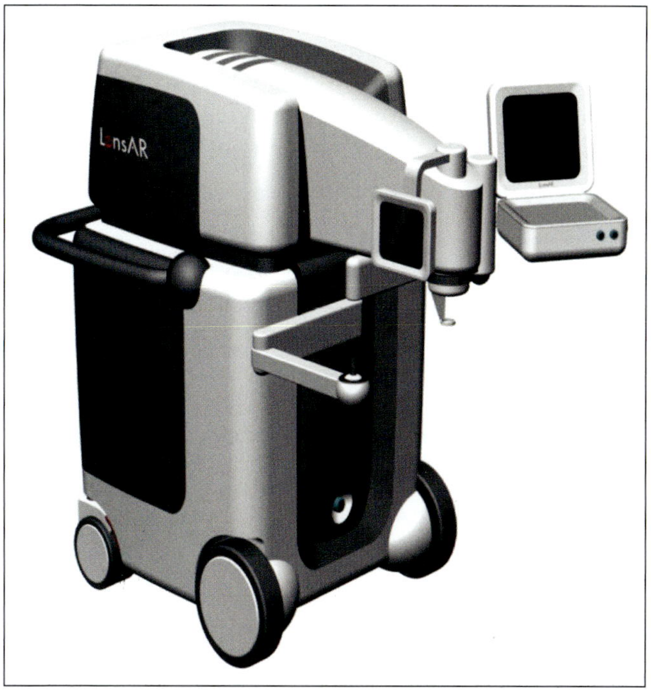

Figure 9. The LensAR laser system.

target tissue. Similar to the Catalys system, it also uses a liquid patient interface. Due to the docking characteristics of this patient interface, characteristic procedure times with this system are approximately 4 to 5 minutes. There are numerous LensAR installations both in and outside of the United States.

The Victus laser by Bausch + Lomb–Technolas Perfect Vision AG is shown in Figure 10. This machine has a small footprint and uses a built-in nondetachable patient bed. It has a solid glass curved patient interface controlled by intelligent pressure sensors that have a radius of curvature of 9.5 mm. This curved patient interface touches the cornea only at the apex. It employs a liquid layer in between the curved glass and the cornea to avoid corneal wrinkles. Additionally to cataract procedures, corneal flap cutting was also demonstrated with the machine. The majority of the Victus installations are in Europe.

There are numerous clinical papers published with all four competing technologies showing excellent clinical outcomes. In fact, all technologies have demonstrated 100% or nearly 100% free-floating capsulotomies and excellent lens fragmentation with significant reduction of the phacoemulsification power. All competitors agree that the most effective "femto-emulsification" can be achieved by chopping the lens up into small cubes. The strong competition in the field has resulted in a rapid development of all four cataract femtosecond laser technologies benefiting the patients and users with better and safer surgical procedures.

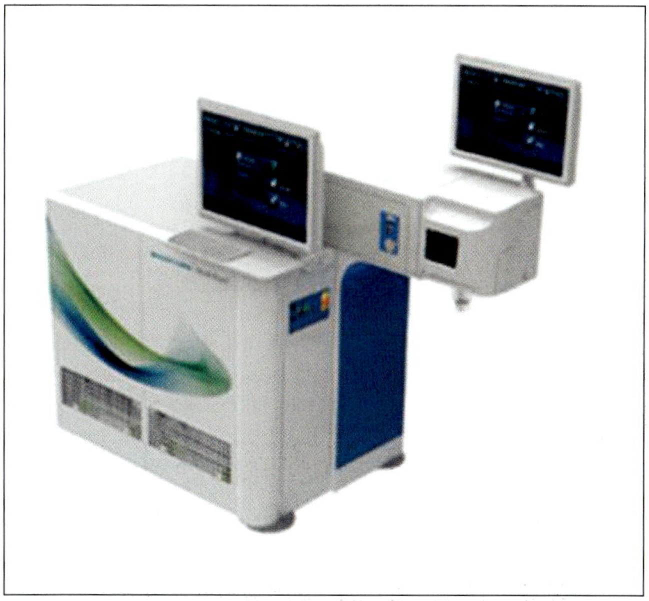

Figure 10. The Victus laser system by Bausch + Lomb–Technolas Perfect Vision AG.

Conclusion

Strong competition among the developers of cataract femtosecond lasers has resulted in a rapid development of femtosecond laser technology for cataract surgery. Basic operating principles and design parameters of such lasers are discussed in detail in this chapter. Differences and similarities between corneal and cataract femtosecond lasers are revealed, and design challenges of a combined femtosecond laser platform are discussed. Finally, the basic characteristics of all currently commercially available competing cataract lasers are briefly listed. The ophthalmic community will benefit from this diversity and no doubt will drive continued development of femtosecond laser cataract technologies in the years to come.

References

1. Bloembergen N. Laser-induced electric breakdown in solids. *IEEE J Quantum Electron.* 1974;10:375-386.
2. Fujimoto JG, Lin WZ, Ippen EP, Puliafito CA, Steinert RF. Time-resolved studies of Nd:YAG laser-induced breakdown. *Invest Ophthalmol Vis Sci.* 1985;26:1771-1777.
3. Zysset B, Fujimoto JG, Puliafito CA, Birngruber R, Deutsch TF. Picosecond optical breakdown: tissue effects and reduction of collateral damage. *Lasers Surg Med.* 1989;9:193-204.
4. Vogel A, Hentschel W, Holzfuss J, Lauterborn W. Cavitation bubble dynamics and acoustic transient generation in ocular surgery with pulsed neodymium:YAG laser. *Ophthalmology.* 1986;93:1259-1269.
5. Glezer EN, Scaffer CB, Nishimura N, Mazur E. Minimally disruptive laser induced breakdown in water. *Optics Letters.* 1997;23:1817.
6. Voegel A, Schweiger P, Freiser A, Asio MN, Birngruber R. Intraocular Nd: YAG laser surgery: light-tissue interactions, damage-range and reduction of collateral effects. *IEEE J Quantum Electron.* 1990;26:2240-2260.
7. Habib MS, Speaker MG, Shnatter WF. Mass spectrometry analysis of the byproducts of intrastromal photorefractive keratectomy. *Ophthalmol Surg Lasers.* 1995;26:481-483.
8. Steinert RF, Puliafito CA. *The Nd:YAG Laser in Ophthalmology.* Philadelphia, PA: Saunders; 1985.
9. Loesel FH, Niemz MH, Bille JF, Juhasz T. Laser-induced optical breakdown on hard and soft tissues and its dependence on the pulse duration. *IEEE J Quantum Electron.* 1996;32:1717-1722.
10. Juhasz T, Loesel FH, Kurtz RM, Horvath C, Bille JF, Mourou G. Corneal refractive surgery with femtosecond lasers. *IEEE J Select Topics Quantum Electron.* 1999;5:902-910.
11. 2009 comprehensive report on global single-use ophthalmic surgical product market. *Market Scope.* 2009;Aug.
12. Leaming DV. Practices styles and preferences of ASCRS members: 2003 survey. *J Cataract Refract Surg.* 2004;30:892-900.
13. Leaming DV. Practices styles and preferences of ASCRS members: 2001 survey. *J Cataract Refract Surg.* 2002;28:1681-1688.
14. Marques FF, Marques MV, Osher RH, Osher JM. Fate of anterior capsule tears during cataract surgery. *J Cataract Refract Surg.* 2006;32:1638-1642.
15. Dick HB, Pena-Aceves A, Mannis A, Krummeanauer F. New technology for sizing the continuous curvilinear capsulorhexis: prospective trial. *J Cataract Refract Surg.* 2008;34:1136-1144.
16. Norrby S. Sources of error in intraocular lens power calculation. *J Cataract Refract Surg.* 2008;34:368-376.
17. Hollick EJ, Spalton DJ, Meacock WR. The effect of capsulorhexis size on posterior capsular opacification: one-year results of a randomized prospective trial. *Am J Ophthalmol.* 1999;128(3):271-279.
18. Can I, Takmaz T, Cakici F, Ozgül M. Comparison of Nagahara phacochop and stop-and-chop phacoemulsification nucleotomy techniques. *J Cataract Refract Surg.* 2004;30:663-668.
19. Vogel A, Schweiger P, Frieser A, Asiyo M, Birngruber R. Intraocular Nd:YAG laser surgery: light-tissue interaction, damage range, and reduced collateral effects. *J Quantum Electron.* 1990;26:2240-2260.
20. Juhasz T, Kastis G, Suárez C, Turi L, Bor Z, Bron WE. Shockwave and cavitation bubble dynamics during photodisruption in ocular media and their dependence on the pulse duration. In: Jacques SL, ed. *Laser-Tissue Interactions VII. Proceedings of SPIE.* 1996;2681:428-436.
21. Kurtz RM, Liu X, Elner VM, Squier JA, Du D, Mourou G. Photodisruption in the human cornea as a function of laser pulse width. *J Cataract Refract Surg.* 1997;13:653-658.
22. Seitz B, Langenbucher A, Homann-Rummelt C, Schlötzer-Schrehardt U, Naumann GOH. Nonmechanical posterior lamellar keratoplasty using the femtosecond laser (femto-PLAK) for corneal endothelial decompensation. *Am J Ophthalmol.* 2003;136:769-772.
23. Slade SG, Durrie DS, Binder PS. A prospective, contralateral eye study comparing thin-flap LASIK (sub-Bowman keratomileusis) with photorefractive keratectomy. *Ophthalmology.* 2009;116(6):1075-1082.
24. Sutton G, Hodge C. Accuracy and precision of LASIK flap thickness using the IntraLase femtosecond laser in 1000 consecutive cases. *J Refract Surg.* 2008;24:802-806.
25. Sekundo W, Kunert K, Russmann C, et al. First efficacy and safety study of femtosecond lenticule extraction for the correction of myopia: six-month results. *J Cataract Refract Surg.* 2008;34(9):1513-1520.
26. Ruiz LA, Cepeda LM, Fuentes VC. Intrastromal correction of presbyopia using a femtosecond laser system. *J Refract Surg.* 2009;25(10):847-854.
27. Steinert RF, Ignacio TS, Sarayba MA. "Top hat"-shaped penetrating keratoplasty using the femtosecond laser. *Am J Ophthalmol.* 2007;143(4):689-691.
28. Nagy Z, Takacs A, Filkorn T, Sarayba M. Initial clinical evaluation of an intraocular femtosecond laser in cataract surgery. *J Refract Surg.* 2009;25(12):1053-1060.
29. Shin YJ, Nishi Y, Engler C, et al. The effect of phacoemulsification energy on the redox state of cultured human corneal endothelial cells. *Arch Ophthalmol.* 2009;127(4):435-441.
30. Murano N, Ishizaki M, Sato S, Fukuda Y, Takahashi H. Corneal endothelial cell damage by free radicals associated with ultrasound oscillation. *Arch Ophthalmol.* 2008;126(6):816-821.
31. Storr-Paulsen A, Norregaard JC, Ahmed S, Storr-Paulsen T, Pedersen TH. Endothelial cell damage after cataract surgery: divide-and-conquer versus phaco-chop technique. *J Cataract Refract Surg.* 2008;34(6):996-1000.
32. Richard J, Hoffart L, Chavane F, Ridings B, Conrath J. Corneal endothelial cell loss after cataract extraction by using ultrasound phacoemulsification versus a fluid-based system. *Cornea.* 2008;27(1):17-21.
33. Juhasz T, Kastis GA, Suarez C, Bor Z, Bron WE. Time-resolved observations of shock waves and cavitation bubbles generated by femtosecond laser pulses in corneal tissue and water. *Lasers Surg Med.* 1996;19:23-31.
34. Schumacher S, Sander M, Stolte A, Doepke C, Baumgaertner W, Lubatschowski H. Investigation of possible fs-LASIK induced retinal damage. In: Södergerg PG, Ho A, Manns F, eds. *Ophthalmic Technologies XVI. Proceeding of SPIE.* 2006;6138:I1-I9.

Face-Off Femtosecond Laser Cataract Surgery

Zoltán Z. Nagy, MD, PhD, DSc

Background

For decades phacoemulsification and more recently microincisional catarct surgery have been a normal part of everyday ophthalmological surgical care. The change in surgical technique also drove a rapid development in artificial lens design. The technology became safe and effective, all kinds of refractive errors can be compensated for, and even near vision can be restored due to different types of intraocular lenses (IOLs). Due to the aging population and safety of the method, a substantial increase in cataract surgeries can be expected in the near future. More and more patients want surgery earlier than ever before; some of them only seek compensation for presbyopia.

According to the data of the World Health Organization in 2010, the number of cataract operations was nearly 20 million globally; by 2020 this number might increase to 32 million worldwide.[1]

Young patients usually want to achieve emmetropia, even if they had myopic, hyperopic, or astigmatic refractive errors preoperatively. The responsibility of treating surgeons and also of the industry has increased tremendously. Presently, according to statistical data, 64% to 70% of patients have a 0.5 D or higher preoperative astigmatism and 15% to 29% have higher than 1.25 D astigmatism.[2,3] The predictability of refractive results are still higher in refractive surgery than during cataract surgery. Therefore, there is room for development in preoperative diagnostics, surgical technique, and IOL design.

Problems With Current Technique of Phacoemulsification

Cataract surgery is a well-established procedure; the phacoemulsification technique was invented and introduced by Charles Kelman in the 1980s. Phacoemulsification itself may cause difficulties during the procedure, which can cause a cascading negative effect on surgical outcome. Wound creation and capsulotomies are in the first line of surgical problems. If something goes wrong at the beginning, then it is difficult to compensate for it during the remainder of the surgery. A wound may rupture or leak, causing delay of postoperative healing, or it may cause vision-threatening endophthalmitis, which should be avoided by all means.

The capsulotomy may be too large, too small, or off center; may have an oval, irregular shape; or anterior rupture may occur, which may propagate to the posterior capsule as well. Determining the effective lens position (ELPo) and the size and centration of the capsulotomies are of paramount importance. This is especially valid for premium lenses, such as multifocal, accommodating, toric, aspheric, etc.

The anterior capsule should cover circumferentially the posterior chamber lens by 0.25 to 0.5 mm. If it is larger, complete coverage is out of the question. The lens may be tilted, creating significant higher-order aberrations, or may shift anteriorly, rendering the postoperative refraction toward myopia. If it is too small, the lens may shift posteriorly, causing a hyperopic shift compared to preoperative biometry calculations. Off-centered lenses may cause an increase of higher-order aberrations and unwanted regular or irregular astigmatism.[4]

The occurrence of anterior capsular tear is around 0.8% with experienced surgeons. On the other hand, during residency programs and as performed by inexperienced surgeons, it is increased 7.5 times.[5,6] Therefore, regular and centralized capsulotomies have a high level of importance.[4,7]

Femtosecond Lasers in Cataract Surgery

Technical Aspects of the Femtosecond Laser Systems

Femtosecond lasers provide a new, innovative technology for ophthalmologists and patients. First, femtolasers have been used for corneal lamellar incisions to increase the safety and predictability of LASIK procedures. It has been shown that flap thickness is more

Nagy ZZ, ed. *Femtosecond Laser-Assisted Cataract Surgery: Facts and Results* (pp 11-20).

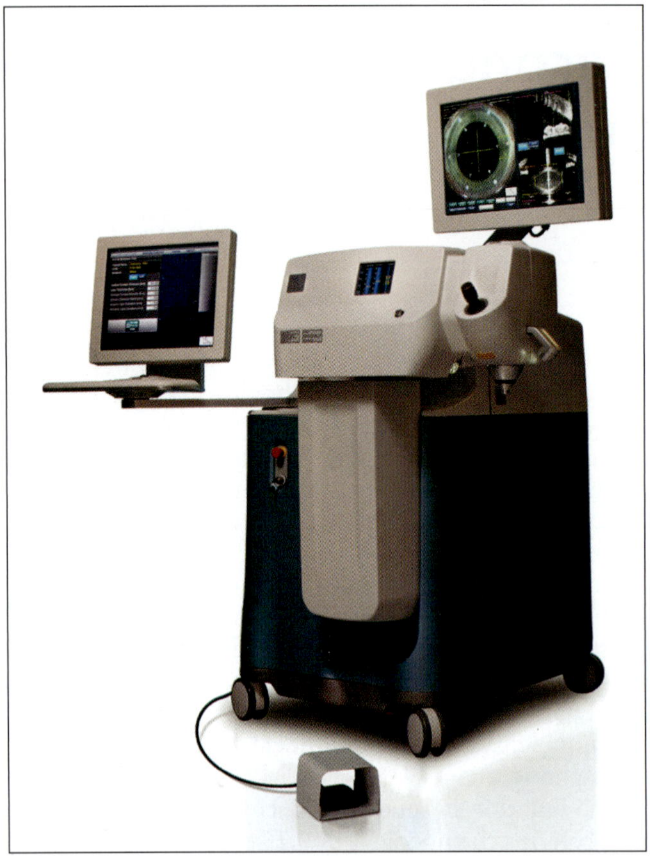

Figure 1. The LenSx laser system.

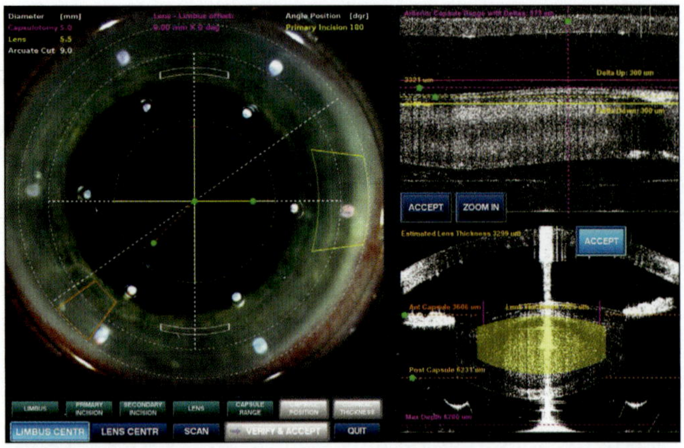

Figure 2. The screen for the surgeon: HD-OCT measurement during femtolaser pretreatment.

accurate with femtolasers compared to mechanical microblades. When other lamellar corneal procedures, such as lamellar keratoplasty, penetrating keratoplasty, and intracorneal ring segment procedures, also became available, femtolasers gained an immediate acceptance by ophthalmologists.

Femtolasers operate with a solid-state laser source that produces thousands of femtosecond pulses per second. Laser pulses are delivered via a sophisticated beam delivery system to the eye. It includes an articulated arm and a series of different optical lenses, scanners, and monitors. The femtosecond lasers are working in the near-infrared range of the electromagnetic spectrum, with a wavelength of 1053 nm. With optical focusing, the laser beam focuses precisely within the corneal tissue, and it is also possible to travel through optical media and to focus the laser beam onto the anterior capsule and within the crystalline lens. This feature has made femtolasers very useful in cataract surgery during the past few years. The process occurs within the tissue of the eye, called photodisruption, which generates plasma formation of free electrons and ionized molecules. These molecules rapidly expand and then collapse, causing the (micro) cavitation bubbles and acoustic shock waves, which eventually separate and incise the ocular tissue.

The first part of femtosecond surgery is the docking procedure; the surgeon uses a curved contact lens or a fluid-containing patient interface integrated with a sterile limbal suction ring. The tubing uses a vacuum system for fixating the patient's eye. The patient interface is easy to dock, and it provides the viewing and surgical diameter range, which allows most types of femtolasers to perform the peripheral corneal wounds and arcuate keratotomy incisions as well. The patient interface usually elevates intraocular pressure no more than 20 to 25 mm Hg; therefore, ocular perfusion and visual perception are maintained during the femtolaser pretreatment.

Femtolasers usually have a live video and proprietary optical coherence tomography (OCT) to assist with the docking and surgical pattern localization.

The laser is guided by sophisticated optical tools, in most cases by HD-OCT (in the Alcon LenSx femtolaser); in other cases, the Scheimpflug camera (OptiMedica, Victus, LensAR) is used to target the precise depth of the tissues. OCT uses the same optical path as the laser beam and is fully integrated and calibrated. OCT covers the whole anterior segment, up to the posterior capsule of the crystalline lens, and is able to assess the lens density as well. The surgical pattern is automatically performed; however, the surgeon has the ability to alter the automatically offered treatment parameters, such as centration of anterior capsulotomy, depth cut within the lens (distance from posterior and anterior capsule), and position of corneal cuts (Figs 1 through 3).

OCT measurements effectively combine the circular and linear scans, which results in better depth and tilt information. The femtosecond laser produces a 100-µm shock wave; therefore, a minimum of 500 µm (rather 700 µm) safety distance is recommended from the posterior capsule.

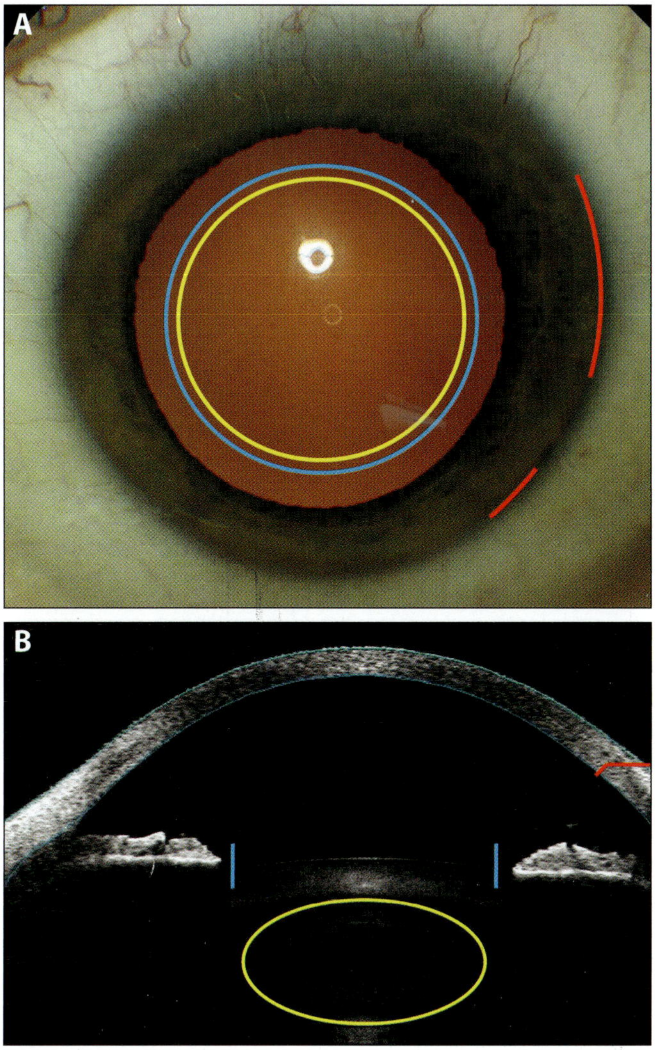

Figure 3. The surgical pattern is automatically performed; however, the surgeon has the ability to alter the automatically offered treatment parameters, such as centration of anterior capsulotomy, depth cut within the lens (distance from posterior and anterior capsule), and position of corneal cuts.

The first-ever human femtosecond laser-assisted cataract surgery was performed in 2008 at Semmelweis University, Budapest, Hungary, by Prof. Nagy.[8] The technology rapidly developed and now has become an accepted procedure for cataract removal in patients by ophthalmologists. As with new and expensive technology, the price and costs are still debated during international meetings, but the fact that it renders cataract surgery to be a more safe, effective, and highly predictable procedure is usually not questioned. The first experiences of our working team with femtosecond laser-assisted refractive cataract surgery have been published in 18 peer-reviewed articles.[4,7-23]

Femtosecond laser-assisted cataract surgery helps to automate critical steps of manual phacoemulsifications and helps to avoid cascading negative effects if something goes wrong during manual cataract removal. It is debated if surgeon skill is still needed or not; however, to achieve the best result, the surgeon must have a proper dexterity because other steps of surgery (eg, lens and cortex removal, lens implantation, avoiding wound damage) cannot be automated. All surgeons must learn manual phacoemulsification before starting the femtolaser method.

Based on the initial results and experiences, the Food and Drug Administration (FDA) approved and cleared the four main steps of femtosecond laser-assisted cataract surgery—capsulorrhexis, lens fragmentation (liquefaction), corneal incisions, and arcuate incisions—in 2009 for the LenSx femtolaser.

Other companies with different femtolasers for cataract surgery, such as the Catalys (OptiMedica), the LensAR (LensAR Inc), and the Victus (Bausch + Lomb–Technolas GmbH) appeared on the market and received FDA clearance for their femtolasers following LenSx. LenSx was acquired by Alcon in 2011 and became Alcon LenSx. The Aliso Viejo, California, production site remains the same (as before acquisition by Alcon).

Today's patient expects perfect postoperative visual acuity following cataract surgery with excellent visual quality and spectacle independence regarding far and near vision. Femtolaser technology offers automated steps during the critical phases of cataract surgery with consistent results that increase predictability.

During the past few years, many things have been changed, such as the shape and geometry of the patient interface, the energy level, the spot size, and the spot separation parameters.

Femtosecond lasers may help in three critical phases of cataract removal—corneal wound creation, capsulotomy, and lens fragmentation and liquefaction. Besides these, the laser is able to treat and control preoperative corneal astigmatism by creating arcuate keratotomy incisions. Unique features are the controllable incision depth, the unprecedented exactness of incisions, the low energy level used during femtolaser pretreatment, and the customizable steps regarding corneal incisions, lens fragmentation pattern, and creating precise size and centered capsulotomies. During arcuate incisions, the surgeon may adjust the incision depth to achieve an 80% or even 90% incision at the corneal periphery without perforating the cornea.

The method is named by different terminology in the literature: femtolaser refractive cataract surgery, femtolaser-assisted cataract surgery, femtolaser cataract surgery, femtolaser lens removal, etc. Currently, the name femtolaser-assisted cataract surgery is gaining a wider acceptance.

The method is refractive in a way because surgeons also change the refraction of the eye during surgery. Cataract removal and refractive surgery have tended to merge in recent years. The reason is that we operate on younger and younger patients, sometimes only for compensating for presbyopia, without the patient having an actual cataract.

Demography shows that in the upcoming decades the need for cataract removal will increase significantly due to the aging of the population. Also, there is an increasing need for earlier lens exchange due to presbyopic changes. The higher refractive errors in myopia and especially in hyperopia render cataract surgery also more popular. Surgeons have to face ever-growing patient demands, with almost compulsory guarantee of surgical predictability and excluding almost all possible complications.

Rationale for Using Femtolasers in Cataract Surgery

Irregular shape of manual capsulotomy may cause lens tilt, anterior or posterior shift, or changing the attempted refraction; long phacoemulsification with high cumulative dissipated energy (CDE) and high effective phaco time (EPT) may cause delayed visual recovery and significant decrease in endothelial cell number.

Femtolaser pretreatment, therefore, may increase the predictability and may help the CDE and EPT by creating perioperative fragmentation lines or liquefying the lens nucleus. Femto-fragmentation also helps to divide the nucleus into 2-4-8 pieces without grooving techniques with the phaco piece.

Irregular wounds may cause leakage and postoperative infection, complications that should also be avoided. Postoperative surgically induced corneal astigmatism should also be minimized during surgery.

Femtolaser pretreatment renders the critical steps of phacoemulsification into a consistent and predictable procedure. This is not a technology to replace good surgeons by automated machines or ophthalmic technicians. Surgical wisdom is still needed, possibly even more so. Of course femtolaser treatment should be started when phacoemulsification is already mastered by the surgeon. In the future it may change as a starting procedure, but for years the supremacy of phacoemulsification will remain in the first line of our surgical armamentarium.

Advantages of Femtolaser-Assisted Cataract Surgery

The main advantages of the method are a better quality of incision with any desired geometry, position, and incision number[16,22]; increased reliability and reproducibility of capsulotomies; increased stability and central position of the implanted posterior chamber lenses[4,7,9,15]; and reduction of the CDE and EPT during phacoemulsification.[8,24]

There is still a lack of prospective, randomized studies to prove the superiority over the manual technique. The superiority of postoperative refraction is also debated by several authors. This is natural because the method is not substantially new, as was the case with the shift from extracapsular cataract removal to phacoemulsification. But it should be remembered that it also had a price with decompensated corneas, rupture of the posterior capsule, sinking the crystalline lens into the vitreous, need for vitrectomy, need for intravitreal phacoemulsification, new techniques for lens implantation in case of capsular complications (suturing the lens, glued IOL technique, etc), need for corneal transplants, and treating postoperative cystoid macular edema.

Femtolaser pretreatment was invented to help the steps of phacoemulsification and to increase safety, consistency, and predictability. Usually when femtolaser-assisted cataract surgery and manual phacoemulsification are being compared, the results of uneventful and successful surgeries are examined. The chance of avoiding possible complications and the rate of real complications are usually not evaluated or done so very infrequently. This is driven mostly by comparing the costs of the manual and femtolaser-assisted procedures. It has a certain reasoning because cataract removal became much more safe and more predictable during the past 2 decades. Therefore, financers think that financing can also be decreased. This is not the opinion of ophthalmic surgeons, and professional debates can be misled by this problem. Our team tried to evaluate more deeply the possible results, advantages, and disadvantages of the method on a broader base than has been done so far during the international meetings. Herewith, we try to summarize our most important steps and results with femtolaser-assisted refractive cataract surgeries.

Steps of Femtolaser-Assisted Cataract Surgery

Docking

The procedure for stabilizing the eye during femtolaser-assisted cataract surgery is called docking. A modified patient interface is used with the Alcon LenSx femtolaser. This is a curved interface that follows the contour of the cornea with a 12.5-mm diameter. Between the surface of the patient interface and the patient's eye, a soft contact lens is applied in order to avoid direct contact and drying of the corneal surface. With the soft contact lens there are no corneal folds, which was the case with first-generation patient interfaces. Corneal folds may have caused irregular capsular contour and required higher laser energy during the whole femtolaser pretreatment.

The rise of intraocular pressure (IOP) is less than 20 mm Hg, which can be tolerated by elderly patients with sometimes compromised vascular structures of the posterior pole due to sclerosis, glaucoma, etc. Higher IOP rise usually occurs during femtolaser LASIK procedures because the cornea should be completely flattened in the treatment area (9.0 mm of central cornea). This pressure rise may go up to 80 mm Hg during the flap procedure. To avoid ischemic retinal and neuropathic injury of the optic nerve by decreased ocular blood flow, during femtolaser-assisted cataract surgery a curved patient interface is used with significantly less IOP rise. Other systems use two-piece noncorneal contact fluid-filled patient interfaces (Victus, Catalys, LensAR). With the fluid-filled patient interfaces, reaching the peripheral cornea to create the corneal wounds is more difficult.

On the other hand, with the liquid immersion interface the increase of IOP was found to increase by 16.6 mm Hg, with the curved patient interface by 32 mm Hg.[25] With the SoftFit patient interface (soft contact lens between the patient interface and the patient's eye) the increase is below 20 mm Hg.[18] Kerr et al found an IOP rise of 11.4 mm Hg with the Catalys laser system during vacuum build-up and a peak of 36 mm Hg immediately following laser capsulotomy and lens fragmentation. The IOP started to decrease after patient interface removal but remained above baseline values.[26] It seems that unwanted IOP rise is no longer a problem during the docking and femtolaser pretreatment.

Corneal Incisions

Self-sealing incisions are very important to prevent wound leakage and postoperative vision-threatening endophthalmitis. Clear corneal nonsutured incisions have been reported to increase the rate of bacterial endophthalmitis.[27] Square incisions were found to be more stable and cause less leakage.[28] If the wound has a trapezoid structure and the inner lip is narrower than the outer, it helps to keep the corneal wound tightened. With femtolaser technology, any kind and any geometry of wound can be created with the desired size, location, and number. The peripheral localization is very important to avoid surgically induced astigmatism (SIA).

At the beginning of femtolaser wound creation, the wounds were more central than expected, causing an unwanted increase in SIA. The smaller diameter size yet the larger surgical field of the SoftFit patient interface provides a better visibility and availability of peripheral corneal incisions, so surgeons may induce less SIA. It is quite difficult manually to precisely control the length and structure of the corneal wound. Masket et al studied femtolaser-created corneal incisions and found that femto-wounds were more stable and easier to reproduce. A multiplanar geometrical wound structure could be achieved easily.[29]

Femtosecond laser–created corneal wounds are self-sealing; they need not be hydrated at the end of the surgery. The reasons are the wound structure and geometry and less stress, less phacoemulsification time, and less CDE during surgery. Theoretically, better wound structure and better stability cause less postoperative endophthalmitis and less SIA. This is needed to be proven by peer-reviewed multicenter studies in the future.

Femtolaser Capsulotomy

The importance of lens displacement regarding postoperative refraction has been extensively studied. It has been shown that 1-mm anterior displacement of the posterior chamber lens causes a 1.25-D myopic shift. In cases of a posterior displacement, hyperopia occurs with the same diopter magnitude. If the capsulotomy is too small, anterior capsule fibrosis (capsular phimosis) may occur implanting a single-piece posterior chamber lens. If the capsulorrhexis is too large, not overlapping the posterior chamber lens will cause tilt, decentration, increase of higher-order aberrations, optical aberration, and posterior capsule opacification.[23,30-35]

In spite of the most sophisticated lens calculation formula, ELPo within the capsular bag is mostly dependent on capsular size, shape, and centration of capsulotomy. Therefore, inaccuracy of ELPo is the major cause in IOL power calculation errors.[36,37]

Our team and others have established that femtosecond laser capsulotomies are more precise, consistent, and better centered compared to manual capsulorrhexis.[4,9,24,38] Due to better overlapping with a 0.25- to 0.5-mm anterior capsule over the posterior chamber lens optics result in less tilt and decentration compared to manual continuous curvilinear capsulorrhexis (CCC).[12] Horizontal IOL decentration was found to be significantly higher in the manual CCC group performing 4.5-mm capsulotomies. Femtolaser capsulotomy resulted in a complete and regular overlap in 89% of cases, while this could be achieved only in 72% of the cases with manual CCCs.[9] The importance of capsulotomy size is of utmost importance in high myopic eyes, where manual capsulorrhexis tends to be larger than 6.0 mm due to the larger size of the eyes and larger pupillary diameter.[4,9]

Lens Fragementation, Liquefaction

In the first published article about femtolaser-assisted cataract surgery, the authors established that femtosecond laser fragmentation decreases the effective phacoemulsification energy and EPT as well.[8] At first, a cross-pattern lens fragmentation was applied, which allowed to halve and then to divide into four quadrants of the nucleus. Later, other patterns, such as cake pattern or pizza pattern (six to eight cut lines), were created by software changes. A hybrid pattern means that the central 3.0-mm part of the lens is liquefied by cylindrical pattern and then a cross or pizza pattern fragmentation can be applied.

Fragmentation of the crystalline lens is recommended above grade 2.0 nuclear opacities according to the Lens Opacities Classification System. Presently, lens fragmentation is recommended up to grade +4.0 nuclear cataracts. Below 2.0 grade, liquefaction is recommended with a cylindrical pattern (concentric rings arising from the back of the crystalline lens toward the anterior lens part). A cubicle pattern may be used to soften the nucleus, thereby minimizing the necessary phacoemulsification energy and time.

Nagy et al reported a 43% reduction in CDE and a 51% reduction in EPT already in the first-ever published article about femtolaser-assisted cataract surgery.[8] Palanker et al reported a 39% decrease in CDE using the Catalys system.[24] Similar results have been reported by Conrad-Hengerer et al (29% decrease in CDE).[39]

Depending on the cataract grade and fragmentation patterns, a significant decrease in CDE and EPT can be achieved with femtolaser technology, which in turn may increase the safety of the method regarding postoperative corneal swelling, loss of endothelial cells, etc. New prospective, randomized studies are necessitated to establish the real value of femtolaser-assisted cataract surgery in fragmentation and long-term safety.

Endothelial Cell Loss

Following manual phacoemulsification, an average of 8.5% cell loss 12 months following surgery has been reported in the literature. The majority of cell loss occurs during the first 6 weeks, which is about 7.5%, followed by a 1% increase during the rest of the first postoperative follow-up year.[12]

Takács et al performed a prospective, randomized study with femtolaser-assisted cataract surgery compared to manual phacoemulsification. The authors concluded that on the first postoperative day femtolaser-treated eyes showed significantly less corneal thickness compared to the manual group, while this difference had disappeared 1 week and 1 month following surgery.[12]

Similarly, Abell et al found no difference in endothelial cell loss 3 weeks after femtolaser-assisted cataract surgery or manual phacoemulsification.[40]

From a safety point of view, it is very important that femtolaser-assisted cataract surgery itself does not compromise the endothelial cell number and corneal thickness compared to manual phacoemulsification. The reduced phaco energy requirement may be of greater importance in eyes with compromised endothelial cell number like Fuchs' endothelial dystrophy, low endothelial cell number for any reason, uveitis, etc. Larger studies are still needed to establish the role of fragmentation pattern, chop technique and lens density on the postoperative endothelial cell number, and corneal thickness.

Macular Changes Following Femtolaser-Assisted Cataract Surgery

There are a limited number of articles in the literature regarding femtolaser-assisted cataract surgery and macular morphology. Ecsedy et al established that femtolaser-assisted cataract surgery–related postoperative cystoid macular edema is not worse compared to manual phacoemulsification. On the other hand, regarding the inner macular ring, results seem to be more favorable in the femtolaser group, mainly due to shorter treatment time and less CDE.[10,11]

Other Safety Issues

The femtolaser-assisted cataract surgery procedure certainly requires a learning curve. This is definitely shorter than during the shift from extracapsular cataract extraction to phacoemulsification. All of our major complications occurred during the first 100 cases. It should also be emphasized that femtolaser-assisted cataract surgery was under continuous development from 2008. Therefore, the learning curve should not be longer than the first 50 cases.

Anterior tear of the capsule may cause a cascading effect during surgery. The rate of anterior tear among experienced and inexperienced surgeons is very different—from 0.8% can be increased to 5.6%.

My personal advice is to follow the contour of the anterior laser capsulotomy; this is highly recommended to avoid anterior tears. Capsular complications and how to manage them is discussed in detail by Nagy et al in the *Journal of Cataract & Refractive Surgery*.[18]

A gentle hydrodissection should be applied. In case of abrupt hydrodissection, the gas bubble within the crystalline lens may leave the crystalline lens toward the posterior capsule (capsular block syndrome), which may disrupt and the nucleus may sink into the vitreous cavity.[41-43] In cases of gentle hydrodissection with the "rock and roll technique" (gently pressing the nucleus down and turning it around), the gas bubble will leave the eye toward the anterior chamber and through the corneal wound. Rupture of the posterior capsule is the most serious complication of femtolaser-assisted cataract surgery, which is mainly due to technical problems during hydrodissection. It is advised that one person from a team should start femtolaser treatment, and after having completed the learning curve, may teach the other members of the team. By this way, many complications can be avoided.

Femtosecond Laser Cataract Surgery in Difficult Cases

Nagy et al's team reported successful femtolaser application in cases of trauma with anterior capsular rupture. Femtolaser capsulotomy helps to create a central and round-shaped capsulotomy without propagating the traumatic capsular rupture to the posterior capsule, thus enabling the surgeon to implant the posterior chamber lens into the capsular sack; this way a more favorable visual outcome can be expected.[19]

Femtolaser technology was also successfully applied in eyes with angle closure glaucoma attack; in the reported case, the anterior chamber depth was 1.1 mm. With the aid of the in-built OCT, a safe and guaranteed size of capsulotomy could be achieved with efficient fragmentation. In cases of nondilating glaucomatous pupil, a Malyugin ring was first used in the literature to increase pupil size.[20] Dick also reported a favorable outcome with nondilating, small pupil cases using the Malyugin ring; in those cases femtosecond laser treatment may provide considerable benefits for patients.[44]

Femtosecond laser capsulotomy is also possible in eyes having penetrating keratoplasty in their anamnesis. The circular scar line of penetrating keratoplasty usually does not disturb femto-capsulotomy, because the scar line is around 7.0 mm in diameter and the capsulorrhexis is below 5.0 mm. The docking procedure is also not more complicated compared to the primary femtolaser-assisted cataract surgery procedure.[21]

Femtolaser capsulotomy is also applicable in eyes with keratoconus, even in advanced cases (Nagy, personal communication).

Schultz et al reported a successful femtolaser-assisted cataract surgery procedure in a cataractous decentered lens of a child with Marfan syndrome. The advantage of femtolaser capsulotomy in this case was clear and has a life-long importance.[45]

Pediatric Cataract

Pediatric cataract might be another important field of application of the femtolaser due to the high elasticity of pediatric crystalline lens. A well-centered and predictably size capsulorrhexis is of high importance, and posterior capsulotomy may render the method even more useful. Dick and Schultz reported successful pediatric cataract cases with four infants. The authors measured the capsulotomy diameter slightly larger than expected due to the higher elasticity of infant capsule.[46]

Nagy and colleagues also have had favorable experience with pediatric cataract and posterior capsulotomy (Nagy, personal communication).

Refractive Outcome

Expectations regarding refractive outcome are very high with the femtolaser-assisted cataract surgery procedure. It should be emphasized that the laser surgery is not substantially different from phacoemulsification; only the key steps are more consistent and automated. Long-term patients and ophthalmologists may expect better refractive outcomes due to more regular capsulotomy, better ELPo, possibly less posterior capsule opacification rate,[23] and reduction of postoperative astigmatism. The technical development should be followed by new technology among diagnostic tools, new lens design, new materials, etc, to use all the benefits offered by femtolaser technology in the surgery of the crystalline lens.

According to Filkorn et al, in a prospective, randomized study, results showed a significantly lower mean absolute error after femtolaser-assisted cataract surgery. This was more significant in eyes with shorter and longer axial length. There was no statistically significant difference regarding refractive outcome of femtolaser-assisted cataract surgery and manual phacoemulsification.[22] Roberts et al also found no statistically significant difference for refractive outcome.[42] Palanker et al also found a similar refractive outcome.[24]

Szigeti et al found that the 5.5-mm central femtolaser-assisted capsulorrhexis tilt and decentration group was better compared to the 6.0-mm diameter group.[17] The authors implanted a 5.0-mm diameter single-optic accommodating Crystalens AT-50AO IOL. The study showed no difference with uncorrected and best-corrected near and far visual acuities.

Lawless et al studied of a cohort of 60 eyes operated with femtolaser-assisted cataract surgery and 29 eyes with manual phacoemulsification. A diffractive multifocal IOL (Restor SN6AD1) was implanted. The results showed no difference in the mean postoperative spherical equivalent refraction between the two patient groups.[47]

Limitations of Femtosecond Laser Technology in Cataract Removal

Docking might be difficult with narrow palpebral fissure and in cases of significant pterygia and loose conjunctiva.

Extensive corneal opacities may render the procedure difficult because it may interfere with photodisruption during capsulotomy and fragmentation. Smaller, rather transparent corneal opacities do not create any problems. The surgeon should consider it and should possibly use a higher energy level for capsulotomy and fragmentation.

Adequate pupillary dilatation is a prerequisite for successful capsulotomy; the pupil should be at least 6.0 mm before femtolaser treatment. If the iris is hit by the laser beam, unexpected bleeding or further constriction may occur. Inflammatory cytokines and prostagladin E2 may be produced by the iris, which may lead to further constriction of the pupil and postoperative inflammation. Therefore, nonsteroid anti-inflammatory drops should be added to the preoperative regimen before starting the femtolaser pretreatment.[48]

In case of a nondilating pupil, a Malyugin ring may offer a solution and may allow the use of femtolaser technology.[20,44] In that case, after the blade-created corneal wound, the anterior chamber should be filled with viscoelastic, then the Malyugin ring can be implanted. After the removal of viscoelastic, the wound should be sutured with 10/0 nylon X-suture, and femtolaser capsulotomy and lens fragmentation can be easily performed. Intracameral epinephrine and viscodilation may also be a solution in case of a smaller pupil, but in case of anterior synechiae a Malyugin ring is the best solution.

Brunescent and black cataracts may be difficult to fragment by the femtolaser beam due to their very hard, compact nucleus. Presently the femtolaser-assisted cataract surgery procedure is recommended until grade +4.0. In cases of white tumescent cataracts, the water content is too high; therefore, photodisruption is not working within the swollen crystalline lens. However, capsulotomy is recommended and helpful in tumescent cases, where manual capsulotomy may run toward the periphery.

Discussion

At present there is a professional debate among ophthalmologists over the advantages of femtolaser cataract surgery vs manual phacoemulsification. There are studies showing better reproducibility and predictability based on guaranteed capsulorrhexis gemometry, diameter, and centration. Other studies show no refractive advantages of the method over manual phacoemulsification. One thing is definite, the method does not replace any method for cataract removal so far used. It helps to maintain consistent results with capsulotomy and posterior chamber lens centration; less phacoemulsification energy and time are used; there is increased safety and creation of desired and customized corneal wounds[49]; and arcuate incision to avoid larger SIA and to control preoperative corneal astigmatism. Thus, the results should not be as different as was the case when the transition occurred from extracapsular cataract extraction to phacoemulsification. But there are differences and steps of cataract surgery that can be customized similarly as has happened in refractive surgery before. With this customization and increased safety and predictability ophthalmologists will be able to use and to provide all the benefits that are offered by the advanced-technology premium lenses to their patients. The main goal is to provide spectacle independence for as many patients as possible who do not have any other ophthalmic pathology besides lens opacities or cataract or presbyopia.

Studies show the importance of capsulorrhexis for providing a more stable anatomical position of the implanted posterior chamber lens regarding rotational, anteroposterior stability (no shift, no tilt), which is of paramount importance with toric and toric multifocal lenses and other presbyopia-correcting lenses.

Studies usually show that the refractive outcome of femtolaser-assisted cataract surgery is similar to the manual technique, but these studies are not discussing the quality of vision. In 2013, the French government initiated a multicenter study based on university eye clinics in order to provide prospective data on femtolaser-assisted cataract surgery procedures.

The decreased amount of ultrasound energy and time is a promising feature of femtosecond laser technology regarding safety and long-term ocular effects. The intraoperative complication rate after the learning curve seems to be lower but at least comparable to standard manual phacoemulsification. Increased safety, promising results with ELPo, higher predictability, and surgical consistency may render the method generally acceptable within the future years.

In the future, compound femtolaser equipment is to be expected that may be applicable for corneal and lens procedures as well. Presbyopia correction was also a promise and is still under investigation. Presently, higher predictability and safety are the main issues of femtolaser-assisted cataract surgery. However, we still have to wait for the results of evidence-based medicine. The effectiveness of phacoemulsification, which was invented in 1967, was proven only by randomized studies 3 decades later.

Similarly, a phase 3 controlled trial should be conducted to establish the real value of femtolaser-assisted cataract surgery. However, the European Society of Cataract & Refractive Surgeons decided in 2013 to launch and conduct a study for the complication rate of femtolaser cataract surgeries during a European-based prospective 1-year study similarly to EUREQUO data collection before. Surgeons and patients alike are eagerly awaiting the results.

REFERENCES

1. Koopman S. Cataract surgery devices. Global pipeline analysis, competitive landscape and market forecasts to 2017. www.asdreports.com/news.asp?pr_id=261. Accessed January 2012.
2. Ferrer-Blasco T, Montes Mico R. Prevalence data for corneal astigmatism before cataract surgery. *J Cataract Refract Surg.* 2009;35:70-75.
3. Hoffmann PC, Hutz WW. Analysis of biometry and prevalence data for corneal astigmatism in 23,239 eyes. *J Cataract Refract Surg.* 2010;36:1479-1485.
4. Kranitz K, Takacs A, Mihaltz K, Kovács I, Knorz MC, Nagy ZZ. Femtosecond laser capsulotomy and manual continuous curvilinear capsulorhexis parameters and their effects on intraocular lens centration. *J Refract Surg.* 2011;27:558-563.
5. Marques FF, Marques DM, Osher RH, Osher JM. Fate of anterior capsule tears during cataract surgery. *J Cataract Refract Surg.* 2006;32:1638-1642.
6. Unal M, Yücel I, Sarici A, et al. Phacoemulsification with topical anesthesia: resident experience. *J Cataract Refract Surg.* 2006;32:1361-1365.
7. Mihaltz K, Knorz MC, Alio JL, et al. Internal aberration and optical quality after femtosecond laser anterior capsulotomy in cataract surgery. *J Refract Surg.* 2011;27:711-716.
8. Nagy ZZ, Takacs A, Filkorn T, Sarayba M. Initial clinical evaluation of intraocular femtosecond laser in cataract surgery. *J Refract Surg.* 2009;25:1053-1060.
9. Nagy ZZ, Kranitz K, Takacs AI, et al. Comparison of intraocular lens decentration parameters after femtosecond and manual capsulotomies. *J Refract Surg.* 2011;27:564-569.
10. Ecsedy M, Mihaltz K, Kovacs I, Takács A, Filkorn T, Nagy ZZ. Effect of femtosecond laser cataract surgery on the macula. *J Refract Surg.* 2011;27:717-722.
11. Nagy ZZ, Ecsedy M, Kovacs I, et al. Macular morphology assessed by optical coherence tomography image segmentation after femtosecond laser-assisted and standard cataract surgery. *J Cataract Refract Surg.* 2012;38:941-946.
12. Takács AI, Kovács I, Mihaltz K, et al. Central corneal volume and endothelial cell count following femtosecond laser-assisted refractive cataract surgery compared to conventional phacoemulsification. *J Refract Surg.* 2012;28:387-391.
13. Nagy ZZ, Filkorn T, Takacs AI, et al. Anterior segment OCT imaging after femtosecond laser cataract surgery. *J Refract Surg.* 2013;29:110-112.
14. Nagy ZZ. Advanced technology IOLs in cataract surgery: pearls for successful femtosecond cataract surgery. *Int Ophthalmol Clin.* 2012;52:103-114.
15. Kranitz K, Mihaltz K, Sandor GL, Takacs A, Knorz MC, Nagy ZZ. Intraocular lens tilt and decentration measured by Scheimpflug camera following manual or femtosecond laser-created continuous circular capsulotomy. *J Refract Surg.* 2012;28:259-263.
16. Alio JL, Abdou AA, Soria F, et al. Femtosecond laser cataract incision morphology and corneal higher-order aberration analysis. *J Refract Surg.* 2013;29:590-595.
17. Szigeti A, Kranitz K, Takacs AI, Mihaltz K, Knorz MC, Nagy ZZ. Comparison of long-term visual outcome and IOL position with a single-optic accomodating IOL after 5.5 to 6.0 mm femtosecond laser capsulotomy. *J Refract Surg.* 2012;28:609-613.
18. Nagy ZZ, et al. Complications of femtolaser assisted cataract surgery. *J Cataract Refract Surg.* In press.
19. Nagy ZZ, Kranitz K, Takacs A, Filkorn T, Gergely R, Knorz MC. Intraocular femtosecond laser use in traumatic cataracts following penetrating and blunt trauma. *J Refract Surg.* 2012;28:151-153.
20. Kranitz K, Takacs AI, Gyenes A, et al. Femtosecond laser-assisted cataract surgery in management of phacomorphic glaucoma. *J Refract Surg.* 2013;29:645-648.
21. Nagy ZZ, Takacs AI, Filkorn T, et al. Laser refractive cataract surgery with a femtosecond laser after penetrating keratoplasty: case report. *J Refract Surg.* 2013;29:8.
22. Filkorn T, Kovacs I, Takacs A, Horvath E, Knorz MC, Nagy ZZ. Comparison of IOL power calculation and refractive outcome after laser refractive catarct surgery with a femtosecond laser versus conventional phacoemulsification. *J Refract Surg.* 2012;28:540-544.
23. Kovacs I, Kranitz K, Mihaltz K, Juhasz E, Knorz MC, Nagy ZZ. The effect of laser capsulotomy on the development of posterior capsule opacification. *J Refract Surg.* 2014;30(3):154-158.
24. Palanker DV, Blumenkrantz MS, Andersen D, et al. Femtosecond laser-assisted cataract surgery with integrated optical coherence tomography. *Sci Transl Med.* 2010;2:58-85.
25. Talamo JH, Gooding P, Angeley D, et al. Optical patient interface in femtosecond laser-assisted cataract surgery. Contact corneal applanation versus liquid immersion. *J Cataract Refract Surg.* 2013;39:501-510.
26. Kerr NM, Abell RG, Voth BJ, Toh T. Intraocular pressure during femtosecond laser pretreatment of cataract. *J Cataract Refract Surg.* 2013;39:339-342.
27. Taban M, Behrens A, Newcomb RL, et al. Acute endophthalmitis following cataract surgery: a systematic revew of hte literature. *Arch Ophthalmol.* 2005;123:613-620.
28. Ernest PH, Lavery KT, Kiessling LA. Relative strength of scleral corneal and clear corneal incisions constructed in cadaver eyes. *J Cataract Refract Surg.* 1994;20:626-629.
29. Masket S, Sarayba M, Ignacio T, Fram N. Femtosecond laser-assisted cataract incisions: architectural stability and reproducibility. *J Cataract Refract Surg.* 2010;36:1048-1049.
30. Laksminarayanan V, Enoch JM, Raasch T, Crawford B, Nygaard RW. Refractive changes induced by intraocular lens tilt and longitudinal displacement. *Arch Ophthalmol.* 1986;104:90-92.
31. Erickson P. Effects of intraocular lens position errors on postoperative refractive error. *J Cataract Refract Surg.* 1990;16:305-311.
32. Atchinson DA. Refractive error induced by displacemnet of intraocular lenses within the pseudophakic eye. *Optom Vis Sci.* 1989;66:146-152.
33. Kozaki J, Tanihara H, Yasuda A, Nagata M. Tilt and decentration of the implanted posterior chamber intraocular lens. *J Cataract Refract Surg.* 1991;17:592-595.
34. Korynta J, Bok J, Cendelin J. Change in refraction induced by change in intraocular lens position. *J Refract Corneal Surg.* 1994;10:556-564.
35. Ravalico G, Tognetto D, Palomba M, Busatto P, Baccara F. Capsulorhexis size and posterior capsule opacification. *J Cataract Refract Surg.* 1996;22:98-103.
36. Cekic O, Batman C. The relationship between capsulorhexis size and anterior chamber depth relation. *Ophthalmic Surg Lasers.* 1999;30:185-190.
37. Norrby S. Sources of error in intraocular lens power calculation. *J Cataract Refract Surg.* 2008;34:368-376.
38. Friedman NJ, Palanker DV, Schuele G, et al. Femtosecond laser capsulotomy. *J Cataract Refract Surg.* 2011;37:1189-1198.
39. Conrad-Hengerer I, Hengerer FH, Schultz T, Dick HB. Effect of femtosecond laser fragmentation on effective phacoemulsification time in cataract surgery. *J Refract Surg.* 2012;28:879-883.

40. Abell RG, Kerr NM, Vote BJ. Toward zero effective phacoemulsification time using femtsecond laser pretreatment. *Ophthalmology*. 2013;120:942-948.

41. Roberts TV, Sutton G, Lawless MA, Jindal-Bali S, Hodge C. Capsular block syndrome associated with femtosecond laser-assisted cataract surgery. *J Cataract Refract Surg*. 2011;37:2068-2070.

42. Roberts TV, Lawless M, Bali SJ, Hodge S, Sutton G. Surgical outcomes and safety of femtosecond laser cataract surgery: a prospective study of 1500 consecutive cases. *Ophthalmology*. 2013;120:227-233.

43. Bali SJ, Hodge C, Lawless M, Roberts TV, Sutton G. Early experience with femtosecond laser for cataract surgery. *Ophthalmology*. 2012;119:891-899.

44. Dick BH, Schultz T. Laser assisted cataract surgery in small pupils using mechanical dilatation devices. *J Refract Surg*. 2013;29:858-862.

45. Schultz T, Ezeanoskie E, Dick HB. Femtosecond laser-assisted cataract surgery in pediatric Marfan syndrome. *J Refract Surg*. 2013;29:650-652.

46. Dick HB, Schultz T. Femtosecond laser-assisted cataract surgery in infants. *J Cataract Refract Surg*. 2013;39:665-668.

47. Lawless M, Bali SJ, Hodge C, Roberts TV, Chan C, Sutton G. Outcomes of femtosecond laser cataract surgery with a diffractive multifocal intraocular lens. *J Refract Surg*. 2012;28:859-864.

48. Schultz T, Joachim SC, Kuehn M, Dick BH. Changes in prostagladin levels in patients undergoing femtosecond laser assisted cataract surgery. *J Refract Surg*. 2013;29:742-748.

49. Schultz T, Tischoff I, Ezeanosike E, Dick BH. Histological sections of corneal incisions in OCT-guided femtosecond laser cataract surgery. *J Refract Surg*. 2013;29:863-864.

Ocular Pharmacology of Femtosecond Laser Cataract Surgery

Zoltán Z. Nagy, MD, PhD, DSc

Pharmacology of femtolaser cataract surgery has an important role because ophthalmic drugs are administered as topical drops or eye ointments prior to femtolaser pretreatment. The pupil should be at least 6.0-mm wide prior to femtolaser surgery, and this pupil size should be maintained during the cataract surgery also. A well-dilated pupil renders surgery much easier and promises less surgical complications. Proper pupil size is of the utmost importance in traditional phacoemulsification also. During femtolaser pretreatment, if the pupil is not widened enough the laser may hit the iris, causing a significant rise in prostaglandin E2 and other kinds of cytokine levels in the aqueous humor. In 1989, Gimbel reported the beneficial effect of nonsteriod anti-inflammatory drug (NSAID) drops in keeping the pupil dilated during phacoemulsification.[1] Bucci and Waterbury reported a rise in prostaglandin E2 level.[2] In 2013, Schultz et al reported a statisically significant increase in prostaglandin E2 level following femtolaser pretreatment.[3] Therefore, preoperative pupillary pharmacology has an important role in achieving all the benefits of femtolaser surgery for both the patient and the surgeon.

Anatomy of Pupil Reactions

The sphincter muscle of the iris runs in a circle around the pupil; when in action the pupil narrows (miosis). The radial fibers of the dilatator muscle enlarge the pupil; this is called mydriasis.

It is important that parasympathetic fibers innervate the sphincter muscle. They come from the Edinger-Westphal nucleus of the oculomotor nuclei and reach the sphincter muscle via the oculomotor nerve (lower branches of the III nerve) first, then the ciliary ganglion, and then the iris.

The sympathetic fibers of the dilatator muscle come from the cervical chain via the carotid artery and the nasociliary nerve.

The pupillary reaction to light and darkness is elicited by the pupillomotor fibers of the retina. Light impulses from the retina are transmitted up toward the pretectal nuclei and from there the oculomotor nuclei are reached.

Miosis can be caused pharmacologically by parasympathomimetic drugs. Mydriasis can be achieved by sympathomimetic drugs and also by parasympatholytic agents (mydriatic drops).

Usually topical tropicamide (0.8%) and phenylephrine (5%) are administered either separately or in combination prior to the start of femtolaser treatment.

With traditional phacoemulsification, pharmacological pupil dilation is started 1 hour before surgery, in combination of the above-mentioned drops, and the patient receives drops every 20 minutes. In femtosecond laser-assisted cataract surgery, pupil dilation should start earlier, at least 1.5 hours before surgery, and NSAID drops also should be added to the preoperative regimen.

The Most Commonly Used Substances During Cataract Surgery

- **Parasympatholytics:** act by blocking acetylcholine receptors of the sphincter pupillae (mydriasis) and the ciliary muscle (accommodation paralysis)
  - **Tropicamide:** effective for approximately 4 to 6 hours
  - **Cyclopentolate:** effective for 12 to 24 hours, more cycloplegic than mydriatic effect
  - **Homatropine:** effective for 1 to 2 days
  - **Atropine:** effective for less than 1 week (longest-acting mydriatic), not used routinely in cataract surgery
- **Sympathomimetics:** act on adrenaline receptors of the dilatator pupillae muscle
  - **Phenylephrine:** effective for 6 hours, onset and duration of action identical to tropicamide; advantage: does not cause accommodation paralysis
  - **Cocaine (4%):** indirect sympathomimetics, inhibits reabsorption of norepinephrine (not used routinely anymore), effective for 6 hours, today used only in diagnostics of Horner syndrome

Nagy ZZ, ed. *Femtosecond Laser-Assisted Cataract Surgery: Facts and Results* (pp 21-22).

NSAID Drops

NSAID drops act primarily as anti-inflammatory agents by inhibiting cyclo-oxygenase and lipo-oxygenase enzymes. This in turn leads to inhibition of prostaglandin-like products and thromboxane, leukotrienes, which may induce inflammation. Usually the use of NSAIDs is safer in ophthalmology than the use of steroid drugs.[4,5]

Topical NSAID drops are potential drugs for adequate pupillary dilation, especially its maintenance during femtolaser cataract surgery. The pharmacological effect on the pupil is lessening intraoperative miosis.[3] A combination of NSAID and pupillary dilation drops prior to femtolaser pretreatment helps to keep the pupil wide.

The usual NSAID drops are diclofenac (0.1%), ketorolac (0.5%), flurbiprofen (0.03%), and indomethacin (1%). According to the literature, topical diclofenac drops should be started at least 24 hours prior to surgery to control perioperative pupil dilation and postoperative inflammation.

What Are the Causes of More Frequent Pupillary Constriction During Femtolaser Cataract Surgery?

During femtolaser treatment, the patient interface exerts a certain pressure. The new generation of femtolasers increases intraoperative pressure only by 16 to 25 mm Hg. The mechanical effect of the patient interface may exert a miotic effect after finishing the femtolaser pretreatment. The patient interface might be a curved interface or a fluid-coupled patient interface. Both have the same effects on the pupil.

A recent article by Schultz et al discusses the increase of prostaglandin E2 level concentration in the aqueous. The authors found an immediate rise of prostaglandin E2 in the aqueous humor using an enzyme-linked immunoassay method.[3] This prostaglandin increase may contribute to the miotic effect that was described in one-third of the cases with experienced surgeons, especially during the learning curve. Besides mechanical pressure effect of the patient interface, the bubble formation in the anterior chamber may also contribute to the mechanical effects in increasing the prostaglandin E2 level in the aqueous humor.

Prostaglandins are high potential bioregulatory substances and are synthesized from the cyclo-oxygenase pathway from arachnoid acid. Within the eye the main sources of prostaglandins are the nonpigmented epithelial layer of the ciliary body. Mechanical and thermal stimuli increase the level of prostaglandins in the aqueous according to Cole and Unger[6] and Mailhöfner et al.[7]

In previous studies, Gimbel found that pupillary constriction was reduced in patients receiving a preoperative NSAID regimen.[1] Bucci and Waterbury found that prostaglandin E2 level is also reduced by using NSAID drops prior to cataract surgery.[2]

Thus, based on the Schultz et al study,[3] it can be presumed that femtolaser pretreatment increases the level of prostaglandin E2 in the aqueous humor so patients should be pretreated with NSAID drops prior to surgery (1 to 2 days), and pupil dilation with combined drops should also be started earlier compared to normal phacoemulsification. In cases of perioperative pupillary miosis, intracameral epinephrine usually is found to be useful for adequate pupil diameter.

References

1. Gimbel HV. The effect of treatment with topical nonsteroidal anti-inflammatory drugs with and without intraoperative epinephrine on the maintenance of mydriasis during cataract surgery. *Ophthalmology.* 1989;96(22):585-588.
2. Bucci FA Jr, Waterbury LD. Aqueous prostaglandin E(2) of cataract patients at trough ketorolac and bromfenac levels after 2 days dosing. *Adv Ther.* 2009;26:645-650.
3. Schultz T, Joachim SC, Kuehn M, Dich BH. Changes in prostaglandin levels in patients undergoing femtosecond laser-assisted cataract surgery. *J Refract Surg.* 2013;29:742-747.
4. Bartlett JD. *Clinical Ocular Pharmacology.* 4th ed. Boston, MA: Butterworth-Heinemann; 2001.
5. Garg A. *Textbook of Ocular Therapeutics.* 2nd ed. New Delhi, India: CV Jaypee; 2002.
6. Cole DF, Unger WG. Prostaglandins as mediators for the responses of the eye to trauma. *Exp Eye Res.* 1973;17:357-368.
7. Mailhöfner C, Schlötzer-Schrehardt U, Gühring H, et al. Expression of cyclo-oxygenase-1 and -2 in normal and glaucomatous human eyes. *Invest Ophthalmol Vis Sci.* 2001;42:2616-2624.

Femtosecond Laser-Assisted Capsulotomy: Advantages in Better Postoperative Intraocular Lens Positioning

Kinga Kránitz, MD; Zoltán Z. Nagy, MD, PhD, DSc

Cataract surgery by phacoemulsification and implantation of an artificial intraocular lens (IOL) has become a safe and effective intervention.[1] In the era of refractive cataract surgery and premium lens implantation, precision in postoperative IOL positioning is the main limitation of customized IOL performance. Prevention or reduction of lens misalignment has become more accurate than ever before.

IOL misalignments worsen visual quality and change planned postoperative refraction through induced astigmatism, myopic or hyperopic shift, higher-order aberrations, reflections, and haloes. The effect of these misalignments depends greatly on the actual combination of these positioning parameters in an eye.[2-4]

Several laboratory tests have been performed to identify the maximum decentration and tilt that still does not worsen the visual outcome of aspheric IOLs. Holladay et al calculated the critical amount of decentration at 0.4 mm and tilt at 5.0 degrees.[5] Piers et al calculated a more permissive range with a maximum in decentration at 0.8 mm and tilt at 10 degrees.[6]

IOL misalignments can be determined by analyzing retroillumination photographs, Purkinje imaging systems, or with a Scheimpflug camera.

IOL decentration is obtained from the distance between the IOL center and the pupillary axis. Positive horizontal coordinates stand for nasal in the right eye and temporal in the left eye. Positive vertical coordinates stand for superior decentrations and negative for inferior ones. Total decentration, determined by trigonometry analysis, shows the magnitude of the result vector of horizontal and vertical decentration. Regarding IOL tilt, positive tilt around the x-axis indicates that the superior edge of the IOL is moved forward, and vice versa for negative tilt. Positive tilt around the y-axis means, in the right eye, nasal tilt and indicates that the nasal edge of the IOL is moved backward, and vice versa for a negative tilt around the y-axis in right eyes. A positive tilt around the y-axis stands for temporal tilt (nasal edge of the IOL moves forward) in left eyes.[7]

More precise postoperative IOL positioning can be achieved through adequate capsulorrhexis on the anterior capsule of the crystalline lens during cataract surgery. In recent years, the most commonly used technique for creating a precise anterior capsulorrhexis during phacoemulsification has been continuous curvilinear capsulorrhexis (CCC). CCC has several surgical and postoperative advantages, but its completion takes vigilant attention and surgical expertise. Obtaining a precise capsulorrhexis is essential to reach demanding refractive results because a properly sized and well-centered capsulorrhexis with a 360-degree overlapping capsular edge prevents optic decentration, tilt, shift toward myopia or hyperopia, posterior and anterior capsular opacification due to symmetric contractile forces of the capsular bag, and shrinkwrap effect. However, an eccentric or irregularly shaped capsulorrhexis with a diameter extending beyond the optic edge may lose these advantages.[8-14]

Capsulorrhexis until now has been a manual procedure. With the advent of femtosecond lasers in ophthalmic surgery, a predictably sized and centered anterior capsulotomy has become possible through a laser–tissue interaction known as photodisruption.

Recently introduced femtosecond laser technology enables a precise and reproducible creation of capsulotomies.

Accuracy of Femtosecond Laser-Assisted Capsulotomy

In an initial study of our research group, we evaluated the use of the femtosecond laser system for creating anterior capsulotomy in human eyes. All laser procedures resulted in successful capsulotomy allowing the surgeon to create a customized capsulotomy individualized for each treatment. A 4.5-mm capsulotomy diameter was chosen to perform capsulotomy in cases of implantation of IOLs with a 6.0-mm optic diameter.

Nagy ZZ, ed. *Femtosecond Laser-Assisted Cataract Surgery: Facts and Results* (pp 23-27).

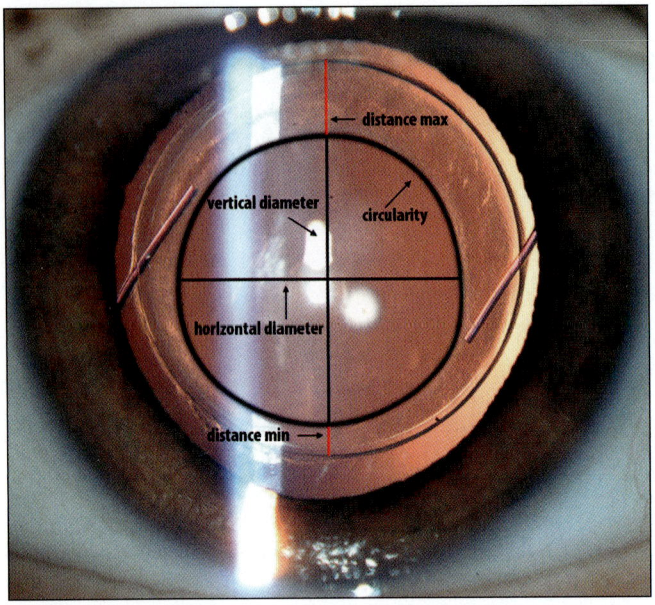

Figure 1. Parameters characteristic to the capsulorrhexis measured by Adobe Photoshop. (Reprinted with permission from Kránitz K, Takacs A, Mihåltz K, Kovács I, Knorz MC, Nagy ZZ. Femtosecond laser capsulotomy and manual continuous curvilinear capsulorrhexis parameters and their effects on intraocular lens centration. *J Refract Surg*. 2011;27[8]:558-563.)

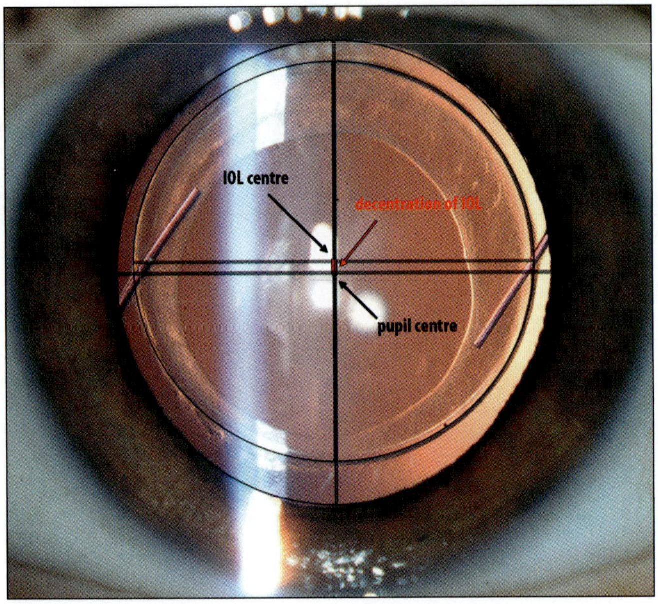

Figure 2. Decentration of the IOL from the pupil center. (Reprinted with permission from Kránitz K, Takacs A, Mihåltz K, Kovács I, Knorz MC, Nagy ZZ. Femtosecond laser capsulotomy and manual continuous curvilinear capsulorrhexis parameters and their effects on intraocular lens centration. *J Refract Surg*. 2011;27[8]:558-563.)

Comparing postoperative accuracy of capsulotomy diameter after femtosecond and manual capsulotomy procedures, only 10% of manual capsulorrhexis achieved diameter accuracy of ±0.25 mm, while femtosecond laser capsulotomy proved to be absolutely precise.[15]

Effect of Circular Femtolaser Capsulotomies on Intraocular Lens Centration

In a prospective, randomized study, postoperative capsulotomy and IOL positioning parameters were analyzed during a 1-year follow-up period according to retroillumination photographs (Figs 1 and 2). We compared femtosecond capsulotomies with conventional, manually performed CCC. Femtosecond laser-assisted capsulotomy and conventional CCC were carried out in 20 eyes of 20 patients, respectively. More regular capsulotomy shape, characterized by better circularity values, was observed 1 week after surgery in the femtosecond capsulotomy group (0.86±0.01 vs 0.83±0.02, $P<.05$). Circularity is a parameter used for determining the regularity of capsulotomy shape according to the following formula: circularity = 4Π (area/perimeter^2). Difference in circularity between the two capsulotomy groups could be explained with disproportion of vertical and horizontal diameter values in the manual capsulorrhexis group. Vertical diameter of capsulotomies proved to be significantly higher 1 week and 1 month after surgery in the CCC group (4.79±0.36 vs 4.51±0.11 and 4.62±0.34 vs 4.47±0.21, respectively, $P<.05$).

In this study, properly sized, shaped, and centered femtosecond capsulotomies resulted in better overlap parameters during the first year (1 week: 0.17±0.19 vs 0.47±0.24; 1 month: 0.24±0.23 vs 0.53±0.25; 1 year: 0.13±0.19 vs 0.54±0.31, $P<.05$). The quotient of the shortest and longest distance between the edge of the capsulorrhexis and the edge of the IOL optic was calculated to determine capsule–IOL overlap (overlap = distance min/distance max). Circularity and overlap values of 1.0 indicate a perfect circle and an absolute regularly overlapping anterior capsule on the optic of the implanted IOL, respectively.

Irregularity of manual capsulorrhexis through asymmetric contractile and vector forces aggravated the centration of implanted IOL over time. In our study, the length of vertical diameter correlated with the overlap of the anterior capsule in the manual capsulorrhexis group (1 week: $r=-0.91$, $P<.01$; 1 month: $r=-0.76$, $P<.01$; 1 year: $r=-0.62$, $P<.01$). Higher values of this parameter are able to lead to irregular anterior capsule overlap.

A 360-degree overlapping capsular edge was thought to be an important factor for standardizing refractive results by keeping the IOL in the desired center position. Our results showed significantly higher horizontal decentration in the manual capsulorrhexis group 1 week and 1 year after implanting IOLs (1 week: 0.28±0.16

vs 0.12±0.11; 1 month: 0.26±0.14 vs 0.13±0.09; 1 year: 0.30±0.16 vs 0.15±0.12, *P*<.05), and there was statistically significant difference in the distribution of dichotomized horizontal decentration values at 0.4 mm between the two study groups 1 week and 1 year after surgery (1 week: 0/20 vs 4/16; 1 year: 0/20 vs 5/15, *P*=.035 and .016, respectively). We found an almost six times higher odds for IOL decentration when capsulorrhexis was performed manually (univariable generalized estimating equation model [odds ratio: 5.95, 95% confidence limit: 1.58-22.22, *P*<.01]). Moreover, it seems that "overlap" captures all characteristics of the capsulorrhexis shape. When predictors of horizontal IOL decentration were explored, only capsulorrhexis overlap showed a significant effect (*P*=.002) among all capsulorrhexis parameters. Our results showed that overlap had significant effect on IOL horizontal decentration representing the importance of precise sizing and centration of capsulotomy.

According to the results of our study, potential clinical advantages can be achieved during refractive cataract surgery through effective prevention of optic decentration with precisely controlled shape, size, and centration of capsulotomy with femtosecond laser.[16]

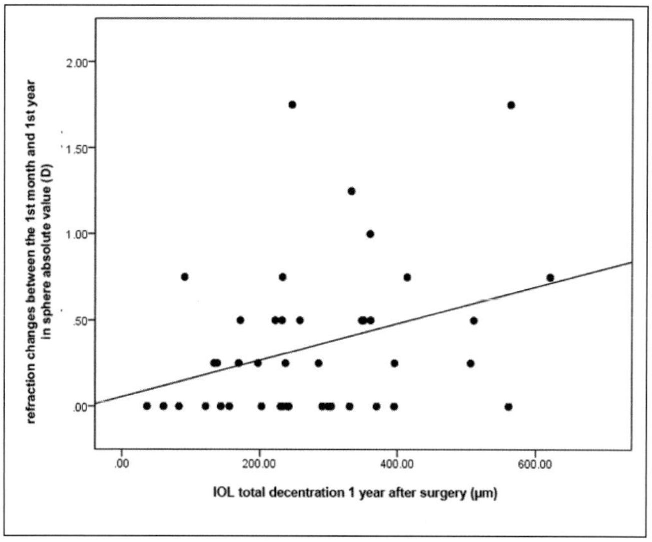

Figure 3. Correlation between the absolute value of IOL total decentration and the total absolute value of changes in manifest refraction spherical equivalent between the first postoperative month and year. Spearman-rank correlation: r=0.33, *P*=.032. (Reprinted with permission from Kránitz K, Miháltz K, Sándor GL, Takacs A, Knorz MC, Nagy ZZ. Intraocular lens tilt and decentration measured by Scheimpflug camera following manual or femtosecond laser-created continuous circular capsulotomy. *J Refract Surg.* 2012;28[4]:259-263.)

Precise Femtolaser Capsulotomies Result in Better Visual Acuity and More Stable Postoperative Refraction Through Decreased Intraocular Lens Misalignment

Our research group evaluated misalignments of implanted IOLs after femtosecond (20 eyes) and conventional manual CCC (25 eyes) by Scheimpflug camera to determine postoperative IOL tilt and to confirm former centration results.

Centration outcomes assessed by Pentacam correlated well with our previous findings: IOLs implanted after manual capsulorrhexis showed significantly higher horizontal and total decentration than in the femtolaser-assisted group (horizontal: 270.83±190.85 µm vs 164.25±113.78 µm, *P*=.034 and total: 334.91±169.67 µm vs 230.27±111.54 µm, *P*=.022).

According to our results, magnitude of both horizontal and vertical tilt also proved to be significantly higher in the manual capsulorrhexis group (horizontal: 2.75±1.67 µm vs 1.53±1.08 µm, *P*=.007 and vertical: 4.34±2.40 µm vs 2.15±1.41 µm, *P*<.001). Since more than 5 degrees of tilt and 0.4 mm of decentration may deteriorate visual outcomes of customized IOLs, clinical significance of femtolaser capsulotomies was examined by comparing the distribution of dichotomized tilt and decentration values between the two study groups. Our results showed statistically significant differences in the homogeneity of dichotomized IOL vertical tilt and both horizontal and total decentration distribution (vertical tilt: 10/25 vs 0/20, *P*=.008 and horizontal decentration: 6/25 vs 0/20, *P*=.036 and total decentration: 8/25 vs 0/20, *P*=.017).

We examined the effect of IOL misalignment on visual acuity and alteration of postoperative manifest refraction. According to our results, IOL decentration influenced the stability of postoperative manifest refraction. There was significant correlation between the absolute value of total decentration and the absolute value of changes in spherical manifest refraction between the first postoperative month and 1 year (r=0.33, *P*=.032) (Fig 3).

In our study, we found a significantly better corrected distance visual acuity (0.92±0.09 vs 0.97±0.06, *P*=.038) associated with lower vertical tilt in the femtolaser group (linear regression analysis: R^2=0.17, β=−0.41, 95% confidence limit: −0.69 to −0.13, *P*=.005). Correlation between visual acuity and tilt values showed that tilt of the IOL from the right anteroposterior position worsens visual quality, supposedly because of induced higher-order aberrations that cannot be corrected with a spectacle.

In this study, we were able to demonstrate that the use of a femtosecond laser to create anterior curvilinear capsulotomy results in less IOL decentration and tilt, better visual acuity, and more stable and predictable postoperative refraction.[17]

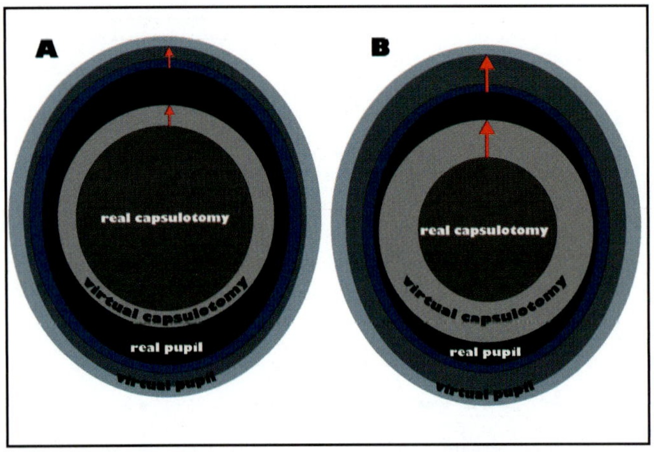

Figure 4. Distortion effect of **A)** myopic and **B)** hyperopic corneas. Red arrows show the magnification effect of the cornea depending on average keratometry values. (Reprinted with permission from Nagy ZZ, Kránitz K, Takacs AI, Mihály K, Kovács I, Knorz MC. Comparison of intraocular lens decentration parameters after femtosecond and manual capsulotomies. *J Refract Surg.* 2011;27[8]:564-569.)

Importance of Femtosecond Laser Capsulotomy in High Myopia

Myopia is a common disorder. In high myopic eyes, often the only solution is implanting an artificial lens after phacoemulsification to correct refractive error. Moreover, these eyes are also more likely to develop cataract.

Completely overlapping anterior capsule on the optic edge of the IOL prevents posterior capsule opacification. Reducing the severity of this disorder is essential in myopic eyes to decrease the risk of retinal detachment due to neodymium:yttrium-aluminum-garnet (Nd:YAG) laser capsulotomy. Complete overlap also results in better IOL centration and less postoperative refractive shift by maintaining the IOL in the proper position.

Our research group examined postoperative IOL positions after femtosecond laser capsulotomies (54 eyes) and conventionally performed CCCs (57 eyes) in high myopia.

Special anatomical characteristics of myopic eyes make cataract surgery a challenge for experienced surgeons as well.

There is no reliable reference marker to aid the surgeon in creating the correct size and shape of CCC. Most commonly, the pupil margin is used as a reference, despite the large variation in pupil diameter. In association with previous articles that reported larger pupillary diameters in myopic eyes under mesopic conditions, statistically significant correlation between axial length and area of pharmacologically dilated pupils was found in our study as well (r=0.19, *P*=.049).

Variable magnification effect of the cornea induces further errors in capsulotomy sizing. The cornea, according to individual anterior segment anatomy, magnifies the anterior capsule approximately 1.15 times. Even an experienced surgeon tends to prepare a larger capsulorrhexis in eyes with larger pupils. The average keratometry value of flatter myopic corneas seems to virtually compensate larger pupil diameters due to the relatively smaller magnification effect (Fig 4). In this study, statistically significant correlation was found between axial length and average keratometry values (r=–0.22, *P*=.018) and between axial length and preoperative anterior chamber depth (r=0.27, *P*=.007). According to our results, the pupillary area correlated significantly with the area of the capsulotomy (r=0.27, *P*=.039), and furthermore, significant correlations were noted between axial length and area of capsulotomy (r=0.278, *P*=.036) and between average keratometry and area of the capsulotomy (r=–0.29, *P*=.033) in the manual capsulorrhexis group, while these parameters did not correlate in the femtolaser group.

As a consequence of all these effects, manual capsulorrhexis is often larger in myopic eyes than is expected. Using a femtolaser during capsulotomy procedure, these errors can be eliminated, creating a precise capsulotomy.

Circularity values similar to our previous results proved to be significantly better in the femtolaser group. The ratio of incomplete overlap proved to be 11% in the case of femtolaser and 28% in the case of manual capsulotomies. This difference between the study groups was statistically significant (*P*=.033). The implantation of an IOL into myopic eyes during conventional cataract surgery may mean a higher risk for IOL decentration due to larger capsular bag and larger capsulorrhexis. We did not find a correlation between IOL centration and axial length in the femtolaser group, but we found one in the manual capsulotomy group (r=0.30, *P*=.026), suggesting that IOL centration is better after a femtosecond laser capsulotomy (Fig 5).[18]

Discussion

Over the past 2 decades, increased demand has led to a marked growth in the number of cataract operations. Surgery is being performed earlier on average because patients' needs and the results that they expect to obtain from the surgery have been raised. To meet these increased visual requirements, increased numbers of different premium multifocal and accommodative IOLs have appeared on the market.

In peer-reviewed papers, our research group demonstrated that femtosecond laser represents an important technological advance in ophthalmic surgery by publishing results of prospective clinical trials implemented in the Department of Ophthalmology, Semmelweis University, Budapest, Hungary.

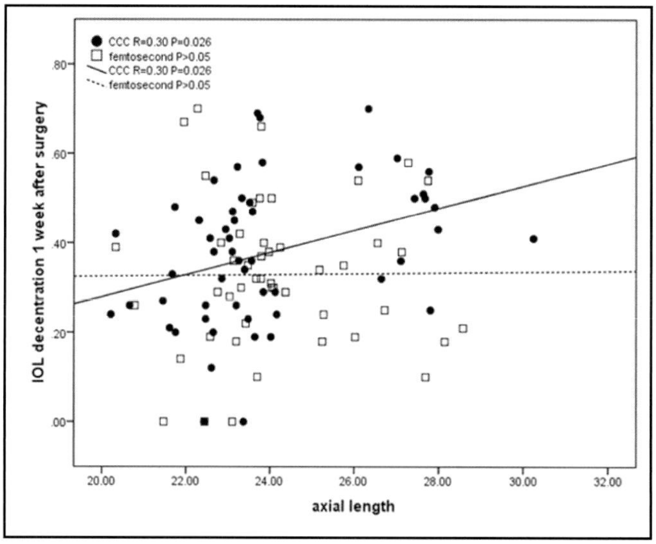

Figure 5. Correlation between axial length and IOL decentration 1 week after surgery. The correlation was significant in the manual capsulotomy group (CCC) (r=0.30, *P*=.026) but not in the laser capsulotomy group (femtosecond) (*P*>.05). (Reprinted with permission from Nagy ZZ, Kránitz K, Takacs AI, Miháltz K, Kovács I, Knorz MC. Comparison of intraocular lens decentration parameters after femtosecond and manual capsulotomies. *J Refract Surg.* 2011;27[8]:564-569.)

Investigating the differences between femtosecond laser capsulotomies and a manual CCC during cataract surgery, capsulotomy size, circularity, and IOL/capsulotomy overlap were evaluated. These parameters correlated well to IOL misalignment, visual acuity values, and postoperative refractive changes.

According to our results, potential clinical advantages could be achieved during refractive cataract surgery with precisely controlled shape, size, and centration of capsulotomy with femtosecond laser.

References

1. 2009 comprehensive report on the global single-use ophthalmic surgical product market. *Market Scope.* August 2009.
2. Baumeister M, Buhren J, Kohnen T. Tilt and decentration of spherical and aspheric intraocular lenses: effect on higher-order aberrations. *J Cataract Refract Surg.* 2009;35(6):1006-1012.
3. Eppig T, Scholz K, Loffler A, Messner A, Langenbucher A. Effect of decentration and tilt on the image quality of aspheric intraocular lens designs in a model eye. *J Cataract Refract Surg.* 2009;35(6):1091-1100.
4. Mihaltz K, Knorz MC, Alio JL, et al. Internal aberrations and optical quality after femtosecond laser anterior capsulotomy in cataract surgery. *J Refract Surg.* 2011;27(10):711-716.
5. Holladay JT, Piers PA, Koranyi G, van der Mooren M, Norrby NE. A new intraocular lens design to reduce spherical aberration of pseudophakic eyes. *J Refract Surg.* 2002;18(6):683-691.
6. Piers PA, Weeber HA, Artal P, Norrby S. Theoretical comparison of aberration-correcting customized and aspheric intraocular lenses. *J Refract Surg.* 2007;23(4):374-384.
7. de Castro A, Rosales P, Marcos S. Tilt and decentration of intraocular lenses in vivo from Purkinje and Scheimpflug imaging. Validation study. *J Cataract Refract Surg.* 2007;33(3):418-429.
8. Ravalico G, Tognetto D, Palomba M, Busatto P, Baccara F. Capsulorhexis size and posterior capsule opacification. *J Cataract Refract Surg.* 1996;22(1):98-103.
9. Aykan U, Bilge AH, Karadayi K. The effect of capsulorhexis size on development of posterior capsule opacification: small (4.5 to 5.0 mm) versus large (6.0 to 7.0 mm). *Eur J Ophthalmol.* 2003;13(6):541-545.
10. Hollick EJ, Spalton DJ, Meacock WR. The effect of capsulorhexis size on posterior capsular opacification: one-year results of a randomized prospective trial. *Am J Ophthalmol.* 1999;128(3):271-279.
11. Ram J, Pandey SK, Apple DJ, et al. Effect of in-the-bag intraocular lens fixation on the prevention of posterior capsule opacification. *J Cataract Refract Surg.* 2001;27(7):367-370.
12. Chang DF, Dewey S, Tipperman R, Wallace RB. Pearls for sizing the capsulorrhexis. *Cataract & Refractive Surgery Today Europe.* 2008;3(9):40-44.
13. Hayashi K, Hayashi H, Nakao F, Hayashi F. Anterior capsule contraction and intraocular lens decentration and tilt after hydrogel lens implantation. *Br J Ophthalmol.* 2001;85(11):1294-1297.
14. Hayashi H, Hayashi K, Nakao F, Hayashi F. Anterior capsule contraction and intraocular lens dislocation in eyes with pseudoexfoliation syndrome. *Br J Ophthalmol.* 1998;82(12):1429-1432.
15. Nagy Z, Takacs A, Filkorn T, Sarayba M. Initial clinical evaluation of an intraocular femtosecond laser in cataract surgery. *J Refract Surg.* 2009;25(12):1053-1060.
16. Kránitz K, Takacs A, Mihàltz K, Kovács I, Knorz MC, Nagy ZZ. Femtosecond laser capsulotomy and manual continuous curvilinear capsulorrhexis parameters and their effects on intraocular lens centration. *J Refract Surg.* 2011;27(8):558-563.
17. Kránitz K, Mihàltz K, Sándor GL, Takacs A, Knorz MC, Nagy ZZ. Intraocular lens tilt and decentration measured by Scheimpflug camera following manual or femtosecond laser-created continuous circular capsulotomy. *J Refract Surg.* 2012;28(4):259-263.
18. Nagy ZZ, Kránitz K, Takacs AI, Mihàltz K, Kovács I, Knorz MC. Comparison of intraocular lens decentration parameters after femtosecond and manual capsulotomies. *J Refract Surg.* 2011;27(8):564-569.

Mechanical Behavior of Capsulotomy Performed With Femtosecond Laser

Gábor László Sándor, MD; Zoltán Kiss, PhD; Zoltán I. Bocskai; Imre Bojtár, PhD, CSc; Ágnes I. Takács, MD; Zoltán Z. Nagy, MD, PhD, DSc

Performing a precise anterior capsulorrhexis is a key part of cataract surgery. An ideal rhexis is circular and well centered, and its edge is intact and free from weak points. These help to maintain proper intraocular lens (IOL) position within the capsular bag and also help to minimize incidence of radial tear. The opening should withstand the stress of maneuvers in surgery because a radial tear may occur at any stage of the operation. A radial tear disrupts the integrity of the capsular bag, thus the appropriate position of an IOL is compromised. As patient demands have increased, the importance of predictable position of IOL has increased dramatically. New technology IOLs, including aspheric, toric, and multifocal, have also driven this need for improved position.

Furthermore, one of the most feared complications during phacoemulsification is posterior capsule rupture. In almost half the cases, posterior tear occurs due to the extension of an anterior tear, often requiring an anterior vitrectomy.[1]

In recent years, the most commonly used technique has been continuous curvilinear capsulorrhexis (CCC).[2] While performing a CCC, the tear presumably runs along natural fibrillar "fault lines," resulting in a very smooth edge of the opening.[3] Extensibility of CCC is superior to other anterior capsulotomy techniques (eg, vitrectorhexis, can-opener, radio frequency diathermy, plasma blade), presumably due to the smooth and regular rim.[4] Other techniques mentioned above may not respect these natural fault lines in collagen architecture, and that may cause an irregular edge.

However, CCC seems perfect from a mechanical viewpoint[5]; it is performed manually and its accuracy and reproducibility are inherently limited by the surgeon's dexterity.

With the introduction of femtosecond laser-assisted cataract surgery, a highly controlled and reproducible capsulotomy became possible through a laser–tissue interaction known as photodisruption.[6] Our study group evaluated and assessed the precise dimensions of the femtosecond laser capsulotomy.[6-8] However, the laser–tissue effect is not fully revealed, thus the mechanical behavior of the capsular opening is not fully understood.

Earlier studies reported a stronger capsulotomy edge performed with femtosecond laser than the edge of manual capsulorrhexis.[6,9-11] However, a multicenter clinical study with a large sample size showed there is a higher incidency of radial tear following femtosecond laser capsulotomy than conventional CCC.[12] Furthermore, scanning electron microscopy (SEM) studies showed microgrooves[9] and perforations[12-14] at the rim of the femtosecond laser capsulotomy. A finite element model shows a jagged edge increases the risk of tear formation, due to unequal stress distribution throughout the rim.[5] Recent SEM studies did not give any answer why femtosecond laser capsulotomy would be stronger than CCC.

A test method was therefore created by our study group for the purpose of evaluation of the mechanical behavior of an anterior capsulotomy performed with a femtosecond laser in a porcine eye model. At this time, a pilot study is underway, thus we are presenting preliminary results in this chapter.

Fresh porcine eyes were included in the study. A femtosecond laser (Alcon LenSx Inc, Aliso Viejo, California) was docked to the eye using the SoftFit patient interface. The exact location of the crystalline lens surface was determined with an integrated optical coherence tomography (OCT) imaging system. A 5.0-mm diameter capsulotomy procedure was performed by scanning a cylindrical pattern starting at least 500 μm below the anterior capsule and ending at least 500 μm above the capsule. Pulse energy of 5.0 μJ, 3.0 μm spot separation, and 4.0 μm layer separation were used for all capsulotomy procedures.

Following the laser procedure, the cornea and iris were removed. After that, the anterior capsule was cut with microscissors around the equator. Using this technique resulted in a ring-shaped capsule specimen.

Nagy ZZ, ed. *Femtosecond Laser-Assisted Cataract Surgery: Facts and Results* (pp 29-31).

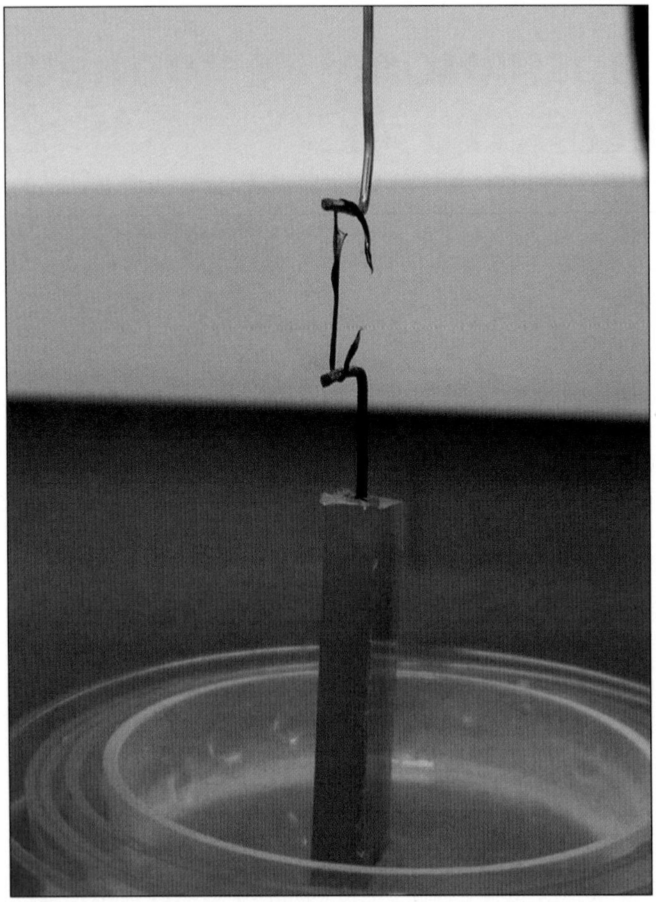

Figure 1. The ring-shaped specimen at the time of rupture. The chamber was removed and the capsule was stained with trypan blue for better visualization. The lower pin is fixed; the upper one is incorporated with the force transducer.

Mechanical testing was carried out with a high-precision testing machine. The specimen support consisted of two polished metal pins. It was submerged into room-temperature balanced salt solution during the test to prevent dehydration of the tissue. The ring-shaped specimen was slipped carefully over the two pins. One pin incorporated a force transducer that was separated from the other one until the capsule ring was torn (Fig 1). The software of the testing machine continuously created a force vs displacement curve.

Figure 2 shows a typical force vs displacement diagram. The curve can be divided into two sections: first, the flat part of the curve presumably reflects a gradual alignment of the collagen network in the direction of stretching; the second, steep part reflects that the molecules become load bearing.[15] Note that the second part of the curve is at least as long as the first one. This suggests that the collagen network remained relatively intact and is able to bear a remarkable load. According to this, the denaturation of collagen caused by thermal damage is not significant. The graph also shows that the rise in force is steep and the curve ends suddenly. This characteristic is useful from a clinical point of view because a surgeon may feel the stretching limit of the capsulotomy during surgical maneuvers.

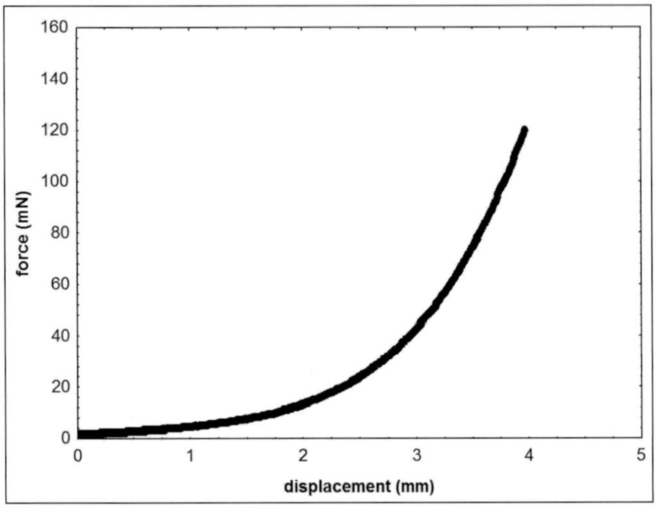

Figure 2. A typical force vs displacement diagram.

The impact of stress concentration at points of microgrooves on mechanical stability of femtosecond laser capsulotomy is unclear at this time. In our opinion, further mechanical and histological examinations should be performed for a correct answer.

Laboratory and clinical studies are controversial, but in summary, they assumed that a capsulotomy created by femtosecond laser differs from manual capsulorrhexis from a biomechanical point of view and this should be taken into consideration by the surgeon. If the surgeon respects the learning curve, it may contribute to the safety of the operation. According to our preliminary laboratory results and own clinical experiences, femtosecond laser capsulotomy has a remarkable strength and stretching capacity and more than adequate resistance for a safe phacoemulsification and a successful IOL implantation.

References

1. Marques FF, Marques DM, Osher RH, Osher JM. Fate of anterior capsule tears during cataract surgery. *J Cataract Refract Surg.* 2006;32(10):1638-1642.
2. Gimbel HV, Neuhann T. Development, advantages, and methods of the continuous circular capsulorhexis technique. *J Cataract Refract Surg.* 1990;16(1):31-37.
3. Luck J, Brahma AK, Noble BA. A comparative study of the elastic properties of continuous tear curvilinear capsulorhexis versus capsulorhexis produced by radiofrequency endodiathermy. *Br J Ophthalmol.* 1994;78(5):392-396.
4. Trivedi RH, Wilson ME Jr, Bartholomew LR. Extensibility and scanning electron microscopy evaluation of 5 pediatric anterior capsulotomy techniques in a porcine model. *J Cataract Refract Surg.* 2006;32(7):1206-1213.

5. Krag S, Thim K, Corydon L, Kyster B. Biomechanical aspects of the anterior capsulotomy. *J Cataract Refract Surg*. 1994;20(4):410-416.
6. Nagy Z, Takacs A, Filkorn T, Sarayba M. Initial clinical evaluation of an intraocular femtosecond laser in cataract surgery. *J Refract Surg*. 2009;25(12):1053-1060.
7. Kranitz K, Takacs A, Miháltz K, Kovács I, Knorz MC, Nagy ZZ. Femtosecond laser capsulotomy and manual continuous curvilinear capsulorrhexis parameters and their effects on intraocular lens centration. *J Refract Surg*. 2011;27(8):558-563.
8. Nagy ZZ, Kránitz K, Takacs AI, Mihaltz K, Kovács I, Knorz MC. Comparison of intraocular lens decentration parameters after femtosecond and manual capsulotomies. *J Refract Surg*. 2011;27(8):564-569.
9. Friedman NJ, Palanker DV, Schuele G, et al. Femtosecond laser capsulotomy. *J Cataract Refract Surg*. 2011;37(7):1189-1198.
10. Naranjo-Tackman R. How a femtosecond laser increases safety and precision in cataract surgery. *Curr Opin Ophthalmol*. 2011;22(1):53-57.
11. Auffarth GU, Reddy KP, Ritter R, Holzer MP, Rabsilber TM. Comparison of the maximum applicable stretch force after femtosecond laser-assisted and manual anterior capsulotomy. *J Cataract Refract Surg*. 2013;39(1):105-109.
12. Abell RG, Davies PE, Phelan D, Goemann K, McPherson ZE, Vote BJ. Anterior capsulotomy integrity after femtosecond laser-assisted cataract surgery. *Ophthalmology*. 2014;121(1):17-24.
13. Mastropasqua L, Toto L, Calienno R, et al. Scanning electron microscopy evaluation of capsulorhexis in femtosecond laser-assisted cataract surgery. *J Cataract Refract Surg*. 2013;39(10):1581-1586.
14. Ostovic M, Klaproth OK, Hengerer FH, Mayer WJ, Kohnen T. Light microscopy and scanning electron microscopy analysis of rigid curved interface femtosecond laser-assisted and manual anterior capsulotomy. *J Cataract Refract Surg*. 2013;39(10):1587-1592.
15. Krag S, Thim K, Corydon L. Diathermic capsulotomy versus capsulorhexis: a biomechanical study. *J Cataract Refract Surg*. 1997;23(1):86-90.

Intraocular Lens Calculation Results and Refractive Outcomes After Femtosecond Laser-Assisted and Conventional Cataract Surgery

Tamás Filkorn, MD; Illés Kovács, MD, PhD; Kinga Kránitz, MD; Ágnes I. Takács, MD; Éva Horváth, MD; Michael C. Knorz, MD; Zoltán Z. Nagy, MD, PhD, DSc

Development of premium intraocular lenses (IOLs) requires more precise refractive outcomes after cataract surgery than ever before. Accurate biometry and IOL calculation are indispensable to achieve good visual acuity. With the advent of new optical biometers, error of IOL calculation procedures decreased due to precise axial length measurements; however, calculation of the effective lens position may serve as a source of further errors.[1,2] IOL tilt, decentration, and anteroposterior movements may induce postoperative refractive error. However, with a femtosecond laser perfectly centered, regular capsulorrhexis can be performed to achieve optimal postoperative IOL position, and surgical trauma could be decreased with nucleus prefragmentation.[3,4]

Intraocular Lens Calculation Results and Refractive Outcomes

In a prospective, randomized study we evaluated IOL calculation results of patients who underwent femtolaser cataract surgery and conventional phacoemulsification and compared refractive outcomes of the two study groups.

Femtosecond laser-assisted cataract surgery was performed on 77 eyes of 77 patients (laser group), while traditional cataract surgery with phacoemulsification was carried out on 57 eyes of 57 patients (control group).

During conventional cataract surgery, 2.75-mm clear corneal incisions, manual continuous curvilinear capsulorrhexis (CCC) with an attempted diameter of 4.5 mm, and phacoemulsification with chop technique were performed followed by monofocal in-the-bag IOL implantation.

Patients in the laser group underwent the femtolaser procedure before phacoemulsification; the integrated real-time optical coherence tomography imaging system enhanced the safety of the procedure by avoiding critical structures. After a user-adjustable centration and depth control of the laser pattern, 2.75-mm clear corneal incisions, 1.0-mm paracentesis, and a 4.5-mm diameter capsulotomy were performed in every patient followed by cross-shape lens fragmentation. After the laser procedure, the closed corneal incisions were opened using a blunt spatula, and the anterior capsule was removed with forceps. The nucleus fragments were removed using phacoemulsification, followed by irrigation-aspiration and implantation of a monofocal IOL into the capsular bag.

Optical biometry measurements were performed using low coherence optical reflectometry (Lenstar LS900, Haag-Streit AG, Koeniz, Switzerland). Third-generation IOL formulas and optimized IOL constants were used for IOL calculation. The Hoffer Q formula was used for short eyes (axial length >22.0 mm), the average of the three formulas was used for eyes with average axial length (between 22.0 and 24.5 mm), the Holladay formula was used for moderately long eyes (axial length between 24.5 and 26.0 mm), and the SRK/T was used for long eyes (axial length >26.0 mm) as recommended in our national biometry protocol.

Postoperative refraction and best-corrected distance visual acuity were ascertained at least 6 weeks after surgery after achieving stable refraction. Only patients with 20/40 or better best spectacle-corrected visual acuity were included in the study to be able to determine correct refraction.

The mean error (ME) was assessed as the difference of the postoperative manifest refraction in spherical equivalent (MRSE) and the predicted postoperative target refraction. The mean absolute error ([MAE] the average of the absolute value of the deviation from predicted postoperative refractive outcome) was used to analyze the accuracy of IOL calculation for different groups. The cumulative proportion of eyes within ±0.25 D, ±0.5 D, ±1.0 D, ±1.5 D, and ±2.0 D of MAE was also expressed to reveal the refractive outcome. Multivariable regression analysis was performed to determine the effect of surgery type on postoperative refractive error.

Nagy ZZ, ed. *Femtosecond Laser-Assisted Cataract Surgery: Facts and Results* (pp 33-35).

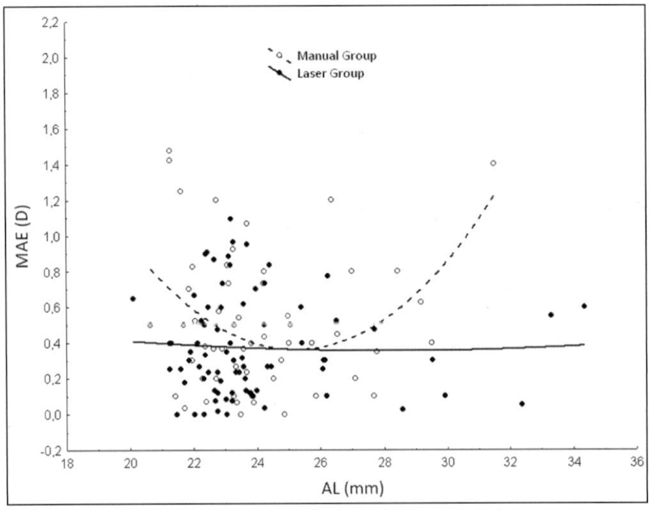

Figure 1. Correlation between the axial length and the MAE in the two groups.

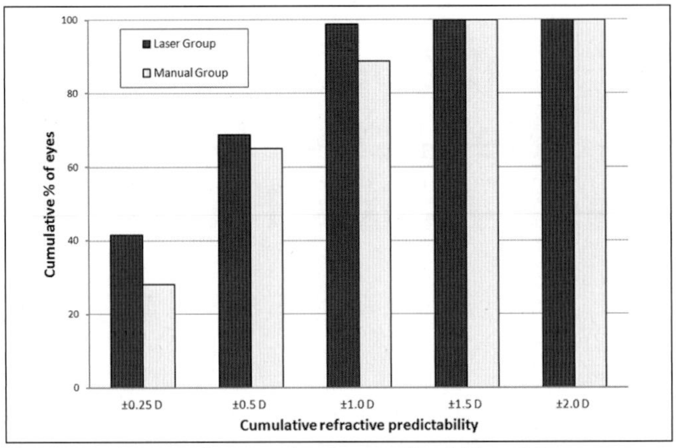

Figure 2. The cumulative refractive predictability of the eyes.

According to our results, eyes with average axial length showed the lowest MAE for all formulas, and IOL calculation error proved to be more significant in long and short eyes.

Using the adequate IOL calculation formula—depending on the axial length—the MAE was 0.38±0.28 D in the laser group and 0.50±0.38 D in the control group. The correlation between the axial length and the MAE in the two groups is shown in Figure 1. Significant cubic correlation was found in the control group (r=0.14, *P*=.011), while no correlation was found in the laser group (*P*>.05).

In multivariable modeling, the type of surgery showed significant effect on the postoperative MAE after adjustment for the effect of axial length and IOL type (*P*=.04). In the laser group, the MAE was lower compared to the control group, with an average difference of 0.12 D. The IOL type had no effect on postoperative refractive error (*P*=.19). The difference between the two study groups was more significant in the case of very short and very long eyes showing the efficacy of femtolaser-assisted surgeries.

Analyzing the ME, there was no statistically significant difference between the two study groups (−0.03±0.47 vs 0.07±0.63, *P*>.05, Mann-Whitney U test). No correlation was found between ME and axial length in the laser group (*P*=.41). In the manual group, there was a weak but significant correlation (r=−0.29, *P*=.03), showing more myopic errors in eyes with long axial length.

Comparing refractive predictability, 41.6% of eyes were within ±0.25 D of target refraction in the laser group, compared to 28.1% of eyes in the manual group. Of the eyes, 68.8% and 64.9% were within ±0.5 D and 98.7% and 87.7% within ±1.0 D, respectively. All eyes were within ±1.5 D in both groups. Figure 2 shows the cumulative refractive predictability of the eyes.

Discussion

Cataract surgery has become a refractive procedure in recent years, making accurate IOL calculation indispensable. These days patients have an increased expectation of better refractive outcome, especially in the case of expensive premium IOL implantation. Besides the inaccuracy of axial length and keratometry measurements, calculation errors are induced mainly by miscalculated postoperative lens position.[2]

Our IOL calculation results are in agreement with previously published large volume studies using ultrasound[5] and partial laser interferometry[6] for IOL calculation.

We found significantly lower postoperative IOL calculation error and better refractive outcomes when femtosecond laser pretreatment was performed before cataract surgery.

The difference between the two methods in IOL calculation errors was the highest in the case of short and long eyes. Presumably, the higher the IOL power (implanted into short eyes), the higher the induced refractive change due to IOL displacement.[7] Moreover, it has been previously shown that IOL tilt, decentration, and anteroposterior movement is higher in long eyes.[4] The precise size, shape, and centration of capsulorrhexis and nucleus prechop technique are the main differences between conventional and femtolaser-assisted cataract surgery that may also influence refractive outcome.

IOL misalignment is a well-known factor that can induce changes in postoperative refraction. The influence of IOL decentration and tilt on postoperative refractive error has been studied by several authors.[7-11] These studies used different methods for IOL calculation but did not differ in conclusions. IOL decentration and tilt induce myopic shift and oblique astigmatism, causing lateral shift of focus. Although an intact CCC can be performed routinely, creating a precisely shaped and centered rhexis in all circumstances may be challenging even for an experienced surgeon. Asymmetric capsular shrinkage increases IOL decentration.[12] Both the size of the capsulotomy and the regularity of anterior capsule overlap influence postoperative IOL position.[13]

Our research group established in previous studies that decentration and tilt of the IOL can be significantly decreased by precise sizing and centration of capsulorrhexis using a femtosecond laser and femtolaser-assisted capsulotomies provided superior results compared to manual CCC.[3,4] Moreover, with femtolaser nucleus prechop the required phaco energy and surgical manipulations could be reduced significantly, presumably decreasing intraoperative zonular stress.[14]

Using femtolaser for cataract surgery, lower postoperative calculation error could be achieved compared to traditional phacoemulsification. The optimal capsulorrhexis and less zonular trauma facilitate stable postoperative IOL position and minimize IOL misalignment compared to precalculated effective lens position. With this technique, better refractive outcomes and higher spectacle independence could be obtained and refractive surprises could be reduced. These results are of particular importance in premium IOL (multifocal and pseudoaccommodative lenses) implantations.

References

1. Olsen T. Sources of error in intraocular lens power calculation. *J Cataract Refract Surg.* 1992;18(2):125-129.
2. Norrby S. Sources of error in intraocular lens power calculation. *J Cataract Refract Surg.* 2008;34(3):368-376.
3. Kránitz K, Takacs A, Mihaltz K, Kovács I, Knorz MC, Nagy ZZ. Femtosecond laser capsulotomy and manual continuous curvilinear capsulorrhexis parameters and their effects on intraocular lens centration. *J Refract Surg.* 2011;27(8):558-563.
4. Nagy ZZ, Kránitz K, Takacs AI, Mihaltz K, Kovács I, Knorz MC. Comparison of intraocular lens decentration parameters after femtosecond and manual capsulotomies. *J Refract Surg.* 2011;27(8):564-569.
5. Gale RP, Saha N, Johnston RL. National Biometry Audit II. *Eye (Lond).* 2006;20(1):25-28.
6. Aristodemou P, Knox Cartwright NE, Sparrow JM, Johnston RL. Formula choice: Hoffer Q, Holladay 1, or SRK/T and refractive outcomes in 8108 eyes after cataract surgery with biometry by partial coherence interferometry. *J Cataract Refract Surg.* 2011;37(1):63-71.
7. Lakshminarayanan V, Enoch JM, Raasch T, Crawford B, Nygaard RW. Refractive changes induced by intraocular lens tilt and longitudinal displacement. *Arch Ophthalmol.* 1986;104(1):90-92.
8. Atchison DA. Refractive errors induced by displacement of intraocular lenses within the pseudophakic eye. *Optom Vis Sci.* 1989;66(3):146-152.
9. Erickson P. Effects of intraocular lens position errors on postoperative refractive error. *J Cataract Refract Surg.* 1990;16(3):305-311.
10. Kozaki J, Tanihara H, Yasuda A, Nagata M. Tilt and decentration of the implanted posterior chamber intraocular lens. *J Cataract Refract Surg.* 1991;17(5):592-595.
11. Korynta J, Bok J, Cendelin J. Changes in refraction induced by change in intraocular lens position. *J Refract Corneal Surg.* 1994;10(5):556-564.
12. Ohmi S. Decentration associated with asymmetric capsular shrinkage and intraocular lens size. *J Cataract Refract Surg.* 1993;19(5):640-643.
13. Nanavaty MA, Raj SM, Vasavada VA, Vasavada VA, Vasavada AR. Anterior capsule cover and axial movement of intraocular lens. *Eye (Lond).* 2008;22(8):1015-1023.
14. Nagy Z, Takacs A, Filkorn T, Sarayba M. Initial clinical evaluation of an intraocular femtosecond laser in cataract surgery. *J Refract Surg.* 2009;25(12):1053-1060.

Corneal Changes Following Femtosecond Laser-Assisted Phacoemulsification Compared to Conventional Cataract Surgery

Ágnes I. Takács, MD; Illés Kovács, MD, PhD; Kata Mihátz, MD, PhD; Tamás Filkorn, MD; Michael C. Knorz, MD; Zoltán Z. Nagy, MD, PhD, DSc

Purpose

The aim of our study was to analyze corneal changes following femtosecond laser-assisted phacoemulsification and compare the results with conventional phacoemulsification regarding corneal thickness, endothelial cell count, and volume stress index.

Materials and Methods

This prospective, computer-randomized study began in February 2010 and ended in February 2011. Seventy-six eyes of 76 patients were included: 38 eyes of 38 patients were operated with femtosecond laser-assisted phacoemulsification (femtolaser group) and 38 eyes of 38 patients were operated with conventional phacoemulsification (phaco group). All surgeries were performed by the same experienced surgeon (Z.Z.N.). Exclusion criteria were dense (grade 4+) or white cataract, corneal scars or opacities, anterior segment abnormalities, floppy iris syndrome, poor pupillary dilation, and low cooperation.

There was no statistically significant difference between the two groups regarding patient age (65.81±12.42 years in the femtolaser group and 66.93±10.99 years in the phaco group), male:female ratio (10:28 in the femtolaser group and 15:23 in the phaco group), and manifest refraction spherical equivalent (−1.0±4.7 D in the femtolaser group and −1.0±5.5 D in the phaco group).

The study design was in accordance with the rules of the university's ethical committee and the tenets of the Declaration of Helsinki. Informed consent was obtained from all of the patients.

Topical anesthesia (proparacaine HCl 0.5%) was applied, and for pupillary dilation, tropicamide 0.5% was instilled every 15 minutes, three times before surgery.

The main steps of the surgeries were performed as follows.

In the phaco group, clear corneal main incisions were performed with a disposable keratome (Alcon Laboratories Inc, Ft Worth, Texas), cystotome and capsular forceps were used to create a continuous curvilinear capsulorrhexis, and the lens material was removed with conventional divide-and-conquer phaco technique.

In the femtolaser group, 4.75-mm capsulorrhexis, cross-pattern lens fragmentation and a 2.8-mm wide two-plane main incision and 1.0-mm wide single-plane side-port incision were performed with the LenSx femtosecond laser system (Alcon LenSx Inc, Aliso Viejo, California). Femtosecond laser–created corneal wounds were opened with a blunt spatula, the edge of the laser-created capsulotomy was identified with a cystotome, and the dissected capsule was removed with a forceps. The four laser prechopped lens quadrants were removed with standard phacoemulsification.

The same type of viscoelastic material (Provisc, Alcon Laboratories Inc) and the same phaco system and settings (Alcon Laboratories Inc, vacuum fixed 380 mm Hg, aspiration rate fixed 35 cc/min, bottle height 110 cm) were used in both patient groups. Following conventional removal of the cortex material, a one-piece hydrophobic acrylic intraocular lens ([IOL] Alcon Laboratories Inc) was implanted for all of the patients. After the removal of the viscoelastic material by irrigation-aspiration, the main corneal incision was closed with gentle hydration in every case.

A complete ophthalmic examination was performed before surgery for all patients, including determination of best-corrected visual acuity, manifest refractive error, intraocular pressure, and slit-lamp examination. Preoperative data of patients are shown in Table 1.

Optical low-coherence biometry (Lenstar LS900; Haag-Streit AG) was performed for IOL calculation. Three-mm central corneal volume and nucleus density (PNS) were measured objectively with a rotating Scheimpflug camera (Pentacam HR; Oculus Optikgeräte GmbH).

A noncontact specular microscope (Konan Noncon Robo NSP-9900; Konan Medical Inc, Hyogo, Japan) was used to measure central corneal endothelial cell count.

Nagy ZZ, ed. *Femtosecond Laser-Assisted Cataract Surgery: Facts and Results* (pp 37-40).

TABLE 1

PREOPERATIVE DATA OF PATIENTS

Preoperative Data	Femtolaser Group	Phaco Group	P Value
Gender (male:female)	10:28	15:23	>.05
Age (years)	65.81±12.42	66.93±10.99	>.05
Axial length (mm)	24.1±3.0	23.9±2.9	>.05
Manifest refraction (D)	−1.0±4.7	−1.0±5.5	>.05
Anterior chamber depth (mm)	2.57±0.39	2.62±0.45	>.05
Lens thickness (mm)	4.5±0.5	4.4±0.5	>.05
CCT (μm)	545±32	550±39	>.05
3 mm CV (mm^3)	3.9±0.2	4.0±0.3	>.05
PNS	2.32±0.97	2.13±1.22	>.05
CECC (cell/ mm^2)	2861±215	2841±215	>.05
Intraocular pressure (mm Hg)	16.0±3.2	15.6±2.9	>.05

CCT = central corneal thickness ; CV = corneal volume; PNS = Pentacam Nucleus Staging; CECC = corneal endothelial cell count

TABLE 2

INTRAOPERATIVE DATA OF PATIENTS

Preoperative Data	Femtolaser Group	Phaco Group	P Value
Phacoemulsification energy (%)	12.7±8.3	20.4±12.6	<.05
Phacoemulsification time (s)	0.56±0.6	0.67±0.65	>.05
Effective phaco time (s)	0.10±0.12	0.12±0.13	>.05

Scheimpflug imaging and specular microscopy were repeated 1 day, 1 week, and 1 month postoperatively.

Volume stress index according to Suzuki et al[1] was calculated as follows: VSI = ΔV/(CDx7.065), where ΔV = V2−V1, V2 is the 3-mm corneal volume after cataract surgery, V1 is the 3-mm corneal volume before cataract surgery, and 7.065 = 1.5x1.5x3.14 (equivalent with a 3-mm diameter area).

Statistica 8.0 (Statsoft Inc) software was used for statistical analysis. Shapiro-Wilks W test showed a normal distribution of the data, so independent sample *t* test was used for further statistical analysis. A repeated-measures analysis of variance was performed to analyze corneal thickness changes. A multivariable regression analysis was used to test the effect of the type of surgery on postoperative central corneal thickness, with incorporation of the following variables: preoperative central corneal thickness, central endothelial cell count, anterior chamber depth, PNS, and effective phaco time. Statistical significance was defined as $P<.05$ in all analyses.

RESULTS

Intraoperatively used phacoemulsification energy was significantly lower in the femtolaser group compared to the phaco group (Table 2).

A statistically significant positive correlation was found between PNS and phacoemulsification time in both groups (r=0.35, $P<.05$ in the femtolaser group; r=0.5, $P<.05$ in the phaco group).

In the multivariable model, in which central endothelial cell count, PNS, preoperative central corneal thickness, and group were included as predictors, the best-fit index was $R^2=0.48$. In this model, type of surgery had a significant effect on central corneal thickness 1 day postoperatively. Preoperative corneal thickness, central endothelial cell count, and PNS also had a significant effect on postoperative central corneal thickness ($P<.05$). Anterior chamber depth and effective phaco time had no effect on postoperative corneal thickness ($P>.05$) according to this model.

Central corneal thickness was significantly lower in the femtolaser group compared to the phaco group 1 day postoperatively (mean difference 29 μm) (Fig 1).

TABLE 3

CENTRAL ENDOTHELIAL CELL COUNT (CELL/MM²) PRE- AND POSTOPERATIVELY IN THE TWO GROUPS (*P*<.05)

Groups	Preop	1 Day	1 Week	1 Month
Femtolaser	2861±216	2860±217	2730±205	2738±245
Phaco	2841±215	2719±350	2669±377	2542±466

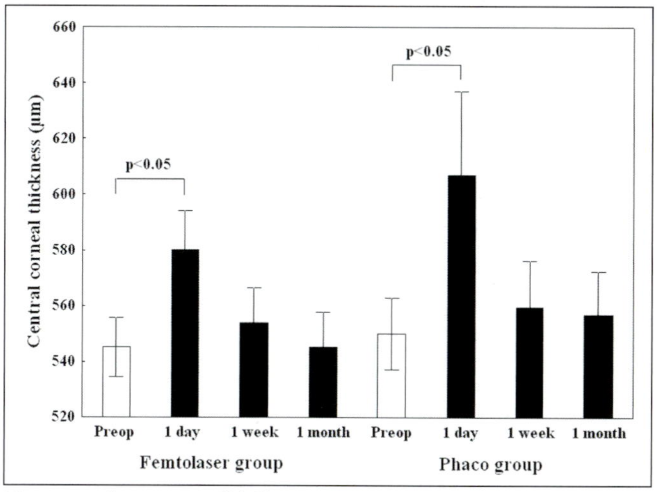

Figure 1. Changes and differences regarding central corneal thickness between the two groups pre- and postoperatively. (Reprinted with permission from Takács AI, Kovács I, Miháltz K, Filkorn T, Knorz MC, Nagy ZZ. Central corneal volume and endothelial cell count following femtosecond laser–assisted refractive cataract surgery compared to conventional phacoemulsification. *J Refract Surg.* 2012;28[6]:387-391.)

There was no statistically significant difference regarding endothelial cell count between the two study groups at any control time point of the study (Table 3).

A statistically significant positive correlation was found between the 3-mm corneal volume increase at 1 day postoperatively and the endothelial cell count 1 month postoperatively in both study groups (Fig 2).

Volume stress index (Fig 3) was statistically significantly lower 1 day following femtosecond laser-assisted phacoemulsification compared to conventional phacoemulsification ($3.0 \pm 2.3 \times 10^{-5}$ and $5.3 \pm 6.0 \times 10^{-5}$, respectively). There was no statistically significant difference between the two study groups 1 month postoperatively regarding volume stress index ($1.7 \pm 3.7 \times 10^{-6}$ in the femtolaser group and $1.7 \pm 3.5 \times 10^{-6}$ in the phaco group).

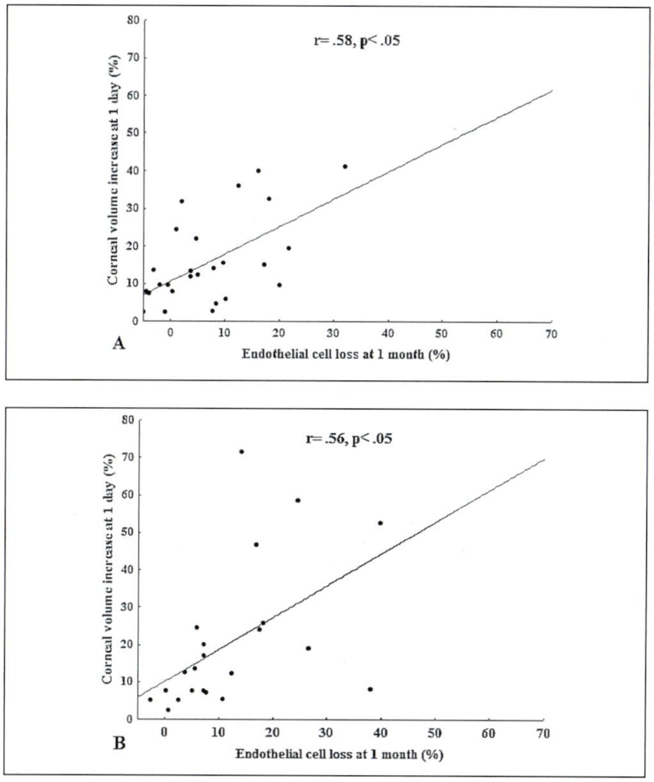

Figure 2. Correlation between 3-mm corneal volume increase 1 day postoperatively and endothelial cell count 1 month postoperatively. **A)** Femtolaser group. **B)** Phaco group. (Reprinted with permission from Takács AI, Kovács I, Miháltz K, Filkorn T, Knorz MC, Nagy ZZ. Central corneal volume and endothelial cell count following femtosecond laser–assisted refractive cataract surgery compared to conventional phacoemulsification. *J Refract Surg.* 2012;28[6]:387-391.)

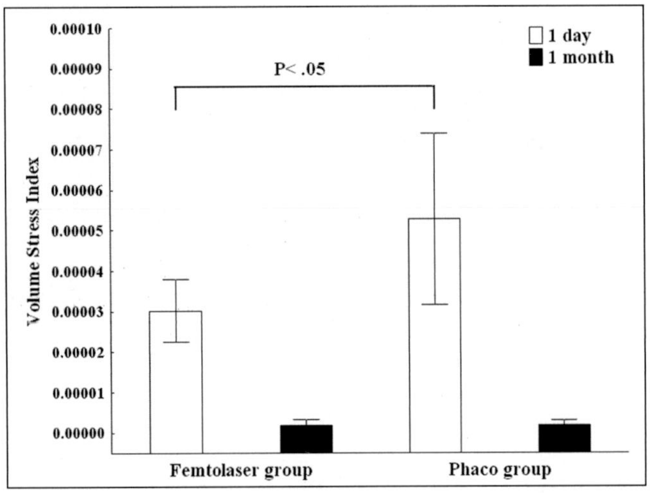

Figure 3. Volume stress index 1 day and 1 month postoperatively. (Reprinted with permission from Takács AI, Kovács I, Mihältz K, Filkorn T, Knorz MC, Nagy ZZ. Central corneal volume and endothelial cell count following femtosecond laser–assisted refractive cataract surgery compared to conventional phacoemulsification. *J Refract Surg*. 2012;28[6]:387-391.)

Reference

1. Suzuki H, Oki K, Takahashi K, Shiwa T, Takahashi H. Functional evaluation of corneal endothelium by combined measurement of corneal volume alteration and cell density after phacoemulsification. *J Cataract Refract Surg*. 2007;33(12):2077-2082.

Femtosecond Laser-Assisted Clear Corneal Wounds and Their Effects on Surgically Induced Astigmatism

Árpád Dunai, MD; Kinga Kránitz, MD; Michael C. Knorz, MD; Zoltán Z. Nagy, MD, PhD, DSc

During the past decade, microincisional cataract surgery using phacoemulsification and artificial intraocular lens (IOL) implantation has become a safe and effective intervention. The changing indications and the high prevalence of cataracts, especially in the aging population, will drive the number of lens extractions to increase. According to the estimates of the World Health Organization, around 20 million cataract surgeries were performed in 2010, and this quantity is expected to reach 32 million by 2020.[1]

Modern cataract patients usually aim to achieve emmetropia. By selecting the appropriate spherical lens power, spectacle independence can be obtained for patients with myopic or hyperopic refractive errors. However, 64% to 70% of them have higher than 0.5 D of preexisting corneal astigmatism, and 15% to 29% have 1.25 D or more.[2-4] Correction of this refractive error allows us to minimize the postoperative ametropy and supports us in reaching higher patient satisfaction.[5] Greater amounts of preoperative corneal astigmatism can be corrected using limbal relaxing incisions. Implantation of toric IOLs is also an efficient method for treating more than 1.5 D of astigmatism.[6] Smaller degrees of cylindrical error can be safely reduced by positioning the clear corneal incisions during cataract surgery.[7] Making an opposite clear corneal incision will lead to an increase in the toric effect of corneal wound healing.[8]

Due to new surgical techniques and IOL designs, surgically induced astigmatism (SIA) decreased significantly and became more predictable.[9] Sutureless clear corneal wounds are now the most common incisions made to perform cataract surgery with phacoemulsification, replacing scleral tunnel and corneoscleral incisions.

Reducing corneal astigmatism is particularly important in the case of implantation of premium IOLs. Incisions for cataract surgery made on the steep axis of the cornea induce flattening, so this effect can be applied to decrease preexisting cylindrical errors.[10] SIA is correlated with incision size, location, and wound construction.[11] With the advent of femtosecond lasers in ophthalmic surgery, properly sized and positioned clear corneal wounds became possible through a laser–tissue interaction known as photodisruption that may help control postoperative corneal astigmatism. According to former reports, both the length and angle of femtolaser corneal incisions remained stable during the first postoperative period, achieving reliable postoperative outcomes.[11-13]

Our research group evaluated and compared the surgically induced corneal astigmatism after femtolaser-assisted cataract surgery and conventionally performed phacoemulsification. In a prospective, randomized study, femtosecond laser-assisted cataract surgery was performed in 20 eyes of 20 patients using a femtosecond laser system (Alcon LenSx Inc, Aliso Viejo, California) to create corneal wounds, capsulotomy, and lens fragmentation, and manual, conventional phacoemulsification was performed in 20 eyes of 20 patients. In the femto group, a biplanar clear corneal tunnel was performed on the steep meridian with an incision width of 2.8 mm. In the manual group, a clear corneal incision was made on the steep axis using a 2.8-mm disposable keratome. In all eyes, a one-piece IOL was implanted using the Monarch injector and a D cartridge (AcrySof SA60AT IOL; Alcon Laboratories Inc, Ft Worth, Texas). All incisions were left sutureless.

To evaluate SIA, topography and wavefront analyses were performed preoperatively and 3 months postoperatively using a rotating Scheimpflug camera (Pentacam HR; Oculus Optikgeräte GmbH, Wetzlar, Germany). Keratometry values in the flat (K1) and steep (K2) meridian with axis, and total, lower-, and higher-order aberrations (RMS values [μm]) of the cornea within the central 9.0-mm zone were measured. The amount and direction of the SIA was calculated using vector analysis as described by Alpins and Goggin.[14]

No statistically significant difference was noted in age, central corneal thickness, preoperative keratometry readings, and preoperative corneal astigmatism between the femto and the manual group (Table 1). No statistically significant difference was found between the two

Nagy ZZ, ed. *Femtosecond Laser-Assisted Cataract Surgery: Facts and Results* (pp 41-43).

TABLE 1

DESCRIPTIVE PREOPERATIVE DATA

	Femtolaser Group ***Mean±SD***	***Manual Group*** ***Mean±SD***	**P**
Age (year)	70.40±11.57	62.27±13.41	.086
K1 (D)	43.37±1.26	44.81±3.13	.107
K2 (D)	44.19±1.36	46.24±5.15	.147
aveK (D)	43.76±1.21	44.69±1.64	.083
Astigmatism (D)	0.93±0.76	0.85±0.77	.763
CCT	543.40±29.96	552.69±30.96	.404

No statistically significant differences were noted in age, central corneal thickness (CCT), preoperative keratometry readings in the steep (K1) and flat (K2) meridian, in average keratometry (aveK) values, and preoperative corneal astigmatism between the femtolaser and the manual groups.

TABLE 2

SURGICALLY INDUCED ASTIGMATISM DATA

	Femtolaser Group ***Mean±SD***	***Manual Group*** ***Mean±SD***	**P***
Magnitude of SIA (D)	0.47±0.13	0.41±0.14	.218
Deviation of SIA axis from planned (degree)	4.47±2.59	7.38±4.72	.048*

There was no statistically significant difference between the two study groups in the amount of surgically induced astigmatism (SIA). Difference of postoperatively measured and planned axis of SIA proved to be significantly higher in the manual study group.
**P<.05*

study groups in the amount of SIA after evaluation of pre- and postoperative elevation-based topography measurements (*P*=.218) (Table 2).

Comparison of the preoperatively planned and postoperatively measured axis of SIA showed a statistically significant difference between the two groups. The deviation of the SIA axis from the previously planned axis was significantly smaller in the femto group than in the manual group (*P*=.048) (Table 2 and Fig). We neither found significant difference preoperatively nor postoperatively between the study groups in corneal aberration data. Within both groups, lower-order and total corneal aberration values remained stable (*P*>.05), but higher-order corneal aberrations increased significantly in both groups (femto group: *P*=.025; manual group: *P*=.002) (Table 3).

Reduction of the magnitude and variability of SIA is essential in the era of modern cataract surgery, particularly in the case of multifocal IOL implantation. Even small amounts of residual astigmatism after surgery with multifocal IOL implantation will reduce the likelihood of spectacle independence.[15,16]

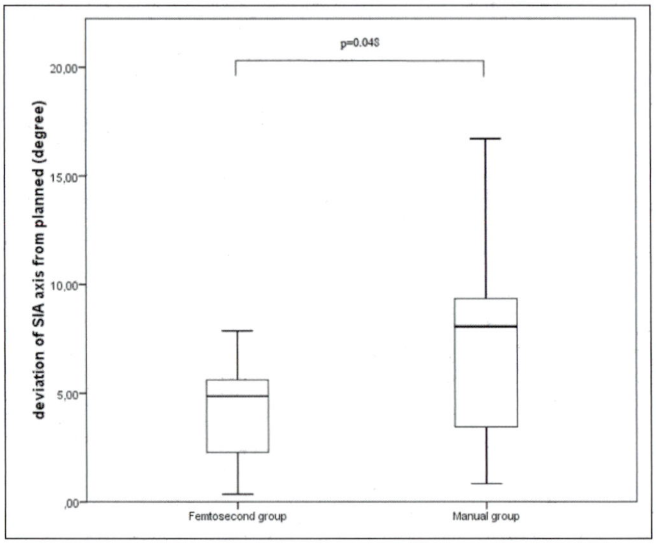

Figure. There was significant difference between the two study groups in regard to the difference of postoperatively measured and planned axis of SIA (*P*=.048).

TABLE 3
CORNEAL ABERRATION DATA

	Femtolaser Group Median±Quartile Range		Manual Group Median±Quartile Range		P*	
	Baseline	3 Months Postop	Baseline	3 Months Postop	Baseline	3 Months Postop
RMS total	0.77±0.56	0.83±0.29	0.63±0.34	0.53±0.18	.293	.065
RMS LOA	0.76±0.57	0.79±0.26	0.61±0.33	0.51±0.18	.283	.072
RMS HOA	0.13±0.09†	0.18±0.12†	0.13±0.05†	0.15±0.05†	.472	.078

Root mean square (RMS) values of lower-order aberrations (LOA), higher-order aberrations (HOA), and total corneal wavefront errors at baseline and 3 months postoperatively.
**P=between groups difference using Mann-Whitney U test. †P<.05 using Wilcoxon paired test.*

Femtosecond lasers facilitate properly sized and positioned clear corneal wounds during cataract surgery.[11,17] According to the results of our study, wavefront analysis of corneal aberrations showed that corneal incisions performed by the femtosecond laser and disposable keratomes did not significantly alter total corneal aberrations. However, in contrast to a former experiment that analyzed induced corneal aberration within the central 4.0-mm zone of the cornea,[11] we found a significant increase in corneal higher-order aberrations in both study groups when using a 9.0-mm analysis zone. Between groups, higher-order aberrations did not differ significantly. There was no difference in the magnitude of SIA between the two techniques. However, in the femto group, significantly lower angular deviation was found between the measured and the planned axis of induced astigmatism compared to the manual group. This effect is possibly the result of the better predictability of location, size, and direction in the femtosecond laser-assisted group.

Favorable characteristics of femtolaser incisions may facilitate the prediction of SIA and minimization of induced corneal aberrations during implantation of premium IOLs.

REFERENCES

1. Koopman S. Cataract surgery devices. Global pipeline analysis, competitive landscape and market forecasts to 2017. www.asdreports.com/news.asp?pr_id=261. Accessed January 2012.
2. Ferrer-Blasco T, Montes-Mico R. Prevalence of corneal astigmatism before cataract surgery. *J Cataract Refract Surg.* 2009;35(1):70-75.
3. Hoffmann PC, Hutz WW. Analysis of biometry and prevalence data for corneal astigmatism in 23,239 eyes. *J Cataract Refract Surg.* 2010;36(9):1479-1485.
4. Guan Z, Yuan F, Yuan YZ, Niu WR. Analysis of corneal astigmatism in cataract surgery candidates at a teaching hospital in Shanghai, China. *J Cataract Refract Surg.* 2012;38(11):1970-1977.
5. Saragoussi JJ. Preexisting astigmatism correction combined with cataract surgery: corneal relaxing incisions or toric intraocular lenses? *J Fr Ophtalmol.* 2012;35(7):539-545.
6. Amesbury EC, Miller KM. Correction of astigmatism at the time of cataract surgery. *Curr Opin Ophthalmol.* 2009;20(1):19-24.
7. Buckhurst PJ, Wolffsohn JS, Davies LN, Naroo SA. Surgical correction of astigmatism during cataract surgery. *Clin Exp Optom.* 2010;93(6):409-418.
8. Ben Simon GJ, Desatnik H. Correction of pre-existing astigmatism during cataract surgery: comparison between the effects of opposite clear corneal incisions and a single clear corneal incision. *Graefes Arch Clin Exp Ophthalmol.* 2005;243(4):321-326.
9. Masket S, Belani S, Wang L. Induced astigmatism with 2.2- and 3.0-mm coaxial phacoemulsification incisions. *J Refract Surg.* 2009;25(1):21-24.
10. Rho CR, Joo CK. Effects of steep meridian incision on corneal astigmatism in phacoemulsification cataract surgery. *J Cataract Refract Surg.* 2012;38(4):666-671.
11. Alió JL, Abdou AA, Soria F, et al. Femtosecond laser cataract incision morphology and corneal higher-order aberration analysis. *J Refract Surg.* 2013;29(9):590-595.
12. Nagy Z, Takacs A, Filkorn T, Sarayba M. Initial clinical evaluation of an intraocular femtosecond laser in cataract surgery. *J Refract Surg.* 2009;25:1053-1060.
13. Nagy ZZ, Kránitz K, Takacs AI, Miháltz K, Kovács I, Knorz MC. Comparison of intraocular lens decentration parameters after femtosecond and manual capsulotomies. *J Refract Surg.* 2011;27:564-569.
14. Alpins NA, Goggin M. Practical astigmatism analysis for refractive outcomes in cataract and refractive surgery. *Surv Ophthalmol.* 2004;49(1):109-122.
15. Kohnen T, Kook D, Auffarth GU, Derhartunian V. Use of multifocal intraocular lenses and criteria for patient selection. *Ophthalmologe.* 2008;105(6):527-532.
16. Hayashi K, Hayashi H, Nakao F, Hayashi F. Influence of astigmatism on multifocal and monofocal intraocular lenses. *Am J Ophthalmol.* 2000;130(4):477-482.
17. Serrao S, Lombardo G, Ducoli P, Rosati M, Lombardo M. Evaluation of femtosecond laser clear corneal incision: an experimental study. *J Refract Surg.* 2013;29(6):418-424.

The Effect of Femtolaser Cataract Surgery on the Macula

Mónika Ecsedy, MD, PhD; Illés Kovács, MD, PhD; Gabor Mark Somfai, MD, PhD; Zoltán Z. Nagy, MD, PhD, DSc

Cataract surgery by phacoemulsification has become the most common intraocular surgery and usually improves the visual outcome. The advent of femtosecond lasers in cataract surgery opened new perspectives since a perfectly sized and located incision, through a tissue reaction known as photodisruption, became possible.[1,2] Initial results of our study group with an intraocular femtosecond laser (LenSx laser system; Alcon LenSx Inc, Aliso Viejo, California) used during phacoemulsification demonstrated higher precision and safety of capsulorrhexis and clear corneal wounds and reduced phacoemulsification power in porcine and human eyes.[3]

However, it is well known that phacoemulsification surgery itself is an inflammatory insult to the eye and in many cases can lead to worsening of pre-existing retinal diseases, such as diabetic macular edema, or development of new diseases, such as Irvine-Gass syndrome.[4-6] In most cases, phacoemulsification does not change the macroscopic funduscopic appearance of the retina, but with novel noninvasive imaging techniques, such as cross-sectional imaging of the retina with optical coherence tomography (OCT), even subtle morphological changes of the macular area can be visualized. In the past decade, studies have found angiographic leakage up to 19% postoperatively[5-8] and an increase of the perifoveal retinal thickness with OCT, which is detectable from the first week up to 6 months and peaks 4 to 6 weeks after surgery, in pseudophakic eyes.[9-11]

During the femtolaser-assisted procedure, a suction ring is also applied to avoid eye movement and laser misdirection, exerting pressure on the pars plana region at the limbus. Previous experimental and clinical studies mainly performed in the investigation of LASIK surgeries demonstrated that the application of a suction ring causes short but considerable fluctuations in intraocular pressure,[12] which can induce several changes in ocular structure, from the deterioration of goblet cells of the conjunctiva up to the retina.[13] During application of microkeratome suction in LASIK, a decrease in the lens thickness and an increase of the vitreous distance were described, suggesting anterior traction on the posterior segment.[14] These alterations can cause posterior hyaloid detachment, transient choroidal circulation abnormalities,[15,16] macular hemorrhage,[17] and even optic atrophy.[18]

After publication of all these data, the incidence of subclinical macular edema after uneventful cataract surgery has become an issue of safety for this frequent operation.[9-11]

The purpose of our study group was to evaluate the safety of this new femtolaser-assisted cataract surgery by comparing its effect on macular thickness and macular morphology to that of traditional phacoemulsification using OCT measurements.

Comparison of Changes in Macular Thickness After Femtolaser-Assisted and Standard Phacoemulsification Cataract Surgery

In a prospective case-control study, we compared the effect of conventional and femtolaser-assisted phacoemulsification cataract surgery on the macula using OCT. Twenty eyes of 20 patients underwent uneventful cataract surgery in both study groups. Macular thickness and volume were evaluated by OCT preoperatively and 1 and 4 weeks postoperatively. Primary outcomes were OCT retinal thickness in three macular areas and total macular volume at 1 and 4 weeks. Secondary outcomes were changes in retinal thickness at 1 week and 1 month postoperatively with respect to preoperative retinal thickness values, effective phaco time, and lens density.

Multivariable modeling of the effect of surgery on postoperative macular thickness showed significantly lower macular thickness in the inner retinal ring in the femtosecond group after adjusting for age and preoperative thickness across the time course (P=.002). In the control group, the inner macular ring was significantly thicker at 1 week (mean: 21.68 µm; 95% confidence limit [CL]: 11.93-31.44 µm, P<.001). After 1 month this difference

Nagy ZZ, ed. *Femtosecond Laser-Assisted Cataract Surgery: Facts and Results* (pp 45-48).

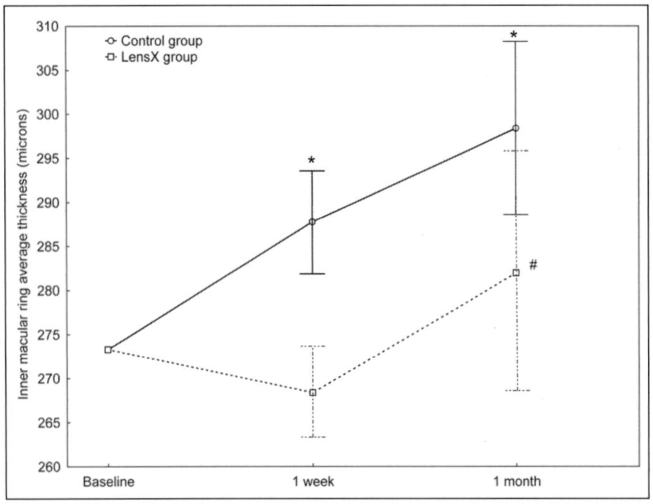

Figure. Mean values of inner macular ring thickness at baseline, 1 week, and 1 month postoperatively in the two study groups, adjusted for age and preoperative inner macular ring thickness. Note: *=*P*<.01, #=*P*<.05 compared to baseline. Whisker: 95% confidence limits of means.

decreased to a mean of 17.56 µm (95% CL: −3.21-38.32 µm, *P*=.09) and became marginally significant.

Macular thickness increased in the control group (mean: 287.76 µm; 95% CL: 282.32-293.20, *P*<.001) but not in the femtosecond group (mean: 268.38 µm; 95% CL: 253.10-273.67, *P*>.05) 1 week after the surgery compared to baseline average (mean: 273.3 µm). After 1 month, mean thickness of the inner macular ring was increased in the femtosecond group also (mean: 281.98 µm; 95% CL: 267.73-296.22, *P*=.02), and further increased in the control group (mean: 298.38 µm; 95% CL: 287.05-309.72, *P*=.003) compared to baseline (Fig).[19]

In our study we could detect the same subclinical parafoveal edema described in the literature[9-11] in the standard phacoemulsification group at 1 week and at 1 month postoperatively with a continuous increase. However, in the femtosecond group, at 1 week the thickness of the inner macular ring did not change and a slight increase was only detectable at 1 month. Based on our results, it is very unlikely that the suction ring used during the positioning of the femtolaser had any harmful effect on macular structure, as 1 week after surgery macular thickening could not be observed in the laser group. The substantially lower vacuum level (up to 40 mm Hg) compared to LASIK (up to 90 mm Hg) used during this procedure could be an explanation for this difference.

The later-detected macular thickening is probably due to the long-term subclinical inflammation triggered by the intraocular tissue (iris) manipulation and mediated by prostaglandins in both groups.[20,21] In concordance with previous reports, we did not find any correlation between macular changes and ultrasound time,[22] suggesting that the blood–retinal barrier is more disrupted during the standard procedure than during femtolaser-assisted cataract surgery. The decreased overall duration of anterior chamber manipulations, the preoperative laser capsulorrhexis, and laser nucleus fragmentation can be an explanation of this phenomenon.

Macular Morphology Assessed by Optical Coherence Tomography Image Segmentation After Femtosecond Laser-Assisted and Standard Cataract Surgery

We also tried to evaluate and compare thickness changes of the different retinal layers in the macula with OCT segmentation software after femtolaser-assisted and traditional phacoemulsification in another prospective case-control study.

Twelve eyes of 12 patients underwent uneventful cataract surgery in the femtolaser-assisted group and 13 eyes of 13 patients in the conventional phacoemulsification group. Total retinal thickness of the macula was evaluated by Stratus OCT (Carl Zeiss Meditec, Dublin, California), preoperatively and 4 to 8 weeks postoperatively. OCT images obtained by Stratus OCT were segmented using OCTRIMA software.[23,24] Regional thickness data in the central area, inner rings, and outer rings were obtained for the retinal layers, and absolute and relative thicknesses of the individual layers compared in the two study groups. Relative thickness was calculated as the ratio of the individual retinal layer and the total retinal thickness.

Statistically significant difference was found between the two groups in terms of absolute outer nuclear layer thickness and relative outer nuclear layer thickness in both inner and outer macular rings. After adjusting for effective phaco time in multivariable modeling, type of surgery showed significantly lower relative outer nuclear layer ratio in the inner (0.26, 95% CL: 0.25-0.27 vs 0.28, 95% CL: 0.27-0.29, *P*=.03) and in the outer retinal ring (0.27, 95% CL: 0.25-0.28 vs 0.29, 95% CL: 0.28-0.31, *P*=.02) in the femtosecond group.

According to our results, after cataract surgery macular edema is detectable mainly in the outer nuclear layer in both groups but is significantly smaller when using the femtosecond laser platform.[25]

Discussion

The development of cystoid macular edema or subclinical macular thickening after uncomplicated phacoemulsification is not fully understood but is thought to be caused by disruption to the blood–retinal barrier allowing fluid to accumulate in extracellular retinal spaces, leading to intraretinal cyst formation or thickening. Iris trauma, postoperative inflammation, prostaglandin release, and tractional force on the macula have been reported as possible causative factors of cystoid macular edema.[26,27] These hypotheses were supported by previous histopathologic specimens displaying retinal capillary dilation, serous fluid in the outer plexiform and inner nuclear layer, and inflammatory cells in the iris–ciliary perivascular complex[28] and OCT studies showing cystic spaces in the outer nuclear layer of the pericentral macula.[7] The mild subclinical perifoveal edema without visual impairment observed after uncomplicated phacoemulsification has been described before in several OCT studies, but its histological morphology was not investigated in detail.[9,25]

In femtosecond laser-assisted cataract surgery, we know even less about this pathology. In our first study we demonstrated that femtolaser-assisted cataract extraction results in a delayed and significantly smaller macular thickening compared to the standard procedure. The possible role of the suction ring used during the positioning of the laser beam could also be excluded based on our results as a cause of subclinical macular changes, as significant retinal thickening was detected only 1 month after the femtolaser-assisted surgery.[19]

As the segmentation of OCT scans is an important tool for the clinician in understanding the pathological processes within the retina, in our second study we aimed to locate the retinal layers involved in the edema formation to permit better detection and follow-up of layer injury, to understand and compare the nature of postoperative retinal changes in both standard and femtolaser-assisted surgical methods.[25]

In our patients, macular edema was mainly detectable as a thickening of the outer nuclear layer in the inner and the outer macular rings in both groups but not the central, foveal area. However, femtosecond laser-assisted surgery resulted in significantly smaller increase of the absolute and relative outer nuclear layer thickness values compared to the standard phacoemulsification method. We used relative retinal layer thickness values as they are more accurate for representing minor changes in macular structure. The significant difference in layer thickness at the same location suggests a similar pathophysiological background in the formation of postoperative subclinical macular thickening in both groups.[25]

In concordance with other data in the literature, we did not find a direct correlation between macular changes and ultrasound time in either of the two studies,[22] suggesting that the blood–retinal barrier is more disrupted during the standard phacoemulsification procedure than during femtolaser-assisted cataract surgery. Based on these assumptions, the detected macular thickening is possibly due to the long-term subclinical inflammation triggered by intraocular tissue (iris) manipulation and mediated by prostaglandins. Presumably the decreased overall duration of anterior chamber manipulations after preoperative femtosecond laser capsulorrhexis and nucleus fragmentation could be an explanation of this phenomenon.[19]

Our results suggest that both methods of cataract extraction (femtolaser assisted and standard procedure) are not only equally safe in terms of the effect on the macula, but femtosecond laser-assisted cataract surgery may even provide an option for less traumatic surgery because of the reduced postoperative inflammation and the smaller chance of macular edema development.[19,25] This may be of high importance in patients with diabetes and diabetic retinopathy or even in patients with uveitis. However, further research is warranted to prove this promising feature of femtosecond laser-assisted cataract surgery.

References

1. Dick HB, Pena-Aceves A, Manns A, Krummenauer F. New technology for sizing the continuous curvilinear capsulorhexis: prospective trial. *J Cataract Refract Surg*. 2008;34(7):1136-1144.
2. Krueger RR, Kuszak J, Lubatschowski H, Myers RI, Ripken T, Heisterkamp A. First safety study of femtosecond laser photodisruption in animal lenses: tissue morphology and cataractogenesis. *J Cataract Refract Surg*. 2005;31(12):2386-2394.
3. Nagy Z, Takacs A, Filkorn T, Sarayba M. Initial clinical evaluation of an intraocular femtosecond laser in cataract surgery. *J Refract Surg*. 2009;25(12):1053-1060.
4. Chew EY, Benson WE, Remaley NA, et al. Results after lens extraction in patients with diabetic retinopathy: Early Treatment Diabetic Retinopathy Study report number 25. *Arch Ophthalmol*. 1999;117(12):1600-1606.
5. Gass JD, Norton EW. Cystoid macular edema and papilledema following cataract extraction. A fluorescein funduscopic and angiographic study. *Arch Ophthalmol*. 1966;76(5):646-661.
6. Irvine SR. A newly defined vitreous syndrome following cataract surgery. *Am J Ophthalmol*. 1953;36(5):599-619.
7. Mentes J, Erakgun T, Afrashi F, Kerci G. Incidence of cystoid macular edema after uncomplicated phacoemulsification. *Ophthalmologica*. 2003;217(6):408-412.
8. Lobo CL, Faria PM, Soares MA, et al. Macular alterations after small-incision cataract surgery. *J Catarct Refract Surg*. 2004;30(4):752-760.
9. Biro Z, Balla Z, Kovács B. Change of foveal and perifoveal thickness measured by OCT after phacoemulsification and IOL implantation. *Eye (Lond)*. 2008;22(1):8-12.
10. Jagow B, Ohrloff C, Kohnen T. Macular thickness after uneventful cataract surgery determined by optical coherence tomography. *Graefes Arch Clin Exp Ophthalmol*. 2007;245(12):1765-1771.
11. Hee MR, Izatt JA, Swanson EA, et al. Optical coherence tomography of the human retina. *Arch Ophthalmol*. 1995;113(3):325-332.
12. Bissen MH, Suzuki S, Ohashi Y, Minami K. Experimental observation of intraocular pressure changes during microkeratome suctioning in laser in situ keratomileusis. *J Cataract Refract Surg*. 2005;31(3):590-594.

13. Davis RM, Evangelista JA. Ocular structure changes during vacuum by the Hansatome microkeratome suction ring. *J Cataract Refract Surg.* 2007;23(6):563-566.
14. Alireza M, Kohnen T. Effect of microkeratome suction during LASIK on ocular structures. *Ophthalmology.* 2005;112(4):645-649.
15. Luna JD, Artal MN, Reviglio MP, Diaz H, Juarez CP. Vitreoretinal alterations following laser in situ keratomileusis: clinical and experimental studies. *Graefes Arch Clin Exp Ophthalmol.* 2001;239(6):416-423.
16. Smith RJ, Yadarola MB, Pelizzari MF, Luna JD, Juarez CP, Reviglio VE. Complete bilateral vitreous detachment after LASIK retreatment. *J Cataract Refract Surg.* 2004;30(6):1382-1384.
17. Moshfeghi AA, Harrison SA, Reinstein DZ, Ferrone PJ. Valsalva-like retinopathy following hyperopic laser in situ keratomileusis. *Ophthalmic Surg Lasers.* 2006;37(6):486-488.
18. Conway ML, Wevill M, Perez AB, Hosking SL. Ocular blood-flow hemodynamics before and after application of a laser in situ keratomileusis ring. *J Cataract Refract Surg.* 2010;36(2):268-272.
19. Ecsedy M, Miháltz K, Kovács I, Takács Á, Filkorn T, Nagy ZZ. The effect of femtolaser cataract surgery on the macula. *J Refract Surg.* 2011;27(10):717-722.
20. Frank RN, Schulz L, Abe K, Lezzi R. Temporal variation in diabetic macular edema measured by optical coherence tomography. *Ophthalmology.* 2004;111(2):211-217.
21. Lobo CL, Bernardes RC, de Abreu JRF, Cunha-Vaz JG. One-year follow-up of blood–retinal barrier and retinal thickness alterations in patients with type 2 diabetes mellitus and mild non-proliferative retinopathy. *Arch Ophthalmol.* 2001;119(10):1469-1474.
22. Cagini CF, Iaccheri B, Piccinelli F, Ricci MA, Fruttini D. Macular thickness measured by optical coherence tomography in a healthy population before and after uncomplicated cataract phacoemulsification surgery. *Curr Eye Res.* 2009;34(12):1036-1041.
23. Cabrera Fernández D, Salinas HM, Puliafito CA. Automated detection of retinal layer structures on optical coherence tomography images. *Opt Express.* 2005;13:10200-10216.
24. Cabrera DeBuc D. A review of algorithms for segmentation of retinal image data using optical coherence tomography. In: Ho P-G, ed. *Image Segmentation.* Shanghai, China: InTech; 2011.
25. Nagy ZZ, Ecsedy M, Kovacs I, et al. Macular morphology assessed by optical coherence tomography image segmentation after femtosecond laser-assisted and standard cataract surgery. *J Cataract Refract Surg.* 2012;38(6):941-946.
26. Flach AJ. The incidence, pathogenesis, and treatment of cystoid macular edema following cataract surgery. *Trans Am Ophthalmol Soc.* 1998;96:557-634.
27. Quinn CJ. Cystoid macular edema. *Optom Clin.* 1996;5(1):111-130.
28. Neal RE, Bettelheim FA, Lin C, Winn KC, Garland JS, Zigler JS. Alterations in human vitreous humour following cataract extraction. *Exp Eye Res.* 2005;80:337-347.

Complications in Femtolaser Cataract Surgery and What to Do

Zoltán Z. Nagy, MD, PhD, DSc

Whenever a new method is introduced (Fig 1), the first question is always what are the complications of the new procedure, how can they be avoided, and are those complications milder than those with the previous method?

Femtolaser-assisted refractive cataract surgery is a relatively new and expensive entity in ophthalmology; expectations are quite high, peer-reviewed data are still missing, and patients and ophthalmologists seek evidence of it being superior over manual phacoemulsification. This is a difficult question because phacoemulsification itself is an established and relatively safe method with good predictability and safety. Is there room for any development? The answer is always yes because there are always newer, advanced technology intraocular lenses (IOLs), and patients want surgery at a younger age than ever before. Thus, expectations are greater from both refractive and safety points of view. Femtolaser technology offers a customized procedure and consistent results in order to maximize the benefit of advanced technology IOLs.[1-6] In this chapter, I will summarize the most important intraoperative complications.

Ophthalmologists generally advise a hard head rest for their patients because with a soft head rest, after insertion of the patient interface, the head could have a lower position due to the soft head rest material. In that case, suction loss is more likely. With a hard head rest, the head cannot be pushed downward and the incidence of suction loss is not increased.

A topical drop anesthesia is recommended. This way the patient can follow the aiming beam provided by the laser in order to properly centrate the patient interface. Cooperation is usually not so high with block or peribulbar anesthesia. Smart and cooperative patients can greatly help the treating ophthalmologists.

Proper docking is a crucial step for having a successful femtolaser treatment. Good centration of the patient interface prevents lens tilt (crystalline lens), allows the use of the nomograms offered automatically by the femtolaser, and usually no adjustment is necessary. In cases of tilt of the crystalline lens, significant adjustment of the femtolaser treatment might be necessary. In those cases, safety might be endangered or compromised.

Possible Intraoperative Complications

Suction Break

Suction break usually occurs in 2% to 4% of cases, usually during the first 100 cases (during the learning curve) intraoperatively. Usually it happens during the capsulotomy part. The possible causes can be improper docking, loose conjunctiva around the limbus, large pterygium, microcornea, megalocornea, and inadvertent movement of the patient's head or eye. Loose conjunctiva in high myopic eyes might also create a problem; in these cases, it is recommended to pull out the conjunctiva with a fine pincette under the patient interface. In our cases, the most frequent causes were inadvertent movement of the patient's eye/head and improper docking. The sudden suction break usually does not cause a complication, and femtolaser treatment can be continued, leaving out the capsulotomy part from the femtolaser treatment. It is not recommended to restart femtolaser capsulotomy with a larger diameter because anterior capsular tear and consecutive postoperative IOL tilt is more likely with a larger capsulotomy diameter.

With early and multiple suction breaks, changing of the patient interface is recommended. Usually femtolaser pretreatment should not be abandoned due to suction break. Patients should be reassured, the head and eye fixed, and patients should be asked to look into the fixating light of the operating microscope.

In conclusion, suction break is usually part of the learning curve. The surgeon should have confidence and should instruct the patient not to move the other eye during the procedure well before the femtolaser treatment even starts. The other important issue to avoid suction break is proper patient interface insertion and good preoperative anesthesia. With a proper speculum, the

Nagy ZZ, ed. *Femtosecond Laser-Assisted Cataract Surgery: Facts and Results* (pp 49-56).

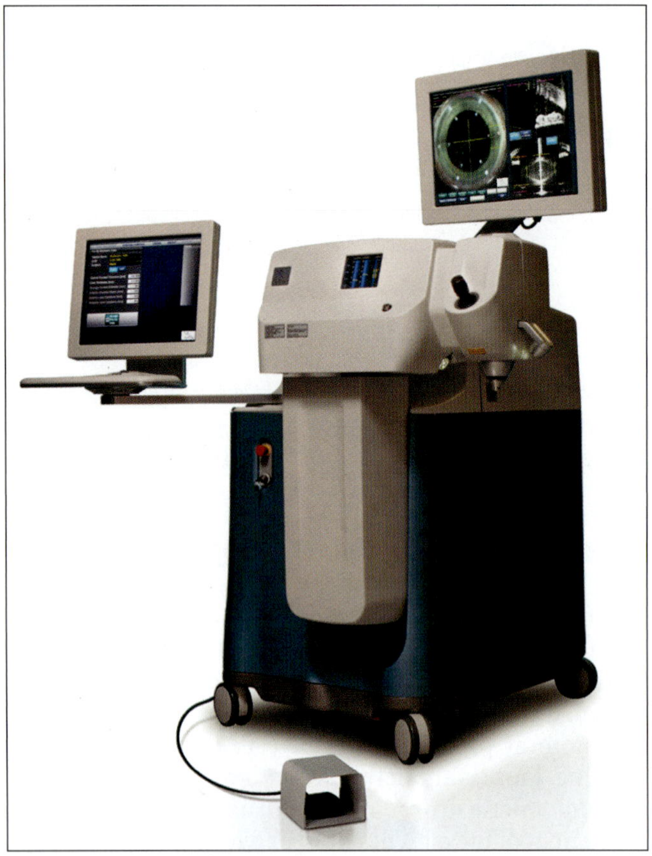

Figure 1. The LenSx femtolaser.

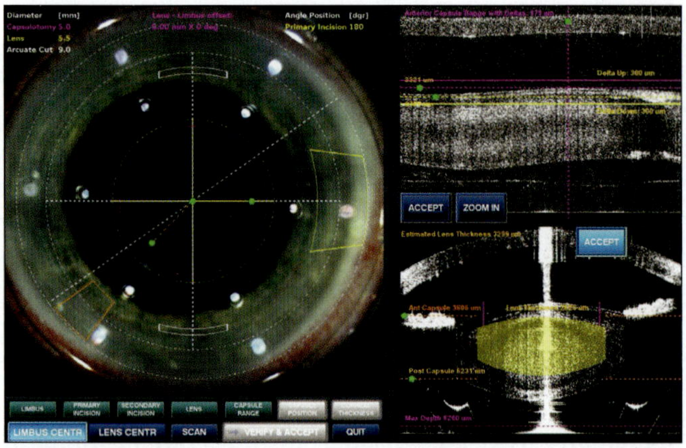

Figure 2. The screen for the surgeon. Note the corneal wounds and the astigmatic incisions. On the right upper part, the OCT identifies the endothelial layer, the anterior capsule (highest and lowest point); on the lower part of the image, OCT identifies the cut within the crystalline lens (yellow area).

palpebral fissure should be opened as large as possible; this also facilitates better patient interface alignment. Changing the patient interface is recommended in cases of early and multiple suction breaks.

> *Possible Causes of Suction Break*
>
> - Improper docking
> - Loose conjunctiva around the limbus
> - Large pterygium
> - Microcornea
> - Megalocornea
> - High myopia/high hyperopia with loose conjunctiva
> - Inadvertent movement of the head or eye (of the patient)

Conjunctival Redness or Hemorrhage

Significant conjunctival redness or hemorrhage was experienced in one-third of the cases, also during the learning curve (treatment of the first 100 eyes). This ratio is relatively stable during later treatments. It is highly recommended that patients should be informed about this completely harmless complication during the preoperative assessment. They typically accept it as a possible consequence of the docking procedure and the suction force of the patient interface. Patients on anticoagulative therapy might be advised to stop anticoagulation unless their general health conditions mandate continued anticoagulant therapy. Conjunctival redness or bleeding usually resolves within a shorter time span (3 to 12 days), leaving behind no mark on the conjunctiva. Administration of vitamin C might be helpful, but preoperative exploration of anticoagulant therapy is mandatory.

Capsular Tags and Bridges

Capsular tags and bridges usually do not cause problems if noticed in time. The new optical coherence tomography (OCT) software programs are able to compensate for the tilt of the crystalline lens (Fig 2). Before this, the occurrence of tags or bridges was approximately 20%, but now with the 97% rate of free-floating capsules, this complication is very rare.

It is advised that during the learning curve the contour of capsulotomy should be closely followed with the rhexis forceps. In that case anterior tears can be effectively avoided. In case of tags or bridges, capsulotomy should be led a bit outside the original laser cut line to avoid further anterior tears.

Tilt compensation by the OCT diagnostic device has a certain limit, of course; with special tilt of the crystalline lens (eg, in Marfan syndrome or traumatic loose zonules), capsular tags might be expected with all types of femtosecond lasers.

Anterior Capsular Tear

Anterior capsular tear is an important safety issue during cataract surgery. Having a regular, circular, and even type of anterior capsulorrhexis provides much higher

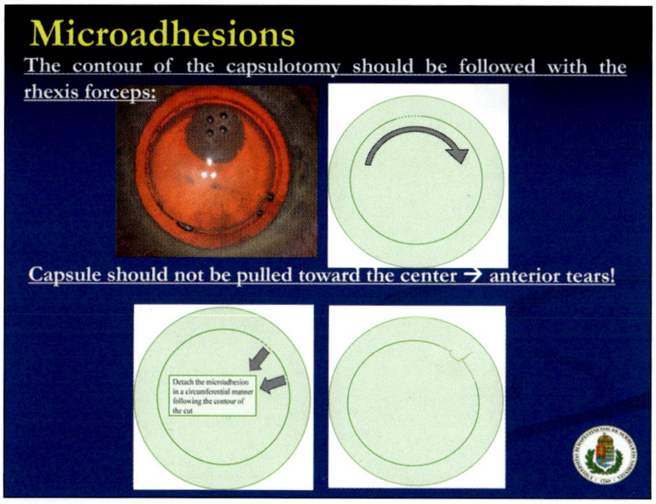

Figure 3. List of femtolaser capsulotomy patterns (complete cut, microadhesion, area of no treatment, complete treatment but not continuous laser cut).

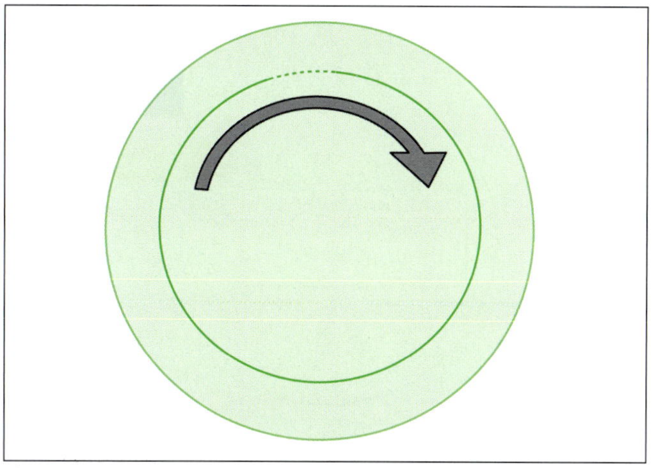

Figure 4. Managing type 2—microadhesions. Tell-tale signs of capsular attachments. As with standard capsulorrhexis, detach type 1 capsulotomy circumferentially.

safety for the surgeon during the operation compared to irregular capsulotomy or capsulotomy with anterior tear or bridges. There are two large studies in the literature discussing anterior tear of the capsule during phacoemulsification. In the first study, authors evaluated more than 2600 eyes. Anterior tear was found in 0.8% of the cases; in 40% of those cases, tear propagated to the posterior capsule and 20% required vitrectomy.[8] The big study evaluated resident experience. In that study, the incidence of anterior tear was found in a much higher number—5.3% of the cases. Irregular anterior capsulorrhexis was found in 9.3% of the eyes and posterior capsular tear with vitreous loss was found in 6.6% of the cases. Thus, with unexperienced surgeons, anterior tear and vitreous loss occurred approximately seven times more frequently.[9]

Anterior tear of the capsule is an important issue that can cause posterior capsular damage with possible sinking of the nucleus into the vitreous cavity. During an earlier study, anterior tear occurred in 4% of our patients (also during the learning curve). None of the cases reached the posterior capsule; therefore, vitrectomy was not needed. With the free-floating capsules, anterior tear is no longer a feared complication of femtolaser pretreatment.

Pearls of Removing Femtosecond Laser-Created Capsulotomies and How to Avoid Possible Complications

Femtolaser-performed continuous central curvilinear capsulorrhexis (CCCC) might be completely continuous, which is called free-floating capsulotomy (type 1). There might be microadhesions (ie, an area of complete cut mixed with minute areas of adhesions [type 2 capsulotomy]). Type 3 shows an area of no treatment (no visible femtolaser cut in the anterior capsule). Type 4 shows a complete cut but it is not continuous.

During the learning curve, it is strongly advised to follow the contour of the femtolaser capsulotomy with the rhexis forceps. The surgeon might also use a cystotome needle to identify the femtolaser cut in the four quadrants. The main aim is to free up the capsulotomy from every direction. Following this maneuver, it can be pulled out easily from the anterior chamber. In case of first users, the capsule might be colored with trypan blue in order to better visualize the anterior capsule. It should be noted the capsular dye such as trypan blue renders the capsule more rigid and vulnerable; therefore, surgery later might be more difficult. A really free-floating capsulotomy might be removed with the suction program of the phacoemulsificator but is recommended only for surgeons with extensive phacoemulsification experience and longer practice with femtolaser cataract surgery.

Managing Microadhesion Areas

In cases of microadhesions (Fig 3), the surgeon should also follow the contour of the femto-capsulotomy. The absence of a gutter and presence of bubbles trapped under the capsulotomy cut serve as tell-tale signs to help the surgeon to identify problems, such as minute remaining capsule attachments (Fig 4). It should be emphasized that during the learning curve, the surgeon should carefully observe the femtolaser capsulotomy with high magnification under the operating microscope. Trypan blue might be of great help during the early phase of the learning curve.

Please note that anterior chamber collapse during CCC might also lead to a radial tear. Therefore, the following should be taken into consideration: never let the

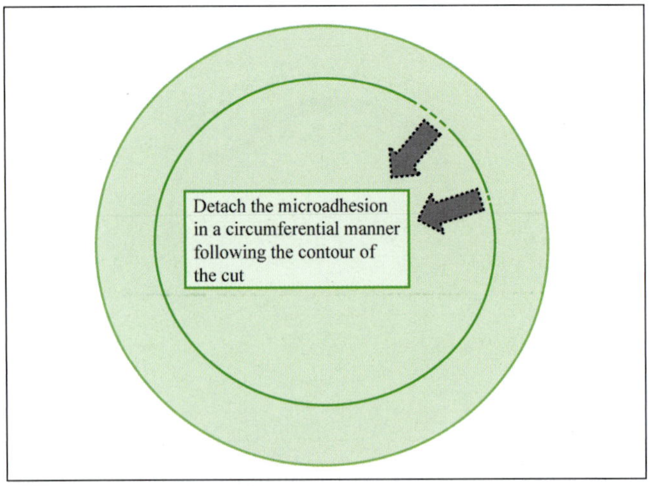

Figure 5. Managing type 2—microadhesions. As with standard CCC, **do not** pull toward the center or amputate the adhesion.

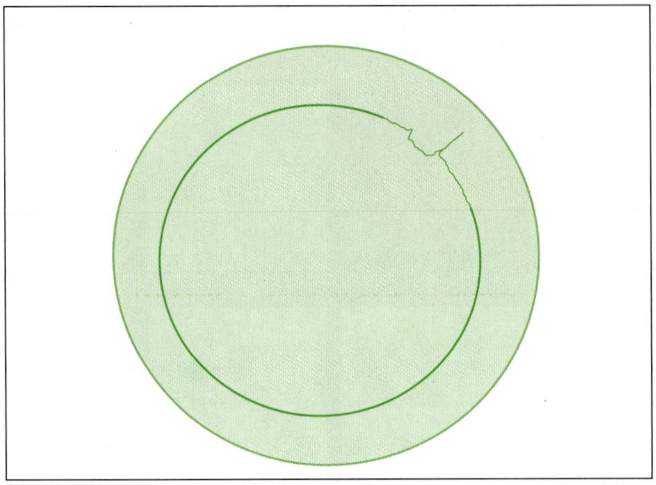

Figure 6. Managing type 2—microadhesions. Do not pull it radially, always pull outward! Pulling it radially could result in a tag or nick that could lead to a tear.

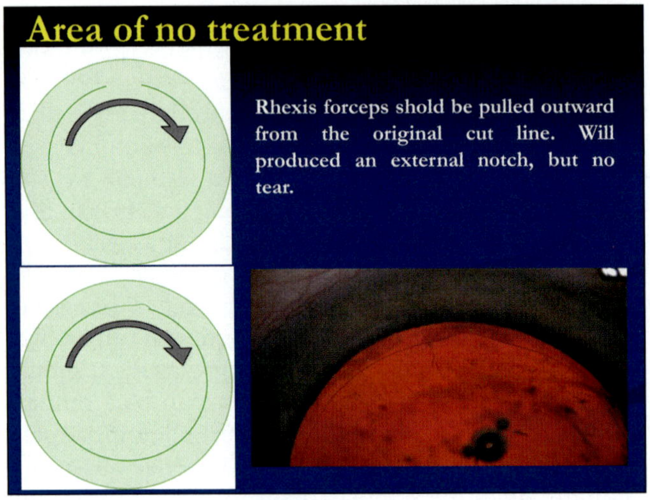

Figure 7. Managing area of no treatment.

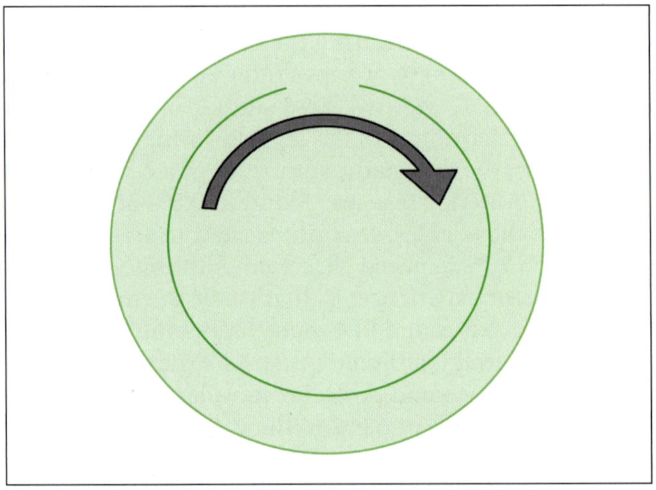

Figure 8. Managing type 3—area of no treatment. As with standard CCC, tear the area of no treatment circumferentially.

anterior chamber collapse, open the paracentesis first, stabilize the anterior chamber with viscoelastic (OVD), only after this open the primary incision, and finally, complete the capsulotomy.

Detach the microadhesion area circumferentially following the contour of the capsulotomy (Fig 5). Never pull toward the center the microadhesion area; in that case it can cause a tag or a nick, which can be responsible for an anterior tear, which might run later toward the periphery (Fig 6). Never amputate the microadhesion area with the capsulorrhexis forceps or capsular scissors because it can cause an irregular shape, which in turn might further increase the vulnerability of the anterior capsule.

Managing Area of No Treatment During Femto-Capsulotomy

In case of no treatment (Fig 7), a circumferential pull is the method of choice (Fig 8). The pulling force should be a bit outside the original femtosecond laser capsulotomy line (Fig 9). In that case, it results in a small external notch with a smooth edge (Fig 10).

Tearing inward can result in a nick in the peripheral capsule that could lead to a real anterior tear propagating toward the posterior capsule. If that happens, the surgeon should be very careful not to exert any vector force on the capsule during phacoemulsification, irrigation-aspiration, and posterior chamber lens (PCL) insertion. The line of capsular injury should be avoided so as not to cause further trauma on the anterior capsule.

Managing the Complete but Not Continuous Capsulotomy Pattern

This (Fig 11) can be caused by an inadvertent and unexpected movement of the patient's head or the eye or the patient interface during femtolaser capsulotomy.

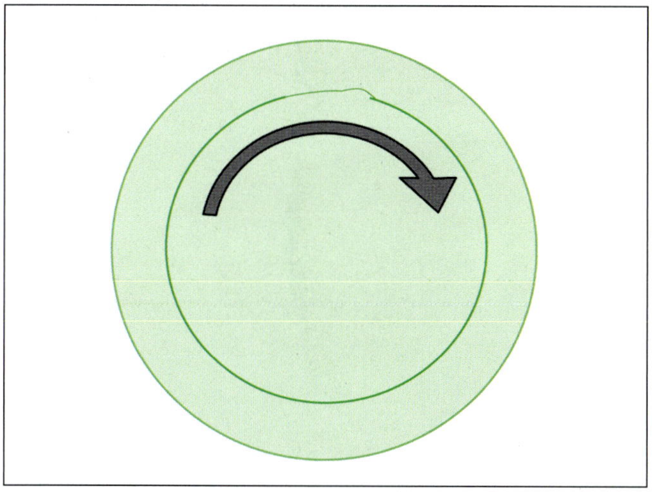

Figure 9. Managing type 3—area of no treatment. Pull circumferentially and possibly outward. It is better to tear outward in cases like this.

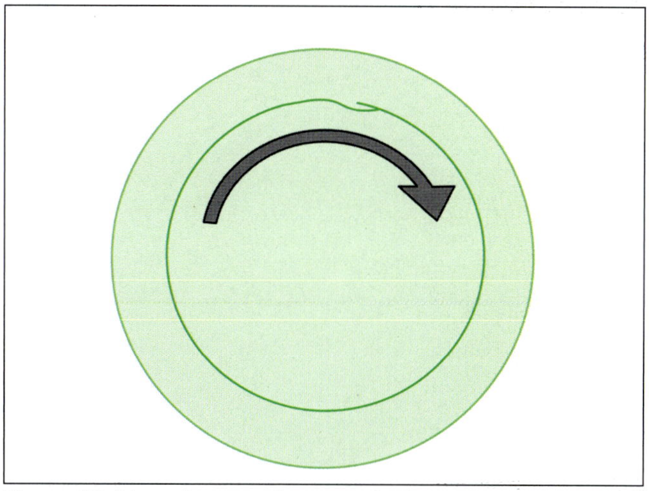

Figure 10. Managing type 3—area of no treatment. Do not pull inward (danger of anterior tear). Do not tear inward; this will leave a nick on the peripheral capsule that could lead to a tear.

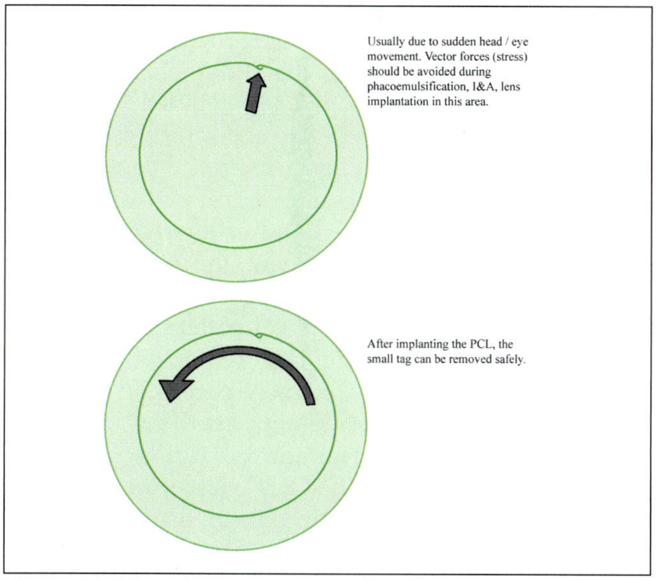

Figure 11. Managing type 4—complete but not continuous capsulotomy.

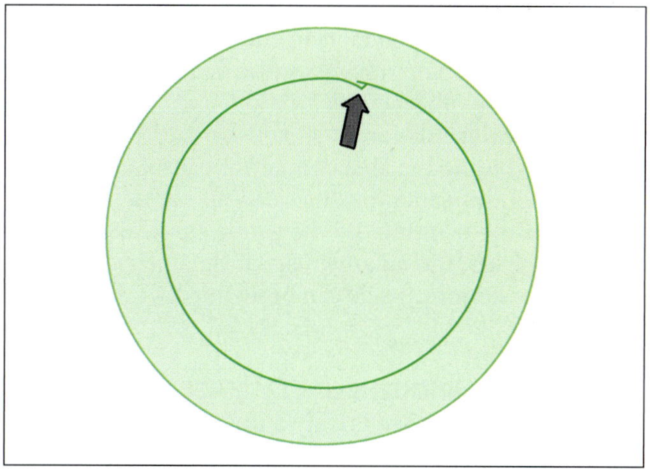

Figure 12. Managing type 4—complete pattern but not continuous. Usually not associated with tear. Can be left alone provided the surgeon does not apply stress along the area during phaco, irrigation-aspiration, and IOL insertion.

This type of irregular capsulotomy is usually not associated with a tear as long as there was no stress applied in this area (Fig 12). For this reason, the surgeon must be careful along this region during phacoemulsification, irrigation-aspiration, or IOL insertion, similar to the previous pattern. After the implantation of the PCL, the surgeon may detach the inner tag with a capsulotomy forceps, but it also may be left alone (Fig 13).

In conclusion, it can be stated that, in cases of capsular tags or bridges during femtolaser treatment, the surgeon should follow the contour of the capsulotomy. When the capsulotomy line reaches the tag, the surgeon should be outside the original cut line. In that case, the capsulotomy diameter will be somewhat larger than the original one, but the anterior tear can be completely avoided. If it is not performed like this, at the point where the laser cut line is reached again, a small tear might appear, which later at hydrodissection or at phacoemulsification might run outside toward the periphery of the lens.

The incidence of anterior capsular tear was low in our series. The cause was gentle surgery, acknowledging that this is a different technique and has a learning curve. The key is to follow the contour of the femtolaser cut. To pull out the whole anterior capsule with a sudden movement of the capsulorrhexis forceps or phacoemulsification head should be avoided during the learning curve, even in seemingly free-floating capsules. Small tags might be hidden for

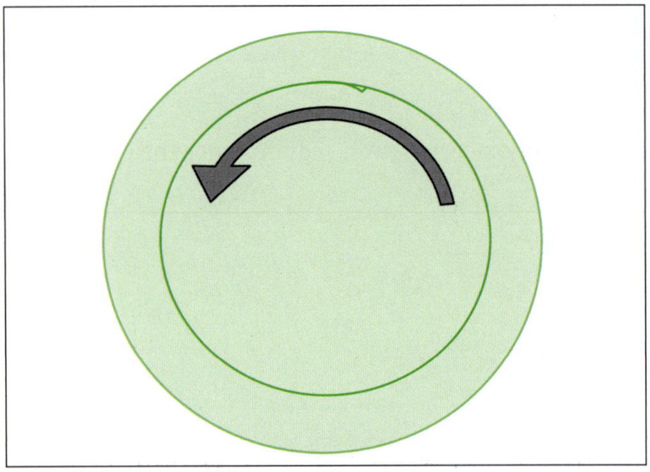

Figure 13. Managing type 4—complete pattern but not continuous. At the end of the surgery, the surgeon may grab and detach the inner tag with a circumferential hand movement under viscoelastic, but the inner tag might be left alone also.

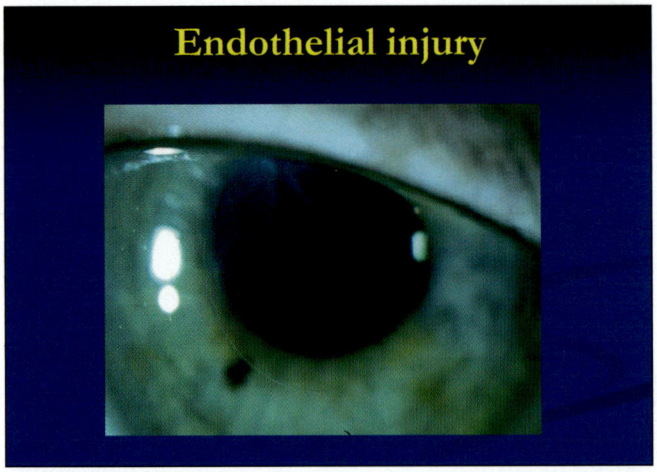

Figure 14. Note the femtolaser-created cut in the endothelial layer due to shallow anterior chamber and not having an OCT, which could have prevented this complication. The patient had no visual problems due to the small partial cut in the endothelial cell layer.

the unexperienced surgeon during the learning curve. In cases of anterior capsular tear, the surgeon should perform a very gentle hydrodissection and phacoemulsification. During phacoemulsification and removing the cortex, gentle vector forces should be exerted (minimal suction), avoiding the area of anterior capsular tear. During the PCL implantation, the leading haptic should be away from the tear line. By the gentle surgical technique and maneuvers, the enlargement of the anterior tear toward the posterior capsule can be avoided.

Endothelial Damage

Endothelial damage is only a potential complication of femtosecond cataract surgery after the invention and introduction of new OCT software. With the new OCT software (Alcon LenSx Inc, Aliso Viejo, California), anterior capsulotomy is possible even if the anterior chamber depth is less than 1.0 mm. Earlier we had a bad experience during the learning curve with not having OCT help during the early study period with the alpha prototype in high hyperopic eyes. The endothelial layer was hit during capsulotomy procedures in three eyes (3/100 eyes); the reason was that the patient interface pushed down the cornea and the safety distance was not enough from the endothelium (Fig 14). We only had the ultrasonic preoperative assessment for judging the anterior chamber depth. Among this series, all eyes were high hyperopic with a smaller anterior chamber depth (endothelial and anterior capsular distance). The surgeon noticed it immediately, so there was no long-term consequence, although the endothelial incision line could be seen even 1 year after surgery.

With the integration of the new OCT device, intraoperative safety has increased and such complications can be completely avoided. From a safety point of view, built-in OCT is a definite benefit for the procedure.

In conclusion, damage of the endothelial layer with the new software can be completely avoided. The Alcon LenSx femtolaser has a live video and screen proprietary HD-OCT to help the docking and surgical pattern localization. The OCT uses the same optical path as the laser beam and is fully integrated and calibrated. The OCT covers the whole anterior segment, up to the posterior capsule of the crystalline lens, and is able to assess the lens density as well. The surgical pattern is automatically performed; the surgeon has the possibility to alter the automatically offered treatment parameters, such as centration of anterior capsulotomy, depth cut within the lens (distance from posterior and anterior capsule), and position of corneal cuts. The OCT measurements effectively combine the circular and linear scans, which results in better depth and tilt information.

Capsular Blockage Syndrome and Posterior Capsular Rupture

During femtolaser treatment of the crystalline lens, intralenticular gas is formed. Therefore, following capsulotomy, the gas bubble should leave the eye from the intralenticular space toward the anterior chamber and through the corneal wound. The first case of capsular blockage syndrome was published in 2011 by Roberts et al.[7] In our series, no blockage syndrome and no posterior capsular rupture occurred due to the fault of the femtolaser. Posterior capsular damage is always a surgical failure. The so-called "rock and roll" technique is advised to avoid this rare but possible serious complication. The surgeon should apply a gentle hydrodissection and then press down gently on the nucleus and turn it around.

During this maneuver, the gas bubble may leave toward the anterior chamber, causing no stress on the posterior capsule. In case of abrupt hydrodissection or not allowing the gas bubble to come forward, the pressure rises within the capsular bag and it can resolve only when the posterior capsule ruptures. The gas bubble should leave the intralenticular space either anteriorly (toward the anterior chamber) or posteriorly (toward the vitreous). The latter has other unwanted complications, such as sinking of the nucleus and filling the anterior chamber by the vitreous, and later, retinal problems such as detachment may appear. Surgeons should take all measures to prevent posterior capsular complications.

> *How to Avoid Capsular Blockage Syndrome*
>
> - Gentle hydrodissection
> - Rock and roll technique with the nucleus according to Nagy
> - Allow the gas bubble to leave toward the anterior chamber

In conclusion, capsular blockage syndrome, and consecutive posterior capsular rupture, is a serious complication of femtolaser-assisted cataract surgery. It is a completely avoidable complication. The surgeon should note that having a good capsulotomy without tags or bridges, which might cause anterior tear, is very important. The hydrodissection should be gentle; do not use a large-diameter cannula and high-speed water jet under the anterior capsule. At the beginning of the hydrodissection, the surgeon should press down gently on the nucleus and move it slowly. This is the "rock and roll" technique, according to Nagy, to allow the air bubble to leave the crystalline lens. When the gas bubble leaves the intralenticular space toward the anterior chamber or leaves the eye completely, there is no further danger to rupture the posterior capsule.

Gas bubble formation eventually can be considered as a useful part of the procedure because it helps to separate the nucleus and the epinucleus. Some surgeons do not use hydrodissection before lens sculpting. Hydrodissection is mandatory in soft lenses and in very hard lenses. In soft lenses, the risk of damaging the posterior capsule during irrigation-aspiration is increased without hydrodissection. The case is similar in dense cataracts. In cases of medium-hard crystalline lenses, hydrodissection can be omitted, but certainly not during the learning curve.

Miosis

Miosis following femtolaser pretreatment occurred in 30% to 50% of the cases during the learning curve. The bubble formation should be minimized because the consequent oxidative stress may enhance the prostaglandin production in the anterior chamber, which in turn causes miosis. The mechanical effect of the patient interface and the shock wave of the femtolaser may also contribute to post-femtolaser miosis. In cases of small pupil, the laser may hit the pupil and consecutive cytokines and prostaglandin products may further decrease the diameter of the pupil.

It is advised that the pupil should be at least 6.0 mm in diameter (optimally at least 8.0 mm) in order to avoid significant constriction after the femtolaser treatment. Changing the preoperative dilating regimen, causing less pupillary constriction, at present the usual miotic reaction is around 20%. Preoperative instillation with dilating drops should be more frequent and nonsteroid anti-inflammatory (NSAID) drops (eg, topical diclofenac) should also be added to the preoperative regimen.

> *How to Avoid Post-Femtolaser Miosis*
>
> - Administer dilating agents earlier and more frequently
> - Preoperatively administer NSAID drops

In conclusion, femtolasers have a shock wave that might affect 1.00 mm of the surrounding area. In the case of a 5.0-mm capsulotomy, the pupil should be at least 6.5-mm wide, while in the case of 4.5-mm capsulotomy, a 6.0-mm diameter is sufficient. Of course the larger the pupil, the less chance to hit the pupillary margin by the laser shock wave. Besides the shock wave, the mechanical effect of the patient interface might insert a miotic effect also. Therefore, thoughtful pupillary dilation (more instillation, possibly starting earlier compared to routine phacoemulsification) and a combination of NSAID drops (diclofenac) are advised. High myopic eyes and eyes with pseudoexfoliation are prone to miotic reaction following femtolaser treatment. Intracameral epinephrine usually helps to overcome this difficulty.

Vitrectomy

In our series, no vitrectomy was needed as a failure of the femtolaser pretreatment. The surgeon should avoid by all means the sinking of the nucleus into the vitreous. If it happens, vitrectomy and intravitreal phacoemulsification should be performed to remove all parts of the crystalline lens to avoid postoperative inflammation. Ketorolac might be used to identify remaining vitreous fibers within the anterior chamber. The surgeon should decide to implant the PCL into the sulcus or to suture/glue it, or whichever other technique is chosen. Multifocal, toric, multifocal-toric, or accommodating lenses should not be implanted. Sometimes shifting to extracapsular technique may prevent sinking of the nucleus. Meticulous 10/0 suture and early suture removal might prevent an increase in postoperative corneal astigmatism.

It can be summarized that to avoid vitrectomy due to sunken nucleus during femtolaser cataract surgery, similar measurements should be made as was recommended in capsular blockage syndrome.

Conclusion

In the first complication study by Bali et al during femtolaser cataract surgery of the first 200 eyes, the four surgeons experienced the following complications: suction break in 2.5% of the treated eyes; a miosis was experienced in 9.5% of the eyes following femtolaser treatment; 10.5% of the eyes had small anterior tags; free-floating capsulotomy was found in 17.5% of the cases; and 13.6% of the laser-created wounds needed a keratome for entry into the anterior chamber. Anterior radial tears were found in 4% (eight eyes), posterior capsular rupture in 3.5% (seven eyes), and a dropped nucleus in 2% (four eyes).[10] Our complication rate was similar to Bali et al's complications, except due to our gentle hydrodissection and using the rock and roll technique, we had no posterior capsular rupture.

Preoperative planning regarding femtolaser treament parameters is very important. The surgeon should meet the patient before femtolaser treatment and should make notes about the treatment plan. The patient should sign the informed consent before starting the procedure.

It is also important that the femtolaser not be far from the main operating room. Then surgery could begin shortly after femtolaser use, the pupil will not constrict, and sterility can be better maintained. Paying patients do not prefer femtolaser pretreatment in another center, due to issues of finding transportation after and longer waiting time between femtolaser treatment and cataract removal. Personnel should also be educated and optimal work flow should be tested during the learning curve to achieve maximal benefits from femtolaser surgery.

Femtolaser-created capsulotomy (CCCC) may provide a lot of benefits for both patients and surgeons. It may enable the use of all the benefits of advanced technology IOLs. The removal of the femtolaser precut capsulotomy is of crucial importance for having a successful femtolaser cataract surgery. The technique was shown previously how to avoid possible later complications, achieving as perfect a capsulotomy as possible. Tell-tale signs of microadhesions (absence of gutter, bubbles under the anterior capsule), area of no treatment, and area of complete but not continuous capsulotomies should alert the surgeon to the possible complications that are completely avoidable following the previously mentioned rules during the early phase of cataract/lens surgeries.

Following the rules; acknowledging that femtolaser cataract surgery seems to be easy and safe, yet there is a learning curve; and understanding the need for different approaches during capsulotomy, lens fragmentation, and wound creation, surgeons might achieve the maximal benefits for patients with advanced technology IOLs. Through this, the overall safety, predictability, and effectiveness of cataract surgery should increase.

References

1. Nagy ZZ, Takacs A, Filkorn T, Sarayba M. Initial clinical evaluation of intraocular femtosecond laser in cataract surgery. *J Refract Surg.* 2009;25:1053-1060.
2. Nagy ZZ, Kranitz K, Takacs AI, et al. Comparison of intraocular lens decentration parameters after femtosecond and manual capsulotomies. *J Refract Surg.* 2011;27:564-569.
3. Kranitz K, Takacs AI, Mihaltz K, Kovács I, Knorz MC, Nagy ZZ. Femtosecond laser capsulotomy and manual continuous curvilinear capsulorhexis parameters and their effects on intraocular lens centration. *J Refract Surg.* 2011;27:558-563.
4. Mihaltz K, Knorz MC, Alio JL, et al. Internal aberration and optical quality after femtosecond laser anterior capsulotomy in cataract surgery. *J Refract Surg.* 2011;27:711-716.
5. Ecsedy M, Mihaltz K, Kovacs I, Takács A, Filkorn T, Nagy ZZ. Effect of femtosecond laser cataract surgery on the macula. *J Refract Surg.* 2011;27:717-722.
6. Takács AI, Kovács I, Miháltz K, Filkorn T, Knorz MC, Nagy ZZ. The effect of femtolaser cataract surgery on the cornea. *J Refract Surg.* In press.
7. Roberts T, Sutton G, Lawless M, Jindal-Bali S. Capsular blockage syndrome associated with femtosecond laser-assisted cataract surgery. *J Cataract Refract Surg.* 2011;37:2068-2070.
8. Marques FF, Marques DM, Osher RH, Osher JM. Fate of anterior capsule tears during cataract surgery. *J Cataract Refract Surg.* 2006;32:1638-1642.
9. Unal M, Yücel I, Sarici A, et al. Phacoemulsification with topical anesthesia: resident experience. *J Cataract Refract Surg.* 2006;32:1361-1365.
10. Bali SJ, Hodge C, Lawless M, Roberts TV, Sutton G. Early experience with femtosecond laser for cataract surgery. *Ophthalmology.* 2012;119:891-899.

ORIGINAL CHAPTER 11

The Effect of Femtosecond Laser Capsulotomy on the Development of Posterior Capsule Opacification

Illés Kovács, MD, PhD; Kinga Kránitz, MD; Zoltán Z. Nagy, MD, PhD, DSc

In the past few years, femtosecond laser-assisted surgery has become an accepted method of cataract removal that enables the creation of a precisely sized and centered anterior capsulotomy with a 360-degree overlapping capsular edge that prevents postoperative intraocular lens (IOL) optic misalignment resulting in good postoperative visual functions.

Currently, posterior capsule opacification (PCO) is the most common late postoperative complication, caused by migration and proliferation of lens epithelial cells that remain in the capsular bag after cataract surgery.[1,2] Creating a precise anterior capsulorrhexis is essential to prevent PCO, since a properly sized and well-centered capsulorrhexis with a 360-degree overlapping capsular edge prevents optic decentration and tilt due to symmetric contractile forces of the capsular bag and shrinkwrap effect.[3] However, eccentric and/or irregularly shaped capsulorrhexis extending beyond the optic edge of the IOL may lose these advantages. A malpositioned IOL with an incomplete anterior capsule overlap may cause a higher incidence of PCO through migration of retained lens epithelial cells because of an incomplete barrier effect.[4,5]

Capsulorrhexis until now has been a manual procedure; however, with the advent of femtosecond lasers in cataract surgery, a predictably sized and centered anterior capsulotomy has become possible. The recently introduced femtosecond laser technology enables the surgeon to create precise and reproducible capsulotomies.[6]

In our previous studies, properly sized, shaped, and centered femtosecond capsulotomies resulted in better overlap parameters during the first year compared to manually performed capsulotomies. A 360-degree overlapping capsular edge was thought to be an important factor for standardizing refractive results by keeping the IOL in the desired center position and preventing IOL tilt.[5,7]

The aim of this study was to evaluate the effect of femtosecond laser–created capsulotomies on the development of PCO in the intermediate term.

Patients and Methods

Patient Population

In this study, the level of PCO was retrospectively evaluated in 79 eyes of 79 cataract patients operated on in the Department of Ophthalmology, Semmelweis University, Budapest, Hungary. All patients with a minimum follow-up time of 18 months were identified in our database of a previous prospective, randomized study on femtosecond cataract surgery, and the data of these patients were processed for further statistical analyses. Finally, 40 eyes of 40 patients were included in which femtosecond laser-assisted capsulotomy was performed, creating a 4.9-mm anterior capsulotomy (FS group). Thirty-nine eyes of 39 patients operated on in the same time period with manual capsulorrhexis with an attempted 4.9-mm capsulotomy served as controls (CCC group). In all cases, an AcrySof hydrophobic acrylic one-piece IOL with a 6-mm optic (Alcon Laboratories Inc, Ft Worth, Texas) was implanted in the capsular bag.

Surgical Technique

Following femtolaser surgery for cataract removal as described previously in all cases, a one-piece hydrophobic acrylic IOL was folded and implanted in the capsular bag with the aid of an injection cartridge through the corneal wound. IOL power was calculated using the SRK/T formula. After IOL implantation, the viscoelastic material was removed from the anterior chamber and capsular bag by irrigation-aspiration. No intra- or postoperative complications occurred. During the first 10 days, all patients received a combination of dexamethasone 0.1% and tobramycin 0.3% drops four times a day.

Posterior Capsule Opacification Analysis

Digital retroillumination photographs were taken under maximal pupil dilation 18 to 26 months after cataract surgery, focusing the camera on the posterior capsule. High-resolution digital retroillumination photographs were taken with a digital camera, and images

Nagy ZZ, ed. *Femtosecond Laser-Assisted Cataract Surgery: Facts and Results* (pp 57-60).

TABLE
DESCRIPTIVE STATISTICS OF THE TWO STUDY GROUPS

Parameter	Femtosecond Group (n=40)		CCC Group (n=39)		P Value*
	Mean	SD	Mean	SD	
Age (year)	65.50	12.94	68.95	10.84	.37
Gender (female:male)	28:12		29:10		.67*
Axial length (mm)	23.25	1.48	23.82	1.93	.31
Follow-up (months)	22.37	4.36	21.74	5.46	.30
Horizontal tilt (degree)	2.01	2.24	2.24	1.36	.69
Vertical tilt (degree)	3.50	2.13	5.10	2.23	.03
Vertical decentration (μm)	106.32	114.66	158.50	101.27	.14
Horizontal decentration (μm)	154.74	126.24	260.50	187.07	.05
Total decentration (μm)	212.01	126.62	320.54	172.07	.03
PCO level (OSCA score)	0.58	0.30	0.84	0.52	.01

CCC = manual continuous curvilinear capsulotomy
**Chi-square test.*

were imported into an open-access software platform for masked, objective evaluation of PCO (OSCA).[8] Two images of one eye photographed from different angles were used to identify and remove light reflections during the PCO analysis. During PCO evaluation, the OSCA software used a location-sensitive entropy-based texture analysis of PCO to calculate PCO score. Validation analyses of this method showed that PCO score provided by OSCA correlates with contrast sensitivity and visual acuity (two important factors that are significantly affected by PCO), thus providing an objective, valid, and reliable method of PCO quantification. The range of possible OSCA scores was from 0 (no PCO) to approximately 15 (practical expected maximum). Typical OSCA values for images with very little or no PCO were around 0.5. Values for patients who were deemed to warrant laser capsulotomy were typically around 4 to 5.[8]

Evaluation of Postoperative Position of Intraocular Lenses

A Scheimpflug imaging system (Pentacam; Oculus Optikgeräte GmbH, Wetzlar, Germany) was used to evaluate IOL tilt and decentration 12 months after cataract surgery. Lens decentration and tilt were measured according to de Castro et al[9] and were described in detail in previous chapters.

Statistical Analysis

Student *t* test for independent samples was used to compare data of the two study groups. To determine the effect of multiple predictors on PCO, multivariable regression analyses were performed via generalized estimating equation (GEE) models by adding axial length and follow-up time as covariates to adjust for their effect on PCO development. GEE models were used to take into account possible dependencies between predictor variables, thus providing reasonable estimates of regression coefficients and standard errors.

RESULTS

Age, gender, and axial length were not statistically significantly different between the two study groups (Table).

In all cases, in both groups a 360-degree overlapping anterior capsulorrhexis was created. However, there was statistically significant postoperative difference in both centration and tilting values between FS and CCC groups. Significantly higher vertical IOL tilt was measured in eyes after manual capsulorrhexis (see Table). There were also higher horizontal and total decentration values in the CCC group than in the FS group (see Table). Finally, the level of PCO was significantly lower in the femtosecond group compared to the manual group (0.58±0.30 vs 0.84±0.52, *P*=.01) (see Table), although no

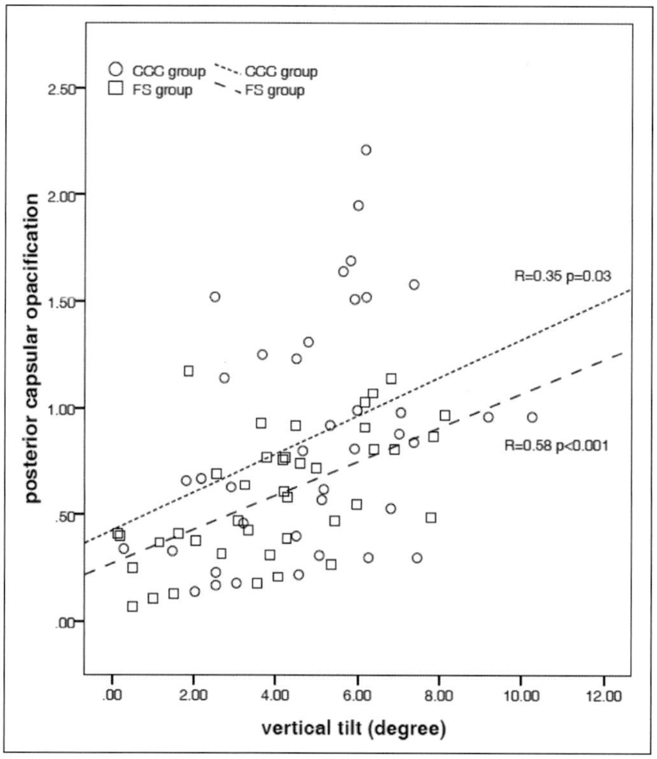

Figure. The correlation between vertical IOL tilt and PCO in the two study groups proved to be significant (r=0.58, *P*<.001 in the femtosecond group and r=0.35, *P*=.03 in the manual group).

capsulotomy procedure had to be performed during the follow-up time in either group.

After adjusting for axial length and follow-up time, manual capsulorrhexis was found to be a significant predictor for the development of PCO in the multivariable regression model (β: 0.33, 95% confidence limit [CL]: 0.01-0.65, *P*=.04). Neither axial length nor follow-up time was a significant predictor of PCO in this model (*P*>.05, for both parameters). Among postoperative IOL position parameters, only vertical tilt showed significant correlation with the level of PCO in both groups (FS: r=0.58, *P*<.001 and CCC: r=0.35, *P*=.03) (Fig). Similarly, in multivariable modeling, vertical tilt was a significant predictor of postoperative PCO after adjusting for the effect of axial length, follow-up time, and type of capsulorrhexis (β: 0.07, 95% CL: 0.01-0.12, *P*=.02).

Discussion

PCO is the most frequent long-term complication following cataract surgery by phacoemulsification with IOL implantation.[1] Although neodymium:yttrium-aluminum-garnet (Nd-YAG) laser capsulotomy is an effective therapy of PCO, known complications include increased intraocular pressure, cystoid macular edema, and retinal detachment.[10]

The development of PCO is a result of multiple IOL- and surgery-related factors. Design and diameter of IOL optics, IOL material, edge profile, and optic–haptic junction have been reported, remarkably influencing its development. Moreover, implantation of an IOL into the capsular bag with complete anterior capsular overlap was found to also have significant preventive effect on PCO development.[5,11-13]

Creation of a properly sized and well-centered capsulorrhexis to achieve a complete anterior capsular overlap is often a surgical challenge. With the advent of femtosecond laser, this crucial step of cataract surgery has become more standardized. According to our previous results, femtosecond laser capsulotomies are round and reproducible, with accurate diameter, whereas manual capsulorrhexis can be irregular in shape and difficult to control its centration.[6] A properly sized and centered anterior capsulotomy results in a complete, circular overlap maintaining the correct postoperative position of the implanted IOL.[4,7] In this study, we found statistically significant difference between the two study groups in IOL positioning parameters. Postoperative vertical tilt and horizontal and total decentration proved to be significantly higher in the manual capsulorrhexis group compared to the femtosecond laser group, confirming our previously published results.

According to multivariable statistical analyses, the type of capsulorrhexis was found to be an independent significant predictor of the PCO after adjustment for the effect of axial length and follow-up time, factors that were already described as predictors of PCO; however, results are inconsistent.[1,14] In our series, after adjustment for axial length and follow-up time, manual creation of anterior capsulotomies increased PCO score by 33% compared to femtosecond laser-assisted capsulotomies. Neither axial length nor follow-up time proved to be a significant predictor of PCO. There was a statistically significant positive correlation between vertical tilt and the severity of PCO. According to multivariable modeling, after adjustment for the effect of axial length, follow-up time, and type of capsulorrhexis, every one degree of IOL tilt resulted in a 7% percent increase in PCO score. These results seem to support the barrier principle in PCO prevention that is based on symmetric contractile forces of a 360-degree overlapping anterior capsular edge pushing the IOL optic consistently to the posterior capsule, which leads to a continuous circular contact between the IOL and the posterior capsule creating an effective barrier to migrating lens epithelial cells. In our study, a 360-degree overlapping anterior capsulorrhexis was created in both groups and there was no difference in irrigation-aspiration technique or time between the two groups.

According to our previously published results, more accurate capsulotomies can be performed with a femtosecond laser than manually not only in emmetropic but in high myopic eyes also.[15] An accurate capsulotomy is especially important in myopic eyes to provide perfect overlap and a continuous, circular barrier for lens epithelial cells preventing PCO because laser capsulotomy has an increased risk for retinal detachment in eyes with longer axial length.[16]

Our results suggest that a well-centered and accurate capsulotomy might have an additive role to IOL edge design and hydrophobic IOL material in the prevention of PCO. In this study, no capsulotomy was required due to severe PCO in either group, and the creation of a capsulotomy using femtosecond laser proved to be a safe procedure not increasing PCO score. In contrast, we observed a slight decrease in PCO formation, which is a supplemental advantage of this method to the improved safety and predictability results that have been published earlier. Further studies are needed to assess the clinical significance of this result, especially in patient groups who are at increased risk for developing PCO.

References

1. Schaumberg DA, Dana MR, Christen WG, Glynn RJ. A systematic overview of the incidence of posterior capsule opacification. *Ophthalmology.* 1998;105:1213-1221.
2. Nishi O, Nishi K, Sakanishi K. Inhibition of migrating lens epithelial cells at the capsular bend created by the rectangular optic edge of a posterior chamber intraocular lens. *Ophthalmic Surg Lasers.* 1998;29:587-594.
3. Ravalico G, Tognetto D, Palomba M, Busatto P, Baccara F. Capsulorhexis size and posterior capsule opacification. *J Cataract Refract Surg.* 1996;22:98-103.
4. Kránitz K, Mih– K, Sándor GL, Takacs A, Knorz MC, Nagy ZZ. Intraocular lens tilt and decentration measured by Scheimpflug camera following manual or femtosecond laser created continuous circular capsulotomy. *J Refract Surg.* 2012;28:259-263.
5. Smith SR, Daynes T, Hinckley M, Wallin TR, Olson RJ. The effect of lens edge design versus anterior capsule overlap on posterior capsule opacification. *Am J Ophthalmol.* 2004;138:521-526.
6. Nagy Z, Takacs A, Filkorn T, Sarayba M. Initial clinical evaluation of an intraocular femtosecond laser in cataract surgery. *J Refract Surg.* 2009;25:1053-1060.
7. Kránitz K, Takacs A, Mihály K, Kovács I, Knorz MC, Nagy ZZ. Femtosecond laser capsulotomy and manual continuous curvilinear capsulorrhexis parameters and their effects on intraocular lens centration. *J Refract Surg.* 2011;27:558-563.
8. Aslam TM, Patton N, Rose CJ. OSCA: a comprehensive open-access system of analysis of posterior capsular opacification. *BMC Ophthalmol.* 2006;23:6-30.
9. de Castro A, Rosales P, Marcos S. Tilt and decentration of intraocular lenses in vivo from Purkinje and Scheimpflug imaging. Validation study. *J Cataract Refract Surg.* 2007;33:418-429.
10. Burq MA, Taqui AM. Frequency of retinal detachment and other complications after neodymium:Yag laser capsulotomy. *J Pak Med Assoc.* 2008;58:550-552.
11. Hollick EJ, Spalton DJ, Ursell PG, et al. The effect of PMMA, silicone, and polyacrylic lenses on posterior capsule opacification 3 years after surgery. *Ophthalmology.* 1998;106:49-54.
12. Schmidbauer JM, Escobar-Gomez M, Apple DJ, Peng Q, Arthur SN, Vargas LG. Effect of haptic angulation on posterior capsule opacification in modern foldable lenses with a square, truncated optic edge. *J Cataract Refract Surg.* 2002;28:1251-1255.
13. Meacock WR, Spalton DJ, Boyce JF, Jose RM. Effect of optic size on posterior capsule opacification: 5.5mm versus 6.0mm AcrySof intraocular lenses. *J Cataract Refract Surg.* 2001;27:1194-1198.
14. Zhao Y, Li J, Lu W, et al. Capsular adhesion to intraocular lens in highly myopic eyes evaluated in vivo using ultralong-scan depth optical coherence tomography. *Am J Ophthalmol.* 2013;155:484-491.
15. Nagy ZZ, Kránitz K, Takacs AI, Mihály K, Kovács I, Knorz MC. Comparison of intraocular lens decentration parameters after femtosecond and manual capsulotomies. *J Refract Surg.* 2011;27:564-569.
16. Dardenne MU, Gerten GJ, Kokkas K, Kermani O. Retrospective study of retinal detachment following neodymium:YAG laser posterior capsulotomy. *J Cataract Refract Surg.* 1989;15:676-680.

The Verion Image Guided System

Zoltán Z. Nagy, MD, PhD, DSc

The Verion Image Guided System by Alcon LenSx (Aliso Viejo, California) was developed after the introduction of femtosecond laser cataract surgery (Fig 1). This is the first system where all the steps between diagnosis and treatment are coupled and helped by the Verion System (Fig 2). Image–Plan–Guide creates a unique system and continuous flow of patient data from the first encounter until the patient's last visit.

The Verion is designed to consistently achieve the desired refractive target. Currently, refractive surgery has a significantly higher predictability; however, patient expectation in cataract surgery has also increased and cataract patients demand similar results as refractive surgical patients.

The Verion System contains a diagnostic unit, which is called the Reference Unit (Fig 3). This consists of a Measurement Module and a Surgical Planner (Fig 4).

The Measurement Unit measures the characteristic data of the patient's eye: K-values, limbus position and diameter, horizontal white-to-white distance, corneal reflex position, pupillometry, and eccentricity of the visual axis. This is a noncontact, preoperative measurement device that captures high-resolution reference images with scleral vessels, limbus, and iris features. All data are auto-imported into the Planner Module of the Reference Unit.

During keratometry, three to five images are captured with a total of 15 to 30 data points to determine spherical power and cylinder.

The Surgical Planner helps to assemble the surgical plan. Data are auto-imported from preoperative measurement information from the Measurement Module. It has a specific program for intraocular lens (IOL) selection and IOL power selection. The surgeon may choose from several formulas, such as Holladay 1, 2, and R; Hoffer Q; SRK/T; and Haigis.

For astigmatism management, the program calculates the diopter and angle of the toric IOL or the position, length, and depth of the relaxing incisions in the case of arcuate corneal incisions. A special feature is the new system for A-constant optimization and the ability to import third-party data (eg, from the HS Lenstar). Other diagnostic tools may also be coupled theoretically to the Verion System.

Another special feature is the Digital Marker for the femtosecond laser (Alcon LenSx) and for the operating microscope. This system helps and guides the surgeon throughout the ophthalmic procedure.

Within the operating microscope, there is an integrated display for the convenience of the surgeon. The Patient Registration System helps to identify the specific characteristics of the treated eyes. It also helps with the Incision Guide (Fig 5) to create the corneal incision in the optimal place and size and length. The Capsulorrhexis Guide (Fig 6) assists the surgeon by projecting the desired diameter and positioned capsulorrhexis circle onto the surface of the cornea during the surgery. During the implantation of the posterior chamber lens (PCL) a so-called Centration Guide helps to correctly center the PCL. The Toric Guide projects where the toric angle of the lens should be positioned at the conclusion of the surgery. The Finalization Check (Fig 7) helps to center the PCL, taking into consideration eccentricity of the visual axis.

The Microscope Integrated Display is optimized for Alcon LuxOR, but is also available for Zeiss, Leica, Möller-Wedel, Takagi, and Topcon operating microscopes. It consists of an integrated camera and display; the light:split ratio is 70:30. It contains the latest green OLED display technology.

The Verion Link is also a new feature; through the Verion Digital Marker M it receives phaco status information from a compatible phaco system (Alcon Centurion) to synchronize workflow.

It should also be noted that the femtosecond laser also receives information from the Reference Unit. To avoid cyclotorsion, it uses the Vessel and Iris Registration data during the docking phase.

Thus, the work flow is from the Reference Unit toward the femtosecond laser, then toward the operating

Nagy ZZ, ed. *Femtosecond Laser-Assisted Cataract Surgery: Facts and Results* (pp 61-65).

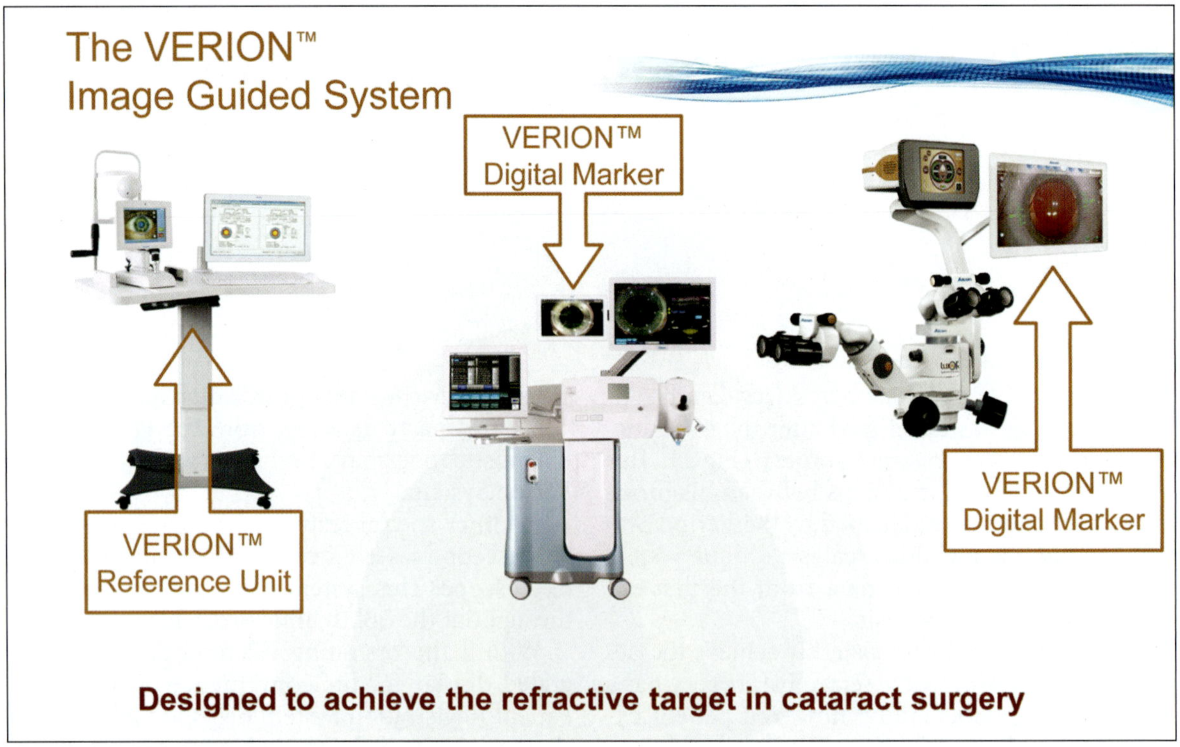

Figure 1. The Verion Image Guided System.

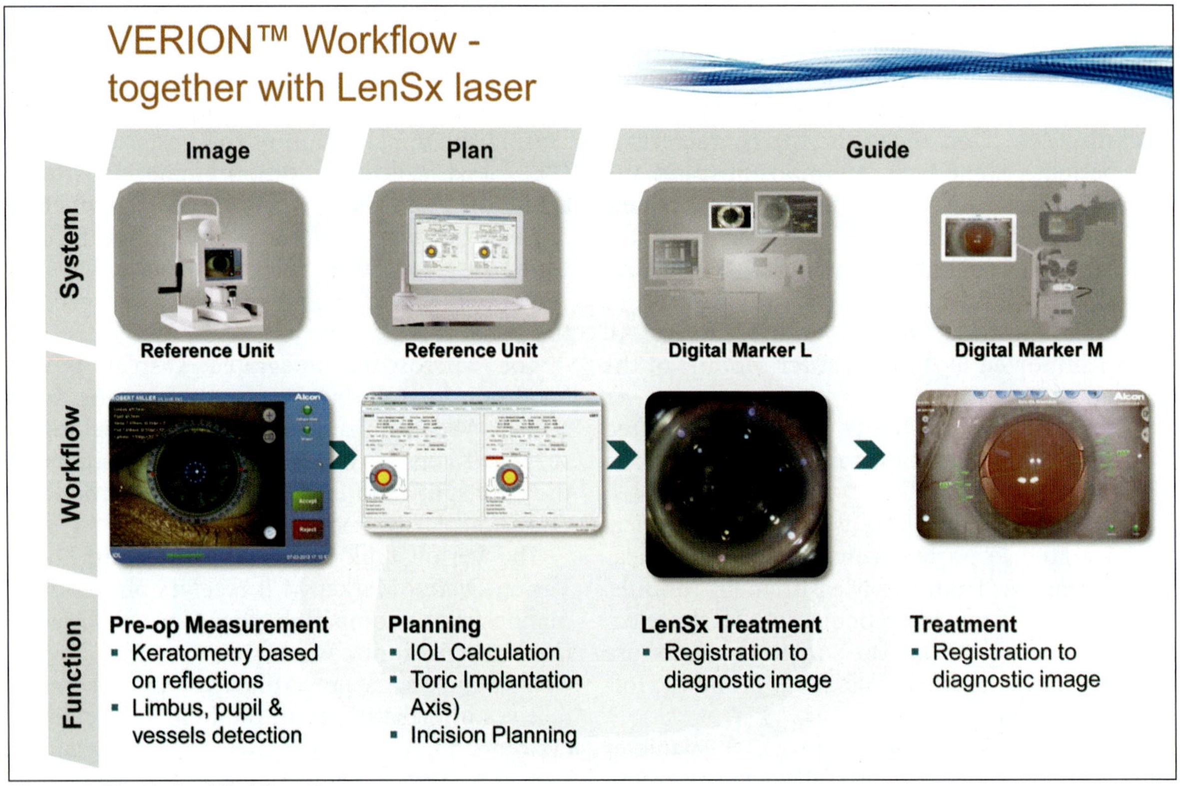

Figure 2. The Verion Workflow System.

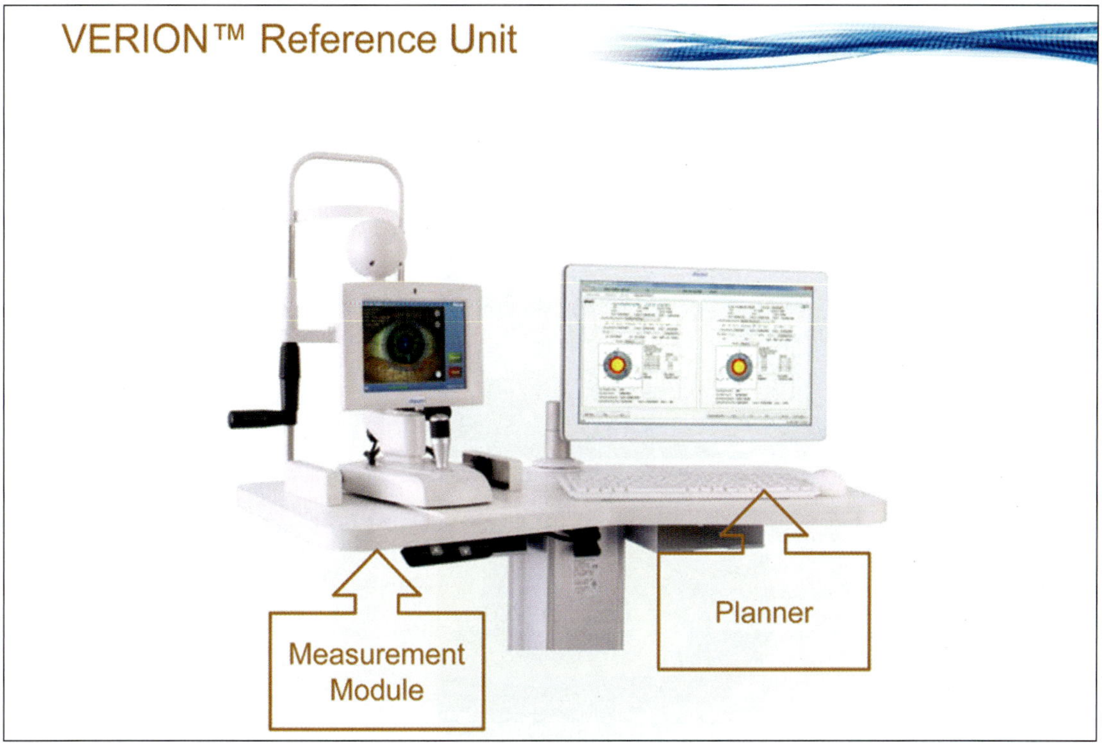

Figure 3. The Verion Reference Unit. The Measurement Module and the Planner.

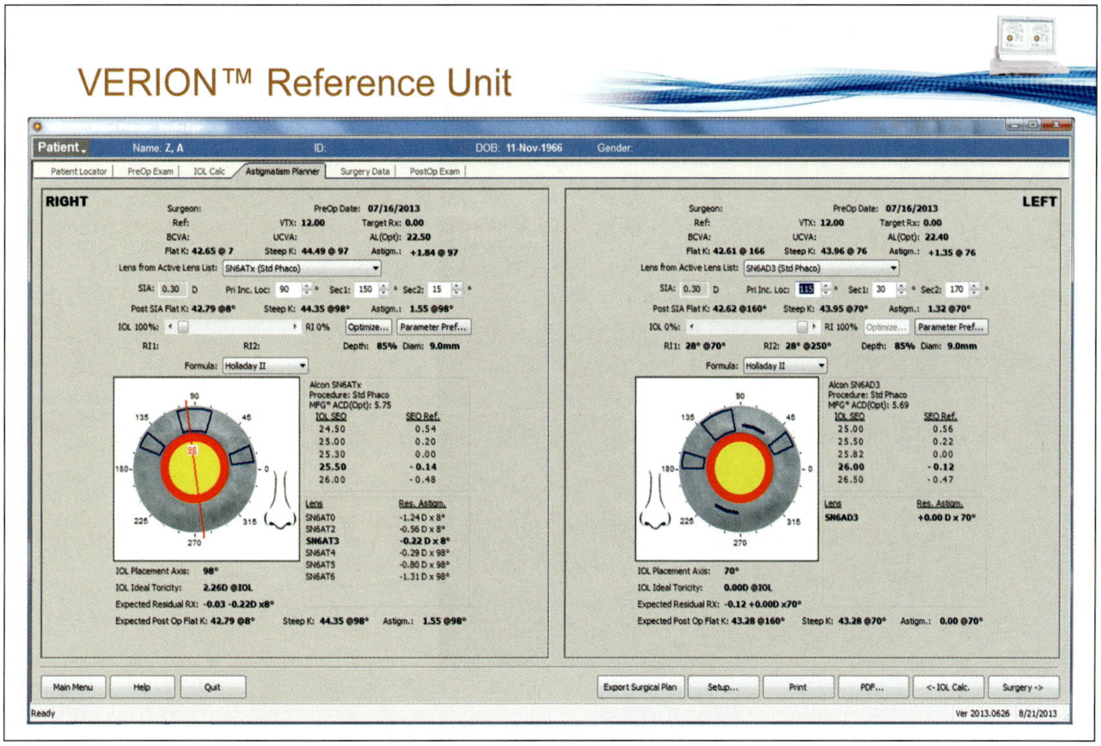

Figure 4. The Planner screen for the surgeon. It shows where to put the incisions and which axis is the most optimal for the toric lens implantation.

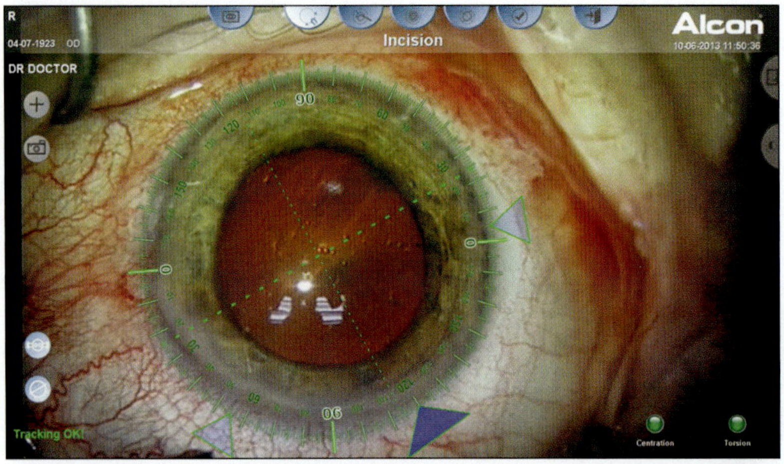

Figure 5. The Incision Guide, which is mounted into the operating microscope.

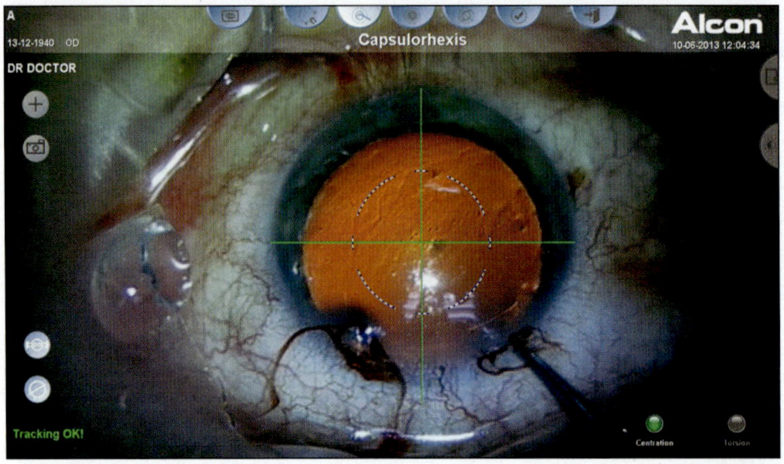

Figure 6. The Capsulorrhexis Guide (for manual capsulorrhexis). In cases of femtosecond laser-assisted capsulorrhexis, the positioning is automatically calculated for the Digital Marker of the femtosecond laser.

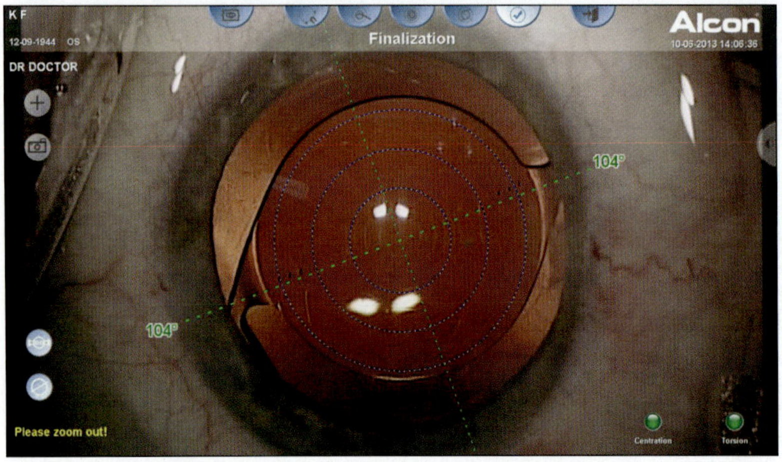

Figure 7. The Finalization Check to check the position of the IOL, the centration, etc.

microscope, and then to the phacoemulsification machine. During postoperative follow-ups, the patient's refractive data are measured again and analyzed by the system. Here the surgeon may create his or her personal surgical data, personalized A-constant, and surgically induced astigmatism data.

The Verion is the first system to combine pre-, peri-, and postoperative data of individual patients to improve the refractive predictability of the cataract procedure. With the femtosecond laser, the surgical steps might be consistent; with the Verion system, preoperative assessment helps to achieve a perfect docking, capsulorrhexis, femto-fragmentation, optimal wound creation, and optimal arcuate incisions to control preoperative astigmatism.

Conclusion

With a convenient desktop interface, the Verion Reference Unit does the following:

- ► During imaging
  - Measures keratometry, pupillometry, and other key preoperative parameters
  - Captures a high-resolution, diagnostic reference image of the patient's eye
  - Autodetects scleral vessels, limbus, pupil, and iris features
- ► During planning
  - Enables surgeons to quickly and efficiently determine an optimized surgical plan
  - Offers multiple advanced formulas for calculations, including lens and power selection
  - Incision and implantation axis planning can be customized for each patient
- ► During guiding it provides
  - Improved data flow via auto-import of patient information and surgery plan into the Alcon LenSx femtosecond laser
  - Advanced imaging by image registration to diagnostic image for automatic marker-less cyclorotation compensation
  - Registration and real-time tracking overlay for precise incision and IOL alignment during femto- and cataract procedures
  - Eliminates the need for manual toric eye markings
  - Supported Microscope Integrated Display microscopes: Alcon LuxOR, Leica, Möller-Wedel, Takagi, Topcon, Zeiss
- ► During treatment
  - Registration to diagnostic image
  - Overlays for incisions, centration, alignment
  - Option: control via Centurion

Flap Creation Using LenSx Femtosecond Multiple-Use Laser System

Éva Juhász, MD; Kinga Kránitz, MD; Ágnes I. Takács, MD; Andrea Gyenes, MD; Zoltán Z. Nagy, MD, PhD, DSc

Background

Since surgical vision correction became possible without significant postoperative pain, corneal flap creation has gained attention. Performing photoablation in the deeper corneal stroma during LASIK procedures results in more rapid visual recovery and less pain compared to the surface ablation technique.[1] The more appropriate and precise the flap creation is, the better the results that can be achieved.

With the use of microkeratomes, even and proper corneal flaps usually could be created; however, several side effects and complications arising from human and mechanical keratome-dependent imperfections were described. It may be unnecessary to emphasize the possible side effects of a poorly constructed corneal flap, such as buttonhole perforation, greater amount of induced higher-order aberrations, or postoperative ectasia as a result of performing uneven and nonuniform surfaces and larger variances between planned and achieved flap thickness.

Several research teams reported that the use of a mechanical microkeratome created thinner central flap thickness than peripheral. If flap thickness is greater at the periphery, the chance of buttonhole flap is increased.[2] Based on peer-reviewed literature, the most significant difference in higher-order aberration induction between surface ablation techniques and LASIK treatments is that LASIK also increases higher-order aberrations of the posterior corneal surface, causing visual disturbances such as glare, halo, and rainbow glare,[3] while photorefractive keratectomy (PRK) does not. If the thickness of the residual corneal stroma is less than 250 μm,[4] postoperative corneal ectasia may occur, resulting in iatrogenic keratoconus.

Development

In the past decade, femtolasers were applied to create corneal flaps instead of using mechanical microkeratomes during LASIK procedures. Later femtolaser systems were introduced for cataract surgery.[5,6] Two different types of femtosecond laser platforms were needed to perform corneal refractive (LASIK) procedures and cataract surgeries that rendered the availability of these methods difficult. According to previous studies, flaps created by femtosecond laser with only one application were more uniform with higher predictable thickness and proved to be more regular and more accurate than those created by a microkeratome.[7,8] With the latest invention of Alcon LenSx, a new generation multifunctional femtosecond laser system that has already been reliably used in femtolaser-assisted cataract surgeries, both operations can be performed by the same device. Outcomes of femto-LASIK surgeries using this new, multifunctional femtolaser system should and proved to be at least as good as the use of the previous monofunctional system as discussed below.

With the introduction of a femtolaser that is applicable not just for intraocular or for corneal-related procedures, but for both, operating costs of an ophthalmic practice can be significantly lowered, contributing to the spread of one of the most advanced technologies in ophthalmology.

Description

The steps of the procedure are partly similar to the steps of femtolaser-assisted cataract surgery. Topical anesthesia drops should be applied three times every 8 to 10 minutes, then eyes are docked to the patient interface applying a corneal suction ring. A modified patient interface (SoftFit) needs to be used to achieve better insertion. With the new SoftFit patient interface, significant reduction in intraocular pressure rise (20%) and increased surgical treatment and visibility zone (from 12.0 to 12.5 mm, 8.5% increase) are provided. After centration of the patient interface and the treatment zone, corneal flaps can be created using the Alcon LenSx femtosecond laser (Alcon LenSx Inc, Aliso Viejo, California). The laser device is in connection with an optical coherence tomography (OCT) device giving live recording of the whole process.

Nagy ZZ, ed. *Femtosecond Laser-Assisted Cataract Surgery: Facts and Results* (pp 67-72).

The Alcon LenSx femtosecond laser system allows the user to make individual flap settings regarding hinge position, spot size, spot separation, energy level, flap thickness, and other parameters.

Flaps can be lifted by a special blunt but quite thin spatula (Slade's spatula) to perform refractive excimer treatment of the tissue beneath, and then they are repositioned.

After flap reposition, the ocular surface needs to be irrigated with chilled balanced salt solution, antibiotic, and steroid drops. Patients can receive transparent protective plastic shields at the end of the surgery in order to protect their eyes from severe trauma.

Relevant Studies of Our Research Team[9,10]

Evaluating Flap Parameters

The purpose of our study was to create corneal flaps during LASIK procedures by applying a new, multi-functional femtosecond laser system (which has already been reliably used in femtolaser-assisted cataract surgeries) prior to excimer laser treatment and to evaluate flap conditions as well as the safety and efficacy of the procedure regarding visual outcomes and flap parameters in myopic and myopic-astigmatic patients consecutively.[11] In 2012, new software was installed to improve results.

Reliability of flap creation using this new-generation multifunctional femtosecond laser was evaluated postoperatively by using anterior segment OCT. Although higher-order aberration induction effect of LASIK procedures is already well known, the same effect of femto-LASIK treatments has not been investigated yet. The aim of this trial was also to evaluate the characteristics of induced corneal higher-order aberrations.

This study was a prospective, single-center clinical trial of Alcon LenSx lasers.[11] Patients were evaluated intraoperatively to assess the ease of flap lifting, the stromal bed quality, and the amount of opaque bubble layer.[11]

In this study, 38 eyes of 20 patients were enrolled with myopia and myopic astigmatism in the range of spherical refractive error from −1.75 D to −6.75 D and cylindrical refractive error from 0.25 D to 2.0 D. The distribution of gender was 50/50 and the average age was 29 (±6.5) years.

All eyes underwent a complete ophthalmological examination and were screened for eligibility. Exclusion criteria were known sensitivity to planned study concomitant medications, participation in any other ophthalmic drug or device clinical trial during the time of this clinical investigation, presentation of any contraindications to femtosecond-initiated LASIK surgeries, corneal thickness values less than 400 μm or that will result in residual bed less than 280 μm when flap creation and excimer ablation are calculated, irregular astigmatism, ectatic corneal disorders (keratoconus, keratoglobus), pregnancy, and lactating women.[11] Exclusion criteria were also age under 18 years, amblyopia, dry eye syndrome, previous history of herpes keratitis, superficial corneal opacities or corneal scars, former refractive surgery, severe diabetes mellitus, and macular disease.

Preoperative uncorrected visual acuity (UCVA) and best spectacle-corrected visual acuity (BSCVA) (median ± quartile range) were 0.1 (±0.07) and 1.0 (±0.0), respectively. Patients underwent femto-LASIK treatment between September 2012 and March 2013 in the Department of Ophthalmology, Semmelweis University, Budapest, Hungary. All surgeries were performed by the same experienced surgeon (Z.Z.N.).

The study was conducted in compliance with the Declaration of Helsinki, as well as with applicable country and local requirements regarding ethics committee/institutional review boards and other statutes or regulations regarding protection of the rights and welfare of human subjects participating in biomedical research. Prior to surgery, a written informed consent was obtained from every patient regarding flap creation using femtosecond laser and refractive treatment. Follow up-time was 3 months.

Visual acuity tests, intraocular pressure measurements, and anterior segment spectral-domain OCT (RTVue; Optovue, Inc) examinations using an additional corneal adapter module were performed postoperatively, 1 day, 1 week, and 1 and 3 months after the surgery. All complications were recorded.

Thickness of the centrum and at points 1.0 and 2.0 mm from the corneal vertex in the vertical and horizontal meridians of the cornea were measured using RTVue's flap-measuring software, which inserts points to the borders of the flap according to different density (Figs 1 and 2). From these measurements, nine thickness data were recorded and analyzed for each flap. Mean values were calculated in each case.[12] Analysis of these points was performed in order to prove planarity of the flaps.

Results

One month after the treatment UCVA was 20/20 in 92.1% and 20/25 or better in 97.4% of patients. Three months after surgery, UCVA was 20/20 in 94.7% and 20/25 or better in 100% of patients (Fig 3). BSCVA remained stable after surgery. BSCVA proved to be 20/20 in 100% of patients 1 and 3 months postoperatively (Table 1).

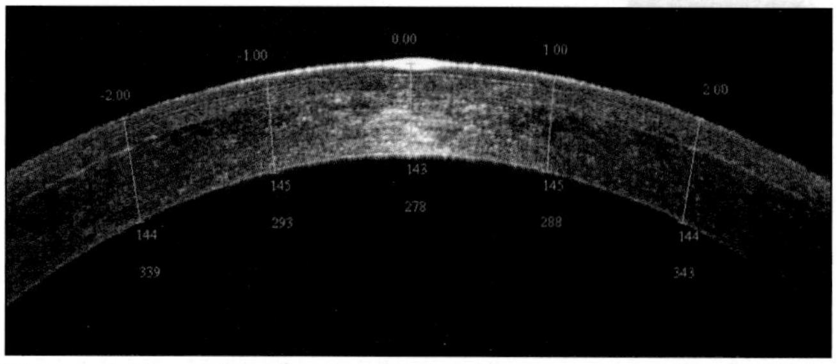

Figure 1. Example of 0-degree meridian cross-sectional RTVue anterior segment spectral-domain OCT image of the cornea.

No complications or adverse events were recorded regarding lost, misplaced, or misaligned flap; corneal ulcer or perforation; or corneal microbial or intraocular infection.

The mean value of postoperatively measured flap thickness was 141.95 (±7.59) μm (Table 2). Flaps had a planar shape, and there was no significant difference between the thickness of the nine points in each cornea (Friedman test, *P*=.058).

There was no statistically significant difference between planned and postoperatively measured flap thickness (preoperatively: 140.00 [±0.0] μm; 3 months postoperatively: 140.28 [±8.0] μm; Wilcoxon test, *P*=.4067). The anterior segment OCT revealed a planar structure of the corneal flap with even thickness in the periphery and in the central part of the cornea. The stromal bed was even and regular in structure. No folds or stromal lines were experienced.

Evaluating Higher-Order Aberrations

Materials and Methods

Our aim was also to compare properties of femto-LASIK and PRK procedures regarding higher-order aberrations of the anterior and posterior corneal surfaces. Sixty eyes of 30 patients with myopia and myopic astigmatism were enrolled in this study. Thirty eyes of 15 patients from the previous femto-LASIK study group were matched to 30 eyes of 15 patients who had undergone PRK treatment using Wavelight Allegretto 400 excimer laser regarding age, gender, and preoperative refractive error (Table 3). Postoperative refractive target was emmetropia in all cases. All eyes underwent a complete ophthalmological examination, just like in the study mentioned previously. Exclusion criteria were also equivalent to ones in the previous study.

There was no significant difference between the two groups in refractive error (*P*=.149), ablation depth (*P*=.105), and UCVA (*P*=.128). Best-corrected visual acuity was 1.0 in all cases.

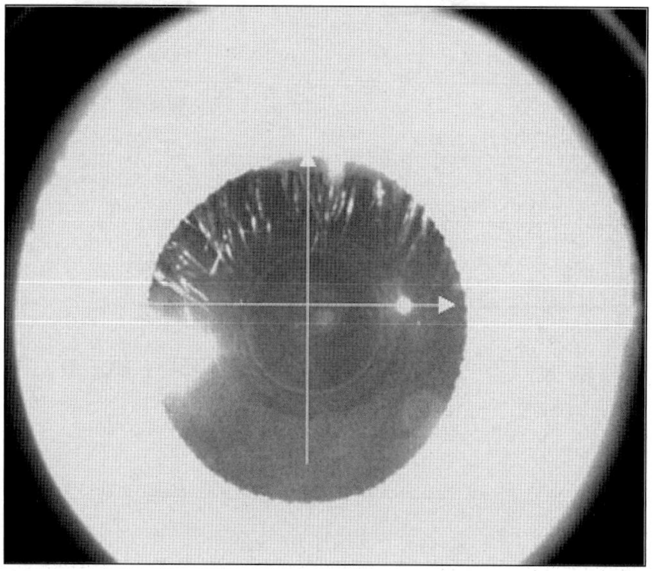

Figure 2. The 0- and 90-degree meridians of the cornea.

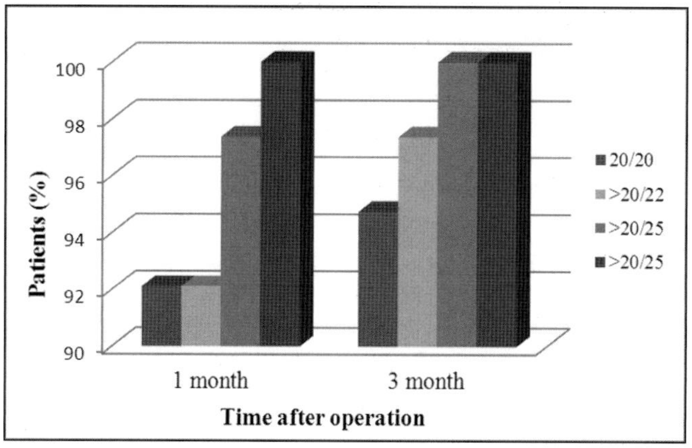

Figure 3. UCVA results.

Corneal wavefront analysis (Pentacam; Oculus Optikgeräte GmbH, Wetzlar, Germany) was performed preoperatively and 3 months postoperatively at 4.5-, 6.0-, and 8.0-mm analysis diameter. Higher-order aberrations of the total cornea (RMS-HOA-total), the anterior surface (RMS-HOA-anterior), and the posterior surface (RMS-HOA-posterior) were analyzed. There was no significant difference in corneal higher-order RMS values in any analysis diameter between the two study groups either.

Results

Three months after surgery, UCVA values increased statistically significantly in both groups (PRK: from 0.1±0.02 to 1.0±0.00; *P*<.001 and femto-LASIK: from 0.1±0.07 to 1.0±0.00; *P*<.001). In the PRK group, UCVA was 0.8 or better in 100% of the cases (30/30), 0.9 or better in 96.67% (29/30), and 1.0 or better in

TABLE 1

PREOPERATIVE CHARACTERISTICS OF PATIENTS

Parameter	Before	3 Months After the Operation	P Value
UCVA			
Median±Quartile	0.1±0.07	1.0±0.0	<.001*
Range	0.04 to 0.3	0.8 to 1.0	
BSCVA			
Mean±SD	1.0±0.00	1.0±0.00	1.0**
Range	1.0	1.0	
SE refraction (D)			
Mean±SD	−4.24±1.53	−0.08± 0.54	<.001**
Range	−7.75 to −2.0	−1.0 to 1.0	
Sphere (D)			
Mean±SD	−3.95± 1.44	−0.01±0.44	<.001**
Range	−6.75 to −1.75	−0.75 to 0.75	
Cylinder (D)			
Mean±SD	−0.59±0.52	−0.14±0.43	<.001**
Range	−2.0 to 0.0	−1.0 to 1.0	

** Wilcoxon test. **Dependent sample paired t test.*

TABLE 2

FLAP THICKNESS OF THE RELEVANT NINE MEASUREMENTS IN THE TWO MERIDIANS (MEAN±SD) AND DEVIATION FROM THE DESIRED FLAP THICKNESS

		Peripheral	Paracentral	Central	Paracentral	Peripheral
0-degree meridian	Mean±SD (μm)	142.32±7.45	141.18±7.54	142.37±7.41	141.58±8.43	142.74±8.1
	Deviation (μm)	−2.32	−1.18	−2.37	−1.58	−2.74
90-degree meridian	Mean±SD (μm)	142.84±7.53	142.03±7.29	142.37±7.41	139.74±18.41	142.76±7.06
	Deviation (μm)	−2.84	−2.03	−2.37	0.26	−2.76

TABLE 3

DESCRIPTIVE DATA

Parameter	PRK Median±Quartile Range	Femto-LASIK Median±Quartile Range	P Value
Age	30.00±7.00	28.00±8.00	.290
Gender (female:male)	8:7	8:7	>.05
Preop refraction (SE)	−3.250±1.625	−3.938±2.625	.149
Preop pachymetry (μm)	552.00±34.00	548.00±48.00	.835
Ablation depth (μm)	71.500±24.000	64.000±33.000	.105

P=between groups difference, P<.05 using Mann-Whitney U test.

TABLE 4

RESULTS OF GENERAL LINEAR MODELS

	P *Preop Refraction*	P *RMS Total Baseline*	P *Group*
RMS total 4.5 mm 3 months	.976	.299	.472
RMS total 6.0 mm 3 months	.02*	.739	<.001*
RMS total 8.0 mm 3 months	<.001*	<.001*	.002*

After adjusting for preoperative refractive error and preoperative RMS values we found statistically significant difference between the two study groups in postoperative higher-order aberrations in 6.0 and 8.0 mm analysis diameters.
**P<.05.*

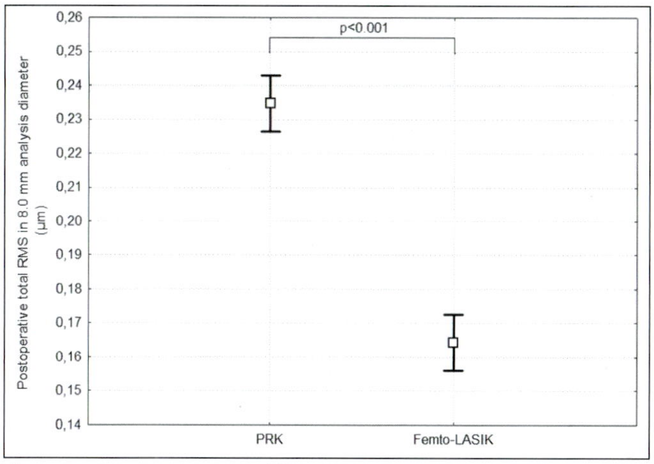

Figure 4. Between groups difference in postoperative total corneal RMS values in 6.0-mm analysis diameter after adjusting for preoperative refractive and wavefront error (*P*<.001).

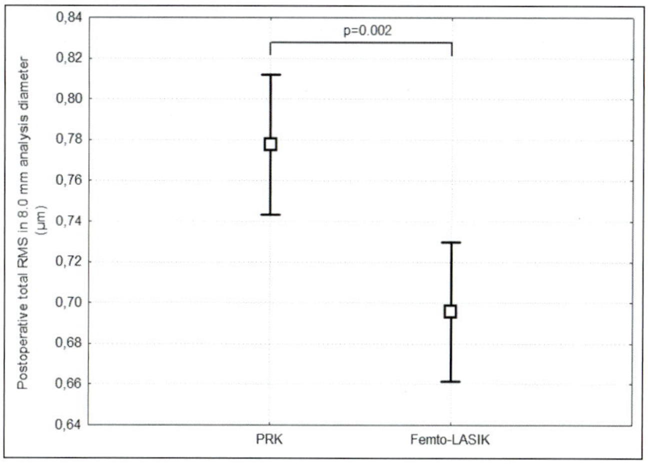

Figure 5. Between groups difference in postoperative total corneal RMS values in 8.0-mm analysis diameter after adjusting for preoperative refractive and wavefront error (*P*=.002).

90.0% (27/30) 3 months after surgery. In the femto-LASIK group, UCVA proved to be 0.8 or better in 100% of the cases (30/30), 0.9 or better in 96.67% (29/30), and 1.0 or better in 93.3% (28/30) 3 months after surgery. BSCVA remained stable and proved to be 1.0 in all cases postoperatively.

Three months after surgery, higher-order RMS values of the anterior corneal surface and the total cornea increased significantly in all analysis diameters (*P*<.001) while higher-order aberrations regarding the posterior corneal surface remained stable (4.5 mm: *P*=.142; 6.0 mm: *P*=.052; 8.0 mm: *P*=.65) in the PRK group. In the femto-LASIK group, higher-order aberrations of the anterior and posterior corneal surface and the total cornea increased significantly in all analysis diameters after the surgical procedure (*P*<.001).

Three months after surgery, there was no statistically significant difference in induced higher-order corneal aberrations in 4.5-mm analysis diameter between the two study groups; however, higher-order RMS values, representing wavefront errors of the anterior corneal surface and the total cornea in 6.0- and 8.0-mm analysis diameters, proved to be significantly higher in the PRK group compared to the femto-LASIK group. We found no statistically significant difference between the two study groups in higher-order aberrations of the posterior corneal surface in these analysis diameters.

After adjusting for preoperative refractive error and preoperative RMS values, general linear models also showed significant difference in postoperative higher-order aberrations in 6.0- and 8.0-mm diameters between the two study groups (RMS total 6.0 mm: *P*<.001; RMS total 8.0 mm: *P*=.002) (Table 4 and Figs 4 and 5).

CONCLUSION

The visual acuity and OCT analysis results mentioned in the studies above showed that safety, efficacy, and reliability of this new, multifunctional femtolaser system during femto-LASIK procedures were proven appropriately.

Despite more postoperative pain and longer recovery, PRK treatment is often preferred over LASIK to avoid greater amounts of induced higher-order aberrations. With the invention of femto-LASIK technique, corneal flaps have become more uniform and regular.[7] Comparison of desired and postoperatively measured flap thickness showed no statistically significant difference demonstrating that flaps could be created reliably and precisely with this new type of femtosecond laser.

There was no statistically significant difference between femto-LASIK and PRK procedures in postoperative higher-order total corneal aberrations in 4.5-mm analysis diameter that corresponds to an average pupil diameter in photopic conditions. However in 6.0- and 8.0-mm analysis diameters, which exceeded the border of the transitional zone of PRK treatment, postoperative corneal aberrations proved to be significantly higher in the PRK group even after adjusting for preoperative aberrations and preoperative refractive error. These results suggest that favorable aberration pattern was available after femto-LASIK than PRK in greater analysis diameters, which includes also the peripheral part of the cornea and represents mesopic or scotopic pupil conditions.

According to former reports, even with the latest advances in femtosecond laser technology, rainbow glare remains a possible optical side effect of femto-LASIK procedures.[13] In our study, patients mentioned no such complaints.

Our results correspond to previous studies in accordance with induced higher-order aberrations on the posterior surface of the cornea. After PRK surgeries no postoperative changes could be detected on the posterior corneal surface; however, femto-LASIK procedures increased posterior corneal aberrations in all analysis diameters supposedly due to thinner residual stromal bed.[14,15] Despite these results, total corneal aberrations were more favorable in the femto-LASIK group.

The outstanding results of this combined device may suggest a wide acceptance of this technology and a new era of femtosecond surgeries.

References

1. Skevas C, Katz T, Wagenfeld L, et al. Subjective pain, visual recovery and visual quality after LASIK, EpiLASIK (flap off) and APRK—a consecutive, non-randomized study. *Graefes Arch Clin Exp Ophthalmol.* 2013;251(4):1175-1183.
2. Zhang XX, Zhong XW, Wu JS, et al. Corneal flap morphological analysis using anterior segment optical coherence tomography in laser in situ keratomileusis with femtosecond lasers versus mechanical microkeratome. *Int J Ophthalmol.* 2012;5(1):69-73.
3. Porter J, MacRae S, Yoon G, et al. Separate effects of the microkeratome incision and laser ablation on the eye's wave aberration. *Am J Ophthalmol.* 2003;136:327-337.
4. Sugar A, Rapuano CJ, Culbertson WW, et al. Laser in situ keratomileusis for myopia and astigmatism: safety and efficacy: a report by the American Academy of Ophthalmology. *Ophthalmology.* 2002;109:175-187.
5. Nagy Z, Takacs A, Filkorn T, et al. Initial clinical evaluation of an intraocular femtosecond laser in cataract surgery. *J Refract Surg.* 2009;25:1053-1060.
6. Palanker DV, Blumenkranz MS, Andersen D, et al. Femtosecond laser-assisted cataract surgery with integrated optical coherence tomography. *Sci Transl Med.* 2010;2:58-85.
7. Cosar CB, Gonen T, Moray M, et al. Comparison of visual acuity, refractive results and complications of femtosecond laser with mechanical microkeratome in LASIK. *Int J Ophthalmol.* 2013;6(3):350-355.
8. Zhai CB, Tian L, Zhou YH, et al. Comparison of the flaps made by femtosecond laser and automated keratomes for sub-bowman keratomileusis. *Chinese Medical Journal.* 2013;126(13):2440-2444.
9. Juhasz E, Filkorn T, Kranitz K, et al. Analysis of planned and postoperatively measured flap thickness after LASIK procedures using the LenSx multifunctional femtosesond laser system. Pending.
10. Nagy ZZ, Juhász E, Kránitz K, et al. Evaluation of induced corneal higher order aberrations after femto-LASIK performed by a multifunctional femtosecond laser and photorefractive keratectomy. Pending.
11. Prospective, single-center clinical trial of subjects scheduled to undergo LASIK surgery requiring an initial corneal flap. Verified March 2012 by Alcon LenSx Inc. ClinicalTrials.gov Identifier: NCT01556893.
12. Stahl JE, Durrie DS, Schwendeman FJ, et al. Anterior segment OCT analysis of thin IntraLase femtosecond flaps. *J Refract Surg.* 2007;23(6):555-558.
13. Gatinel D, Saad A, Guilbert E, Rouger H. Unilateral rainbow glare after uncomplicated femto-LASIK using the FS-200 femtosecond laser. *J Refract Surg.* 2013;29(7):498-501.
14. Juhasz E, Kránitz K, Sándor GL, Gyenes A, Toth G, Nagy ZZ. Wavefront properties of the anterior and posterior corneal surface. *Cornea.* 2014;33(2):172-176.
15. Joung Lee M, Mok Lee S, Ju Lee H, et al. The changes of posterior corneal surface and high-order aberrations after refractive surgery in moderate myopia. *Korean J Ophthalmol.* 2007;21:131-136.

SECTION II

Classic Papers

Initial Clinical Evaluation of an Intraocular Femtosecond Laser in Cataract Surgery

Zoltan Nagy, MD; Agnes Takacs, MD; Tamas Filkorn, MD; Melvin Sarayba, MD

Abstract

PURPOSE: To evaluate femtosecond laser lens fragmentation and anterior capsulotomy in cataract surgery.

METHODS: Anterior capsulotomy and phacofragmentation procedures performed with an intraocular femtosecond laser (LenSx Lasers Inc) were initially evaluated in ex vivo porcine eyes. These procedures were then performed in an initial series of nine patients undergoing cataract surgery. In addition to standard intraoperative assessments (including capsulotomy diameter accuracy and reproducibility), optical coherence tomography was used to evaluate human procedures.

RESULTS: For an intended 5-mm capsulorrhexis in porcine eyes, average achieved diameters were 5.88±0.73 mm using a standard manual technique and 5.02±0.04 mm using the femtosecond laser. Scanning electron microscopy revealed equally smooth cut edges of the capsulotomy with the femtosecond laser and manual technique. Compared to control porcine eyes, femtosecond laser phacofragmentation resulted in a 43% reduction in phacoemulsification power and a 51% decrease in phacoemulsification time. In a small series of human clinical procedures, femtosecond laser capsulotomies and phacofragmentation demonstrated similarly high levels of accuracy and effectiveness, with no operative complications.

CONCLUSIONS: Initial results with an intraocular femtosecond laser demonstrate higher precision of capsulorrhexis and reduced phacoemulsification power in porcine and human eyes. [*J Refract Surg*. 2009;25:1053-1060.] doi:10.3928/1081597X-20091117-04

Originally published in Journal of Refractive Surgery, *December 2009.*

Cataract surgery with intraocular lens (IOL) implantation is the most common ophthalmic surgical procedure worldwide. It is also the most common surgery that corrects refractive error, performed over five times more frequently than corneal refractive surgery.[1] Phacoemulsification is the dominant form of cataract surgery in developed countries, accounting for >90% of procedures.[2,3] Although a number of recent developments have occurred in IOL technology, the basic phacoemulsification procedure has remained largely unchanged over the past 20 years, involving a series of individual steps including corneal incision creation, capsulorrhexis, and phacofragmentation.

Although highly successful, each of these manual steps presents an opportunity for improvement in both safety and effectiveness. For example, manual capsulorrhexis results in capsular tears in approximately 1% of cases and has limited diameter predictability, which can affect IOL centration, postoperative anterior chamber depth, and posterior capsular opacification rates.[4-7] The surgical challenges posed by nuclear chopping techniques have hindered widespread adoption, despite evidence that they reduce ultrasound requirements relative to traditional phacoemulsification.[2,8]

Femtosecond lasers represent an important technological advance in ophthalmic surgery. Combined with computer-controlled optical delivery systems, femtosecond lasers can produce precise surgical incisions without collateral damage to surrounding tissues.[9-13] Since 2001, several femtosecond laser systems have been introduced clinically and more than 2 million ophthalmic procedures have been performed with femtosecond lasers, primarily for creation of a corneal flap in LASIK. The precision of femtosecond lasers exceeds that of highly sophisticated mechanical devices, with fewer likely collateral tissue effects.[14]

Nagy ZZ, ed. *Femtosecond Laser-Assisted Cataract Surgery: Facts and Results* (pp 75-82).

We evaluated a novel intraocular femtosecond laser to perform key steps of the traditional cataract procedure, including capsulotomy and lens fragmentation. Initial procedures were performed in ex vivo porcine eyes, with subsequent demonstration in human patients.

By improving the accuracy of the cataract procedure, this technology has the potential to reduce complications and improve visual outcomes.

Patients and Methods

Ex Vivo Porcine Eyes

Capsulotomy Procedures and Diameter Measurements. The accuracy and reproducibility of femtosecond laser capsulotomy diameters was first compared to those of manual continuous curvilinear capsulorrhexis, with each procedure performed by an experienced cataract surgeon (M.S.) in a series of five ex vivo porcine eyes with an intended 5-mm diameter.

The LenSx laser system (LenSx Lasers Inc, Aliso Viejo, Calif) uses a curved contact lens to applanate the cornea. The location of the crystalline lens surface is determined following applanation using proprietary optical methodology. A 5-mm diameter capsulotomy procedure was performed by scanning a cylindrical pattern starting at least 100 µm below the anterior capsule and ending at least 100 µm above the capsule. Proprietary energy and spot separation parameters, which had been optimized in previous studies, were used for all laser procedures. Following the laser procedure, a corneal incision was created and the cut capsule was removed with forceps under a standard ophthalmic operating microscope.

For manual capsulorrhexis procedures, a round corneal marker was initially used to aid the surgeon in creating the correct size and shape capsulorrhexis. The porcine eye negligibly magnifies images at the pupillary plane (approximately 1.06×) due to its flat keratometry and shallow anterior chamber.[15-17] For this reason, a 5-mm corneal marker was used to guide the planned 5-mm capsulorrhexis. Continuous curvilinear capsulorrhexis was performed with the aid of a standard ophthalmic operating microscope and a cystotome. After creation of the capsulotomy by each method, the cornea was excised and the diameter of the capsular aperture was measured directly using digital calipers (Mitutoyo Corp, Aurora, Ill).

Scanning Electron Microscopy (SEM). The capsular edge morphology of standard capsulorrhexis and femtosecond laser capsulotomy procedures was also compared by SEM. Five procedures were performed with each device as described above, after which, the majority of the anterior lens capsule (inclusive of the capsulotomy) was carefully excised with scissors. This anterior lens capsule specimen was then fixed in Karnovsky Fixative (2% paraformaldehyde/2.5% glutaraldehyde in 0.1 M phosphate buffer). Samples were then subjected to successive dehydration steps and prepared for SEM.

Capsular Edge Strength. To compare capsular edge strength following femtosecond laser capsulotomy and manual capsulorrhexis, the diameter at which rupture occurred was determined for each procedure.[18] Following capsulotomy creation by each method as described above, the lens material was removed using an irrigation/aspiration device (Legacy 2000; Alcon Laboratories Inc, Ft Worth, Tex) in a series of porcine eyes. Castroviejo caliper (Rhein Medical, St Petersburg, Fla) with rounded tips was then introduced into the capsular aperture and the unstretched diameter recorded. Because the capsule aperture created by manual capsulorrhexis was not uniformly circular, the average of x- and y-diameters was used for this analysis. The tips were then slowly opened to stretch the capsular tissue. The diameter at which the capsule edge ruptured was then recorded and the circumference stretching ratio (R) between the stretched and unstretched circumference was computed. Analysis was performed with a minimum of eight eyes for each group, with a planned 5-mm central, anterior capsulotomy aperture.

Lens Fragmentation. Porcine eyes from animals at least 5 years of age were used to compare ultrasonic time and power requirements between traditional divide-and-conquer phacoemulsification methods and phacofragmentation using laser segmentation of the lens nucleus. The lens nucleus in the eyes from these older animals is consistently dense, requiring ultrasound power for complete lens removal. In the first group of eyes (n=12, manual group), grooves were created with an Alcon Legacy 2000 in perpendicular meridians. The lens was then divided into quarters and removed with a combination of phacoemulsification and irrigation/aspiration. In the second group of eyes (n=12, femtosecond group), the lens was subjected to a cross-pattern femtosecond laser treatment to create four equal segments. The laser pattern consists of two ellipsoidal planes (6 mm in length) that intersect at the center at depths starting 1000 µm above the posterior capsule and continuing anteriorly, to less than 1000 µm below the anterior capsule. Proprietary energy and spot separation parameters, which had been optimized in previous studies, were used for all laser procedures. Following introduction of the phacoemulsification probe, the fragmented lens quadrants were removed with a combination of phacoemulsification and irrigation/aspiration, with ultrasonic power and time recorded for each sample.

TABLE 1
BASELINE CHARACTERISTICS OF NINE EYES THAT UNDERWENT FEMTOSECOND LASER CATARACT SURGERY

	Mean±SD	*Median*	*Range*
Spherical equivalent refraction (D)	−0.30±2.60	0.0	−4.70 to 2.50
Axial length (mm)	23.6±1.1	23.5	22.3 to 26.1
Central corneal thickness (μm)	534±30.2	535	491 to 593
Anterior chamber depth (mm)	3.4±0.5	3.5	2.6 to 4.0
Lens thickness (mm)	4.2±0.4	4.3	3.4 to 4.7
Nuclear density	1.7±0.3	1.5	1.5 to 2.0

In Vivo Human Studies

The study was conducted in compliance with the Declaration of Helsinki, as well as with applicable country and local requirements regarding ethics committee/institutional review boards, informed consent, and other statutes or regulations regarding protection of the rights and welfare of human subjects participating in biomedical research.

The objective of this study was to evaluate the ability of the intraocular femtosecond laser to successfully perform an anterior capsulotomy and phacofragmentation during cataract surgery. Nine eyes of nine patients (four men, five women) scheduled to undergo cataract/IOL surgery were enrolled in this preliminary study following preoperative screening for eligibility and informed consent. Patients with active ocular disease, poorly dilated pupils, previous ocular surgery, or known zonular weakness were excluded from the study. Mean patient age was 61 years (range: 48 to 77 years). Preoperative refractive data, axial length, corneal thickness, anterior chamber depth, lens thickness, and lens density (0=very soft, 1=semi-soft, 2=medium, 3=hard, 4=very hard) are shown in Table 1.

After pupillary dilation (1 drop of tropicamide 0.5% every 15 minutes × 3) and instillation of topical anesthesia (proparacaine HCl 0.5%) or retrobulbar anesthesia (using 1.5 to 2.0 cc of 2% lidocaine and 0.5% marcaine 50/50 mixture), the following nine procedure combinations were performed: lens fragmentation only (n=3), anterior capsulotomy only (n=3), and combined lens fragmentation and anterior capsulotomy (n=3). All laser procedures were performed using the LenSx laser system. The lens fragmentation laser pattern consists of two ellipsoidal planes that intersect at the center with the height of the cross-pattern programmed to provide a 1-mm clearance from the posterior and anterior lens surface. The height of the cylindrical pattern to perform capsulotomy was programmed at least 100 μm below and above the anterior capsule, with a diameter setting of 4.5 mm for both patterns. Proprietary energy and spot separation parameters, which had been optimized in previous studies, were used for all laser procedures. After programming, the surgical pattern was centered by the surgeon (Z.N.) in the dilated pupil and initiated using the footswitch, with combined fragmentation and capsulotomy laser procedures performed in approximately 1 minute. Immediately after the laser procedure, patients were evaluated with optical coherence tomography (Visante OCT; Carl Zeiss Meditec, Fremont, Calif) to assess the laser incisions.

The patient was then prepped and draped for surgery, which was performed using standard sterile techniques and instrumentation. Upon removal of the laser-created anterior capsulotomy, the specimen was laid over the cornea and flattened. The diameter was directly measured at two perpendicular axes using a Barraquer caliper (Asico, Westmont, Ill). Standard phacoemulsification was then performed to complete the procedure. In cases where laser phacofragmentation was performed, the nucleus was separated into four pieces using gentle pressure from the phaco probe. For non-lasered lens treatments, a two-section divide-and-conquer nucleofractis technique was performed to allow segmentation into four quadrants and subsequent emulsification. Ultrasound power and time were recorded for each case. Following removal of the lens cortex, an IOL was implanted in the capsular bag.

Patients followed a standardized postoperative regimen consisting of one drop of tobramycin 0.3% and dexamethasone 0.1% ophthalmic suspension four times a day for 7 to 10 days. Postoperatively, patients were seen at the standard intervals following cataract surgery at day 1, 1 week, and 1 month.

TABLE 2

CAPSULOTOMY DIAMETER COMPARISON FOR 5-MM INTENDED CAPSULORRHEXIS IN EX VIVO PORCINE EYES

	Mean±SD (Range) [95% CI]	
Measured Axis	***Manual Capsulorrhexis (n=12)***	***LenSx Femtosecond Laser (n=10)***
X-diameter	5.76±0.72 (4.71 to 6.80) [5.30-6.21]	5.02±0.04 (4.94 to 5.07) [4.99-5.05]
Y-diameter	6.00±0.81 (4.90 to 7.39) [5.48-6.51]	5.02±0.04 (4.94 to 5.07) [4.99-5.05]
Mean diameter	5.88±0.73 (4.88 to 6.83) [5.42-6.34]	5.02±0.04 (4.94 to 5.07) [4.99-5.05]
Mean error (%) (mm)	0.88 (17.6)	0.02 (0.4)

SD = one standard deviation, CI= confidence interval

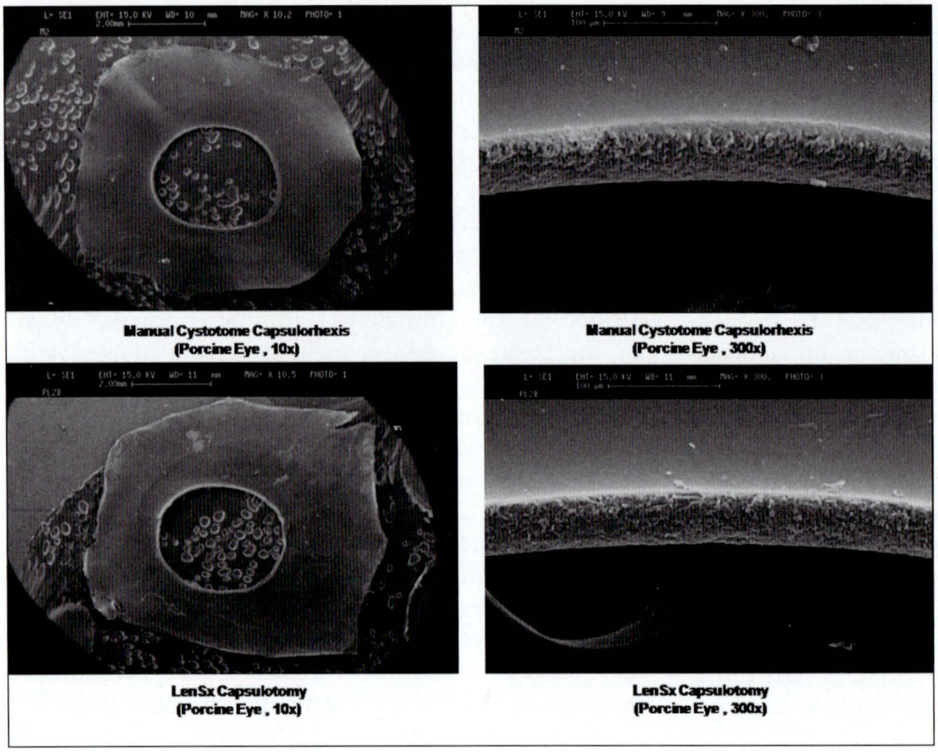

Figure 1. Scanning electron microscopy of capsulotomies in porcine eyes created manually by the surgeon and those created with the LenSx femtosecond laser.

RESULTS

Ex Vivo Porcine Studies

Capsulotomy Diameter Measurements. As shown in Table 2, reproducibility of capsulotomy dimensions created with the LenSx femtosecond laser was significantly higher than that of manual capsulorrhexis ($P<.001$, F-test). This significant difference was found despite physical marking of the desired capsulorrhexis diameter in manual procedures, a step that is generally not performed clinically. Capsulorrhexis produced non-circular capsulotomies, with an average difference of approximately 300 μm between the x- and y- diameters. Capsulotomies created by femtosecond laser were uniformly circular with no measurable difference between the x- and y-diameters. The accuracy of the anterior capsulotomies created with the femtosecond laser was also significantly higher than that for manual capsulorrhexis ($P<.001$).

Scanning Electron Microscopy. Recent studies suggest that edge morphology may predict capsular edge strength and resistance to capsular tears, with smooth regular edges being the most favorable.[18] As seen in Figure 1, which shows representative images of manual capsulorrhexis and LenSx capsulotomies (at 10× and 300× magnifications), the edge features of the laser capsulotomy were at least as smooth as those of the manual capsulorrhexis.

TABLE 3

TISSUE STRETCHING TEST RESULTS IN PORCINE EYES FOR CAPSULE APERTURES CREATED BY MANUAL CAPSULORRHEXIS AND LENSX FEMTOSECOND LASER

Group	Circumference Stretching Ratio (Mean±SD, Range)
Manual capsulorrhexis (n=8)	1.98±0.08 (1.84 to 2.09)
LenSx laser (n=10)	2.13±0.03 (2.07 to 2.17)

Note. More stretching means a stronger capsulorrhexis.

Capsular Edge Strength. Results of the stretching test for both capsulotomy techniques are shown in Table 3. The stretching ratio of capsule apertures created by the LenSx femtosecond laser was greater than that created by manual anterior capsulotomy ($P<.001$), with the values for manual capsulorrhexis similar to those found in other reports.[18]

Phacofragmentation. As seen in Figure 2, average phaco power was reduced 43% ($P<.001$) in eyes undergoing phacofragmentation, with a 51% reduction in effective phaco time ($P<.001$).

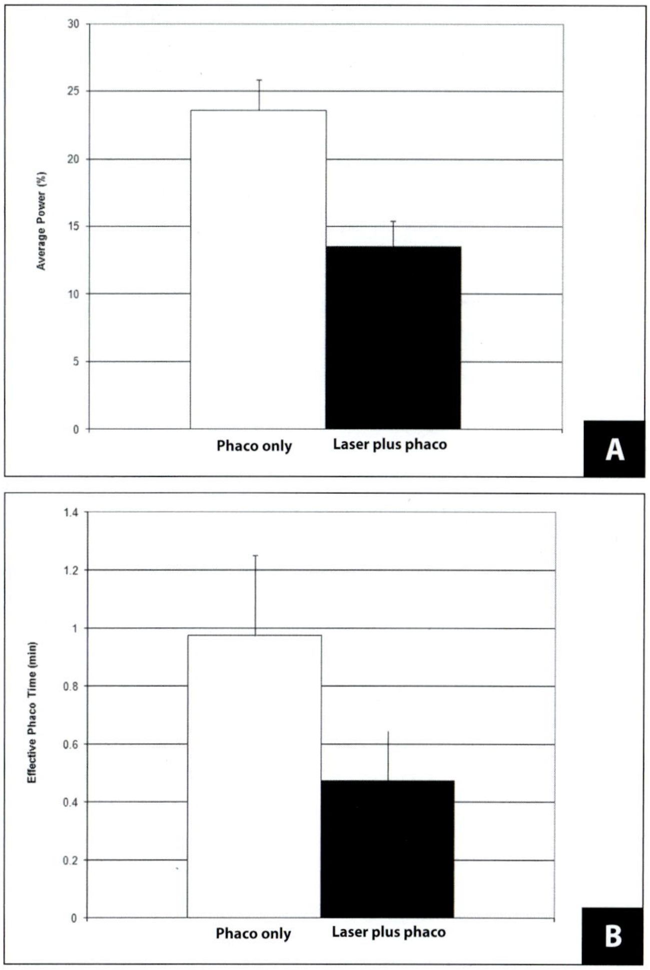

Figure 2. A) Comparison of average phaco power between the two groups of porcine eyes showed a 43% reduction in the eyes pretreated with the LenSx femtosecond laser ($P<.001$). **B)** Comparison of effective phaco time between the two groups of porcine eyes showed a 51% reduction in the eyes pre-treated with the LenSx femtosecond laser ($P<.001$). Error bars indicate one standard deviation.

In Vivo Human Procedures

Capsulotomy Creation. Isolated capsulotomy was performed in three eyes, with an additional three eyes undergoing combined laser capsulotomy and fragmentation procedures. Laser capsulotomy procedures used the same cylindrical pattern as evaluated in porcine eyes. Optical coherence tomography performed immediately after laser treatment revealed a complete cut edge in all scanned meridians, with slight retraction of the cut edge (Fig 3).

The anterior capsulotomy was complete in all eyes and did not require the use of scissors to cut any intact portion. No radial tears were observed after any of the procedures. In all cases, the achieved diameter of the specimen (in both axes) equaled the intended diameter to within the accuracy of the caliper, producing a mean diameter error of 0.0 mm.

Phacofragmentation. Laser procedures were performed in three eyes, with an additional three eyes undergoing combined laser capsulotomy and fragmentation procedures. Laser fragmentation procedures used the same cross-pattern as evaluated in porcine eyes. Optical coherence tomography performed immediately after laser treatment (see Fig 3) demonstrated that the laser fragmentation pattern was effectively delivered, with division of the nucleus into smaller segments easily performed prior to phacoemulsification (Fig 4).

Lens removal was uneventful in all eyes, with successful IOL implantation. The IOL was centered in all study eyes, and no posterior capsule tears were observed. The surgeon determined that all capsulotomies were well-centered based on visual inspection with the operating microscope. Lenses that received laser fragmentation were easily divided into segments, with decreased phaco power/time requirements to complete the lens removal than eyes not undergoing laser phacofragmentation.

Postoperative Slit-lamp Findings. Trace to mild corneal edema was observed in seven of the nine study eyes at day 1, consistent with standard procedures performed by the same surgeon. In each of these cases, edema was completely resolved at 1-week follow-up. No corneal abrasions were observed following the laser procedure or during postoperative follow-up.

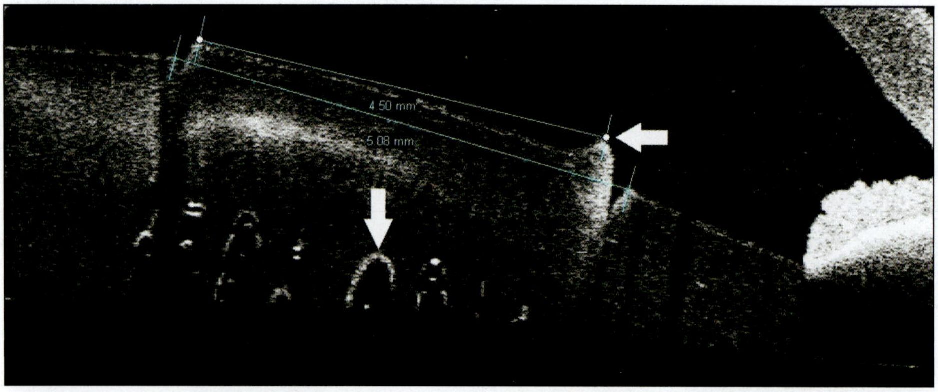

Figure 3. Optical coherence tomography of an eye immediately following femtosecond laser capsulotomy and phacofragmentation with the LenSx laser. Intralenticular bubbles are seen at the nuclear cleavage plane (down arrow). Accurate diameter and complete separation of the anterior capsule without residual adhesion is also shown (left arrow).

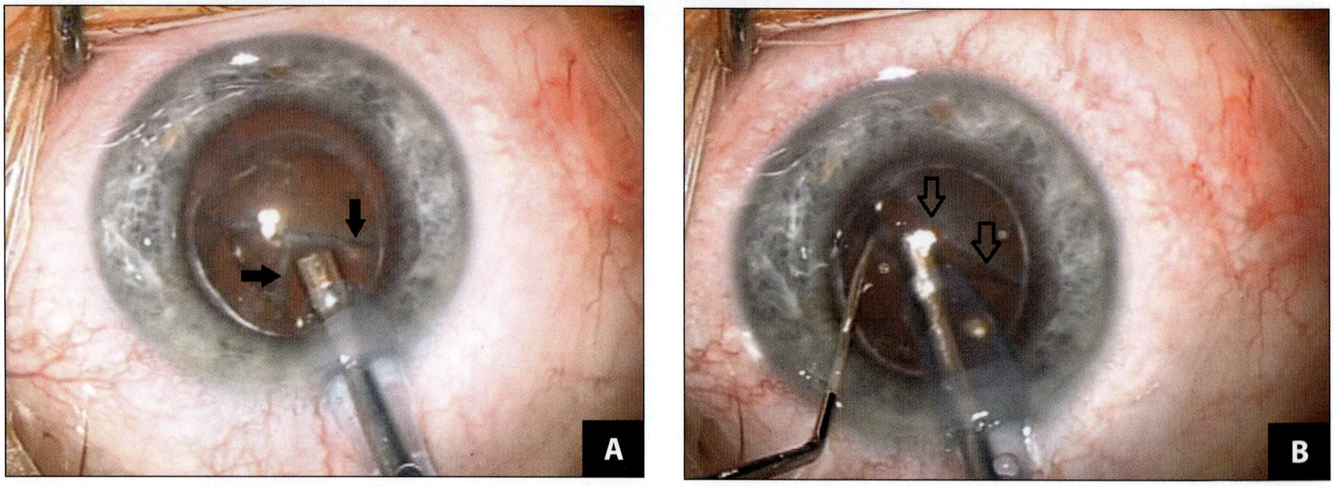

Figure 4. A) Intraoperative image showing the femtosecond laser phacofragmentation X-pattern (arrows) dividing the nucleus into four equal segments. **B)** Spreading of the cut segments demonstrate the straight cleavage (arrows) created by the LenSx femtosecond laser.

Trace anterior chamber cells and flare were present in six eyes at day 1 follow-up. These observations were again consistent with standard procedures performed by the same surgeon, with complete resolution by 1 week in all eyes. Preoperatively and through the course of follow-up, all patients had normal pupil examination, with no evidence of iris damage, atrophy, or transillumination defects observed in any eye during the course of the study.

Postoperative Visual Acuity Results. Visual acuity was measured at baseline and at 1 day, 1 week, and 1 month. Corrected distance visual acuity was 20/40 or better in seven (77.8%) of nine eyes at 1 day and in nine (100%) of nine eyes at 1 week. At 1 month postoperatively, all eyes were 20/20.

Intraocular Pressure (IOP). Mean IOP at baseline for the total population was 13.8 mmHg (range: 10 to 18 mmHg). Mean IOP at 1 day, 1 week, and 1 month was 16.1 mmHg (range: 12 to 19 mmHg), 16.0 mmHg (range: 15 to 18 mmHg), and 14.2 mmHg (range: 11 to 18 mmHg), respectively. None of the eyes had IOP >21 mmHg at any time point.

Complications and Adverse Events. No adverse events or complications occurred during the course of the study.

Discussion

We evaluated the LenSx femtosecond laser for intraocular procedures, including incisions in the lens capsule and fragmentation of the lens nucleus. Laser-created anterior capsulotomies created ex vivo were more uniform, accurate, and predictable than those produced by manual capsulorrhexis. Interestingly, laser capsular edge strength, as indicated by the ratio of maximally stretched to unstretched circumference, was at least as great as that with manual capsulorrhexis. The presented ex vivo studies in porcine eyes also suggest that reductions in phaco power and time may be seen when laser phacofragmentation is performed in conjunction with phacoemulsification.

Initial procedures performed in humans further support the feasibility of the LenSx intraocular femtosecond laser system to enhance the safety and reproducibility of two of the most critical steps in the cataract surgery procedure, anterior capsulotomy and phacofragmentation. In contrast to previous attempts aimed at improving manual capsulorrhexis using physical or virtual calipers,[5,19,20] the precision of laser-created capsular incisions is largely surgeon independent and potentially more flexible in terms of size, shape, and positioning. Although refractive outcome was not the focus of this initial report, the importance of perfectly sized and symmetrically shaped capsulotomy in refractive performance is increasingly being recognized.[5,21,22] In comparison to earlier laser phacofragmentation techniques with Nd:YAG and erbium:YAG laser systems,[23-27] the femtosecond laser procedure can divide the nucleus with low-energy pulses and without the need to physically enter the eye, thereby simplifying the phacoemulsification procedure.

Although additional clinical studies are required to further evaluate the potential clinical advantages and limitations of femtosecond laser technology in cataract surgery, no safety issues were identified in this pilot study. Importantly, the laser wavelength is not absorbed by the cornea. Unlike the large shock and acoustic waves generated by the phacoemulsification device, which can be associated with endothelial cell damage,[28-31] those generated by femtosecond photodisruption dissipate within approximately 100 µm of the targeted lens tissue that is millimeters from the cornea.[9,32-36] Similarly, the maximum retinal fluence from the LenSx is approximately five times less than the multiple shot damage threshold determined by Schumacher et al.[37] These findings are consistent with the safety record established for femtosecond laser corneal surgery in over 2 million procedures over the past decade.

Author Contributions

Study concept and design (Z.N., M.S.); data collection (Z.N., A.T., T.F.); interpretation and analysis of data (M.S.); drafting of the manuscript (Z.N., M.S.); critical revision of the manuscript (A.T., T.F., M.S.)

References

1. 2009 Comprehensive Report on the Global Single-Use Ophthalmic Surgical Product Market. *Market Scope*. August 2009.
2. Leaming DV. Practice styles and preferences of ASCRS members—2003 survey. *J Cataract Refract Surg*. 2004;30:892-900.
3. Leaming DV. Practices styles and preferences of ASCRS members—2001 survey. *J Cataract Refract Surg*. 2002;28:1681-1688.
4. Marques FF, Marques DM, Osher RH, Osher JM. Fate of anterior capsule tears during cataract surgery. *J Cataract Refract Surg*. 2006;32:1638-1642.
5. Dick HB, Peña-Aceves A, Manns A, Krummenauer F. New technology for sizing the continuous curvilinear capsulorhexis: prospective trial. *J Cataract Refract Surg*. 2008;34:1136-1144.
6. Norrby S. Sources of error in intraocular lens power calculation. *J Cataract Refract Surg*. 2008;34:368-376.
7. Hollick EJ, Spalton DJ, Meacock WR. The effect of capsulorhexis on posterior capsular opacification: one-year results of a randomized prospective trial. *Am J Ophthalmol*. 1999;128:271-279.
8. Can I, Takmaz T, Cakici F, Ozgül M. Comparison of Nagahara phaco-chop and stop-and-chop phacoemulsification nucleotomy techniques. *J Cataract Refract Surg*. 2004;30:663-668.
9. Vogel A, Schweiger P, Frieser A, Asiyo MN, Birngruber R. Intraocular Nd:YAG laser surgery: light-tissue interaction, damage range, and reduced collateral effects. *IEEE Journal of Quantum Electronics*. 1990;26:2240-2260.
10. Loesel FH, Niemz MH, Bille JF, Juhasz T. Laser-induced optical breakdown on hard and soft tissues and its dependence on the pulse duration. *IEEE Journal of Quantum Electronics*. 1996;32:1717-1722.
11. Juhasz T, Kastis G, Suárez C, Turi L, Bor Z, Bron WE. Shockwave and cavitation bubble dynamics during photodisruption in ocular media and their dependence on the pulse duration. In: Jacques SL, ed. *Laser-Tissue Interactions VII. Proceedings of SPIE*. 1996;2681:428-436.
12. Kurtz RM, Liu X, Elner VM, Squier JA, Du D, Mourou G. Photodisruption in the human cornea as a function of laser pulse width. *J Cataract Refract Surg*. 1997;13:653-658.
13. Seitz B, Langenbucher A, Homann-Rummelt C, Schlötzer-Schrehardt U, Naumann GO. Nonmechanical posterior lamellar keratoplasty using the femtosecond laser (femto-plak) for corneal endothelial decompensation. *Am J Ophthalmol*. 2003;136:769-772.
14. Juhasz T, Loesel FH, Kurtz RM, Horvath C, Bille JF, Mourou G. Corneal refractive surgery with femtosecond lasers. *IEEE Journal of Selected Topics in Quantum Electronics*. 1999;5:902-910.
15. Szczesna DH, Kasprzak HT. The modeling of the influence of a corneal geometry on the pupil image of the human eye. *Optik*. 2006;117:341-347.
16. Holmen JB, Ekesten B, Lundgren B. Anterior chamber depth estimation by Scheimpflug photography. *Acta Ophthalmol Scand*. 2001;79:576-579.
17. Kim YH, Choi JS, Chun HJ, Joo CK. Effect of resection velocity and suction ring on corneal flap formation in laser in situ keratomileusis. *J Cataract Refract Surg*. 1999;25:1448-1455.
18. Trivedi RH, Wilson ME, Bartholomew LR. Extensibility and scanning electron microscopy evaluation of 5 pediatric anterior capsulotomy techniques in a porcine model. *J Cataract Refract Surg*. 2006;32:1206-1213.
19. Wallace RB III. Capsulotomy diameter mark. *J Cataract Refract Surg*. 2003;29:1866-1868.
20. Tassignon MJ, Rozema JJ, Gobin L. Ring-shaped caliper for better anterior capsulorhexis sizing and centration. *J Cataract Refract Surg*. 2006;32:1253-1255.
21. Ohmi S. Decentration associated with asymmetric capsular shrinkage and intraocular lens size. *J Cataract Refract Surg*. 1993;19:640-643.
22. Cekic O, Batman C. The relationship between capsulorhexis size and anterior chamber depth relation. *Ophthalmic Surg Lasers*. 1999;30:185-190.
23. Kanellopoulos AJ, Dodick JM, Brauweiler P, Alzner E. Dodick photolysis for cataract surgery: early experience with the Q-switched neodymium: YAG laser in 100 consecutive patients. *Ophthalmology*. 1999;106:2197-2202.
24. Kanellopoulos AJ; Photolysis Investigative Group. Laser cataract surgery: a prospective clinical evaluation of 1000 consecutive laser cataract procedures using the Dodick photolysis Nd:YAG system. *Ophthalmology*. 2001;108:649-655.
25. Huetz WW, Eckhardt HB. Photolysis using the Dodick-ARC laser system for cataract surgery. *J Cataract Refract Surg*. 2001;27:208-212.

26. Bowman DM, Allen RC. Erbium:YAG laser in cataract extraction. *J Long Term Eff Med Implants.* 2003;13:503-508.

27. Dodick JM, Lally JM, Sperber LT. Lasers in cataract surgery. *Curr Opin Ophthalmol.* 1993;4:107-109.

28. Shin YJ, Nishi Y, Engler C, Kang J, Hashmi S, Jun AS, Gehlbach PL, Chuck RS. The effect of phacoemulsification energy on the redox state of cultured human corneal endothelial cells. *Arch Ophthalmol.* 2009;127:435-441.

29. Murano N, Ishizaki M, Sato S, Fukuda Y, Takahashi H. Corneal endothelial cell damage by free radicals associated with ultrasound oscillation. *Arch Ophthalmol.* 2008;126:816-821.

30. Storr-Paulsen A, Norregaard JC, Ahmed S, Storr-Paulsen T, Pedersen TH. Endothelial cell damage after cataract surgery: divide-and-conquer versus phaco-chop technique. *J Cataract Refract Surg.* 2008;34:996-1000.

31. Richard J, Hoffart L, Chavane F, Ridings B, Conrath J. Corneal endothelial cell loss after cataract extraction by using ultrasound phacoemulsification versus a fluid-based system. *Cornea.* 2008;27:17-21.

32. Hansen WP, Fine S. Melanin granule models for pulse laser induced retinal injury. *Applied Optics.* 1968;7:155-159.

33. Goldman AI, Ham WT Jr, Mueller AH. Ocular damage thresholds and mechanisms for ultrashort pulses of both visible and infrared laser radiation in the rhesus monkey. *Exp Eye Res.* 1977;24:45-56.

34. Cain CP, Toth CA, Noojin GD, Carothers V, Stolarski DJ, Rockwell BA. Thresholds for visible lesions in the primate eye produced by ultrashort near-infrared laser pulses. *Invest Ophthalmol Vis Sci.* 1999;40:2343-2349.

35. Zysset B, Fujimoto FG, Deutsch TF. Time-resolved measurements of picosecond optical breakdown. *Applied Physics B.* 1989;48:139-147.

36. Juhasz T, Kastis GA, Suárez C, Bor Z, Bron WE. Time-resolved observations of shock waves and cavitation bubbles generated by femtosecond laser pulses in corneal tissue and water. *Lasers Surg Med.* 1996;19:23-31.

37. Schumacher S, Sander M, Stolte A, Doepke C, Baumgaertner W, Lubatschowski H. Investigation of possible fs-LASIK induced retinal damage. In: Södergerg PG, Ho A, Manns F, eds. *Ophthalmic Technologies XVI. Proceeding of SPIE.* 2006;6138:61381I-1 to 61381I-9.

Anterior Segment OCT Imaging After Femtosecond Laser Cataract Surgery

Zoltan Z. Nagy, MD, PhD, DSc; Tamás Filkorn, MD; Ágnes I. Takács, MD; Kinga Kránitz, MD; Tibor Juhasz, PhD, DSc; Eric Donnenfeld, MD; Michael C. Knorz, MD; Jorge L. Alio, MD, PhD

Abstract

PURPOSE: To report the anterior segment imaging characteristics after femtosecond laser assisted cataract surgery.

METHODS: Cataract surgery was performed with the LenSx femtosecond laser (Alcon-LenSx Inc., Aliso Viejo, CA) in 40 eyes of 40 patients. The laser was programmed to perform a 4.5-mm capsulorhexis, a cross-pattern fragmentation of the nucleus, a 2.8-mm main incision, and a 1.0-mm side-port incision. The anterior segment was then analyzed using the Visante OCT anterior segment program (Zeiss-Meditec AG, Jena, Germany).

RESULTS: The preoperatively set treatment parameters correlated well with the achieved results. For the capsulorhexis, the femtosecond laser cut was programmed to start 350 µm behind the anterior lens capsule and OCT measured 377 ± 55.3 µm. Nucleus fragmentation was programmed to start 750 µm in front of the posterior capsule and end 550 µm behind the anterior capsule, and OCT measured 794 ± 111 and 568 ± 147 µm, respectively. The diameter of the capsulorhexis measured by OCT was 4.54 ± 0.2 mm, compared to the 4.5 mm programmed.

CONCLUSIONS: Anterior segment OCT imaging was able to detect the tissue changes within the lens after femtosecond laser capsulorhexis and nucleus fragmentation. The measured values correlated well with the planned treatment parameters.

[J Refract Surg 2013;29:110-112.]

Originally published in Journal of Refractive Surgery, *February 2013.*

Femtosecond laser technology has been widely used in recent years, especially in corneal surgery. The first use in corneal flap creation in LASIK was reported in 2003.[1] The technique was first described by Kurtz et al,[2] and later Vogel[3] and Juhasz[4] contributed.

In recent years, femtosecond laser technology has been introduced for cataract surgery.[5-11] We report the results of anterior segment imaging immediately after femtosecond laser treatment of the lens and the cornea during cataract surgery, with special regard to morphological changes observed within the crystalline lens and in the cornea.

Patients and Methods

Forty eyes of 40 patients with cataract were included in this study. Cataract grade was assessed by the Lens Opacities Classification System III (LOCS III) grading system. All eyes were between LOCS 2.0 and 4.0. Exclusion criteria were dilated pupil size less than 6 mm, corneal scars, lens subluxation, previous eye surgery, and very hard (more than LOCS 4.0) or mature cataract.

Patients gave their informed consent to the femtosecond laser procedure and the study was approved by the Ethical Committee of the University (Semmelweis University, Budapest) and the Regional Ethical Committee. Surgery was performed as detailed elsewhere.[7] In brief, all operations were performed under topical anesthesia (proparacaine hydrochloride 0.5%) by the same surgeon (ZZN). The LenSx femtosecond laser system

Nagy ZZ, ed. *Femtosecond Laser-Assisted Cataract Surgery: Facts and Results* (pp 83-85).

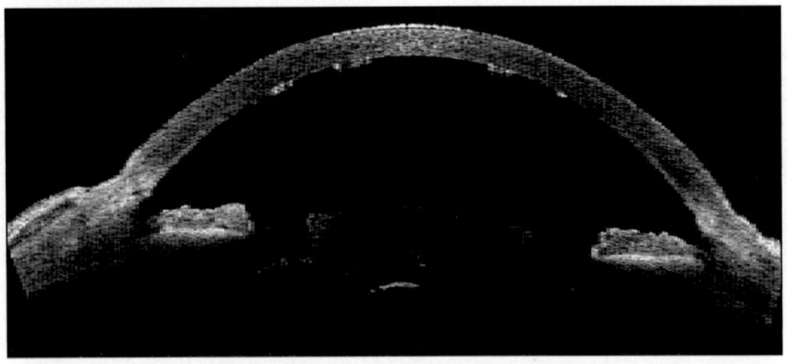

Figure 1. Carbon dioxide bubbles attached to the corneal endothelium (Visante OCT; Zeiss Meditec AG, Jena, Germany).

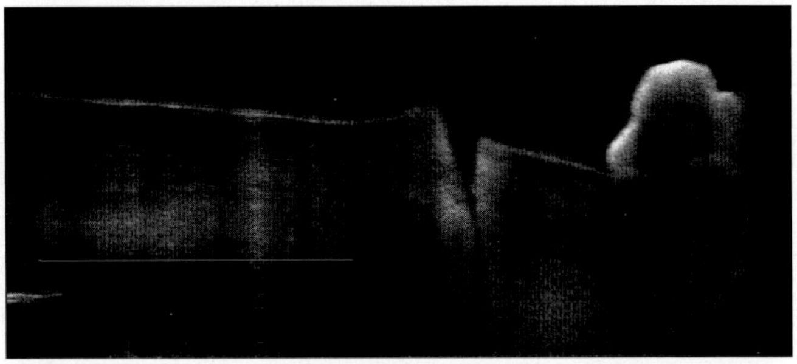

Figure 2. Laser-created continuous curvilinear capsulotomy. In the lower part, the complete capsulorhexis can be seen (Visante OCT; Zeiss Meditec AG, Jena, Germany).

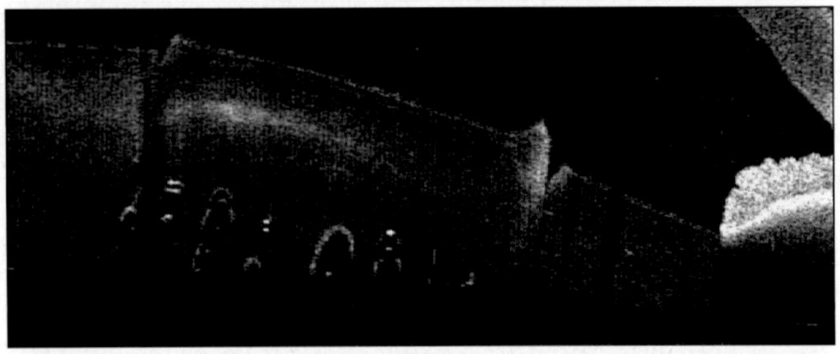

Figure 3. Laser capsulotomy within the anterior capsule (Visante OCT; Zeiss Meditec AG, Jena, Germany).

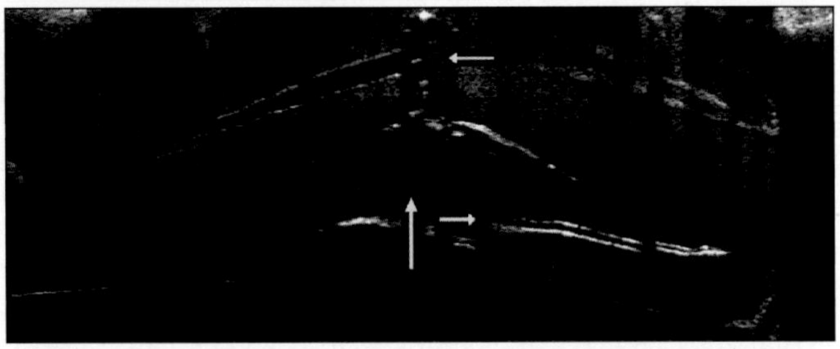

Figure 4. Dissection plane of the femtosecond laser within the lens nucleus (Visante OCT; Zeiss Meditec AG, Jena, Germany).

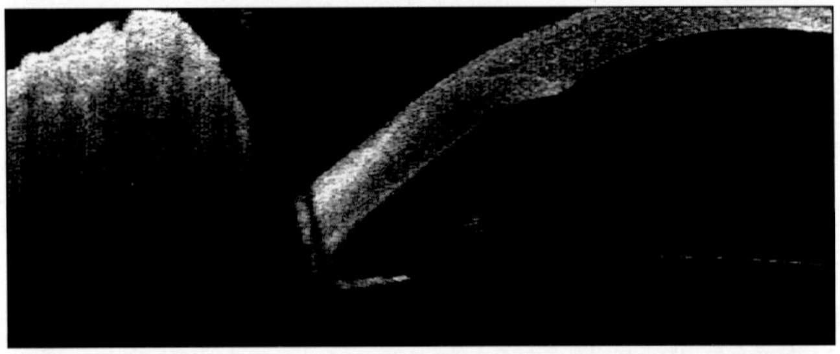

Figure 5. Self-sealing corneal wound created with the femtosecond laser (Visante OCT; Zeiss Meditec AG, Jena, Germany).

(Alcon LenSx Lasers Inc., Aliso Viejo, CA) was used to generate a 4.5-mm capsulotomy, nucleus fragmentation in a cross-pattern with a diameter of 4.5 mm, and two corneal incisions (a 2.8-mm two-plane main incision and a 1.0-mm single-plane side port incision). The capsulotomy laser-cut was programmed to start 350 μm below the anterior lens capsule and end 100 μm above the anterior capsule. The nucleus fragmentation was programmed to start 750 μm in front of the posterior capsule and to end 550 μm behind the anterior capsule.

In all treated eyes, anterior segment imaging was performed using optical coherence tomography (OCT) (Visante OCT; Zeiss Meditec AG, Jena, Germany) immediately after the femtosecond laser procedure. Anterior segment single and high-resolution corneal programs were used for imaging the anterior segment, including the anterior capsule, lens material, and cornea. The Visante software was used to measure the dimensions of the laser-treated area behind the anterior capsule for the capsulorhexis creations, and the distances of the nucleus fragmentation from the anterior and posterior capsule during nucleus fragmentation. The shape and position of the corneal laser incisions were also analyzed.

Results

An intact, round, and complete capsulorhexis was achieved in all eyes. During capsulorhexis creation, carbon dioxide bubbles appeared in the anterior chamber (**Figure 1**).[12] The laser pulses started at a distance of 377 ± 55 μm behind the anterior capsule, as measured with the Visante OCT (**Figure 2**). The diameter of capsulorhexis was 4.54 ± 0.2 mm after femtosecond laser treatment (**Figure 3**).

In all eyes, the cross-pattern fragmentation lines within the lens nucleus were visible in the OCT image. The laser pulses created two vertical planes within the lens, which were perpendicular to each other. In 22 eyes (45%), an additional horizontal plane was formed within the lens (**Figure 4**). This horizontal layer was most likely caused by the carbon dioxide bubbles[12] formed within the nucleus during the laser treatment. The femtosecond laser fragmentation planes extended between 568 ± 147 μm behind the anterior capsule and 794 ± 111 μm from the posterior capsule.

The two corneal incisions (2.8-mm main incision and 1.0-mm side port) were both programmed to be 1.8 mm in length. The measured values (OCT) were similar at 1.84 ± 0.12 mm (**Figure 5**). The planned width of the incisions was 2.8 mm, whereas the postoperative value was 2.71 ± 0.11 mm.

Discussion

To our knowledge, this is the first report on anterior segment imaging immediately after femtosecond laser application for cataract surgery. Femtosecond lasers were first used to produce anterior circular capsulorhexis and phacofragmentation procedures in porcine eyes by Nagy et al.[5]

Initial results demonstrated a higher precision of the laser capsulotomy than a manual capsulorhexis both in porcine eyes[5] and clinically.[6,7]

The femtosecond laser system used in our study uses a built-in OCT to measure the dimensions of the anterior segment, namely the cornea, the anterior and posterior lens capsule, and the nucleus. The laser treatment is planned and performed based on these measurements. In this study, we evaluated the actual treatment location using another anterior segment OCT system immediately after laser treatment and compared the measured values to the planned values. We found that the preoperatively set laser treatment parameters correlated well with the achieved results. This indicates that the built-in OCT system is reliable in measuring the anterior segment and in guiding the laser treatment in laser refractive cataract surgery.

Author Contributions

Study concept and design (JLA, ED, TJ, KK, ZZN); data collection (JLA, TF, ZZN, AIT); analysis and interpretation of data (JLA, TF, MCK, ZZN); drafting of the manuscript (JLA, ZZN); critical revision of the manuscript (JLA, ED, TF, KK, MCK, AIT); statistical expertise (JLA); administrative, technical, or material support (TF, AIT); supervision (JLA, KK)

References

1. Ratkay-Traub I, Ferincz I, Juhasz T, Kurtz RM, Krueger RR. First clinical results with the femtosecond neodymium-glass laser in refractive surgery. *J Refract Surg.* 2003;19(2):94-103.
2. Kurtz RM, Liu X, Elner VM, et al. Plasma mediated ablation in human cornea as a function of laser pulse width. *J Refract Surg.* 1977;13:653-658.
3. Vogel A, Capon MRC, Vogel A, Birngruber R. Intraocular photodisruption with picosecond and nanosecond laser pulses: tissue effects in cornea, lens and retina. *Invest Ophthalmol Vis Sci.* 1994;35(7):3032-3044.
4. Juhasz T, Kastis GA, Suarez G, Bor Z, Bron EW. Time-resolved observations of shock waves and cavitation bubbles generated by femtosecond laser pulses in corneal tissue and water. *Lasers Surg Med.* 1996;19(1):23-31.
5. Nagy ZZ, Takacs A, Filkorn T, Sarayba M. Initial clinical evaluation of an intraocular femtosecond laser in cataract surgery. *J Refract Surg.* 2009;25(12):1053-1060.
6. Nagy ZZ, Kranitz K, Takacs AI, Mihaltz K, Kovacs I, Knorz MC. Comparison of intraocular lens decentration parameters after femtosecond and manual capsulotomies. *J Refract Surg.* 2011;27(8):564-569.
7. Kranitz K, Takacs A, Mihaltz K, Kovacs I, Knorz MC, Nagy ZZ. Femtosecond laser capsulotomy and manual continuous curvilinear capsulorhexis parameters and their effects on intraocular lens centration. *J Refract Surg.* 2011;27(8):558-563
8. Miháltz K, Knorz MC, Alio JL, et al. Internal aberrations and optical quality after femtosecond laser anterior capsulotomy in cataract surgery. *J Refract Surg.* 2011;27(10):711-716.
9. Kránitz K, Takacs A, Miháltz K, Kovács I, Knorz MC, Nagy ZZ. Intraocular femtosecond laser use in traumatic cataracts following penetrating and blunt trauma. *J Refract Surg.* 2012;28(2):151-153.
10. Filkorn T, Kovacs I, Takacs A, Horvath E, Knorz MC, Nagy ZZ. Comparison of IOL power calculation and refractive outcome after laser refractive cataract surgery with a femtosecond laser versus conventional phacoemulsification. *J Refract Surg.* 2012;28(8):540-544.
11. Ecsedy M, Miháltz K, Kovács I, Takacs A, Filkorn T, Nagy ZZ. Effect of femtosecond laser cataract surgery on the macula. *J Refract Surg.* 2011;27(10):717-722.
12. Habib MS, Speaker MG, Schnatter WF. Mass spectrometry analysis of the by-products of intrastromal photorefractive keratectomy. *Ophthalmic Surg Lasers.* 1995;26(5):481-483.

Comparison of Intraocular Lens Decentration Parameters After Femtosecond and Manual Capsulotomies

Zoltán Zsolt Nagy, MD, DSC; Kinga Kránitz, MD; Agnes I. Takacs, MD; Kata Mihâltz, MD; Illés Kovács, MD, PhD; Michael C. Knorz, MD

ABSTRACT

PURPOSE: To evaluate a laser technique and manual technique to perform capsulorrhexis in cataract eyes.

METHODS: Anterior capsulotomy was performed with an intraocular femtosecond laser (LenSx Lasers Inc) in 54 eyes (FS group) and manual continuous curvilinear capsulorrhexis was performed in 57 eyes (CCC group). Circularity and area of capsulotomy and IOL decentration were measured using Photoshop CS4 Extended (Adobe Systems Inc) 1 week after surgery. Average keratometry, axial length, and preoperative anterior chamber depth were examined with the Lenstar LS 900 (Haag-Streit AG).

RESULTS: No statistically significant differences were noted between groups in axial length, preoperative refractive state, and in the area of capsulotomy. Circularity values were significantly better in the FS group (P=.032). We found incomplete overlap of capsulotomies in 28% of eyes in the CCC group and 11% in the FS group (P=.033). Significant correlations were noted between axial length and area of capsulotomy, and between average keratometry and area of the capsulotomy in the CCC group (R=0.278, P=.036; and R=–0.29, P=.033, respectively), but both did not correlate in the FS group (P>.05). In the CCC group, the pupillary area correlated significantly with the area of the capsulotomy (R=0.27, P=.039). Significant correlation was noted between IOL decentration and axial length in the CCC group (R=0.30, P=.026), but there was no correlation in the FS group (P>.05).

CONCLUSIONS: Femtosecond laser capsulorrhexis was more regularly shaped, showed better centration, and showed a better intraocular lens/capsule overlap than manual capsulorrhexis. [*J Refract Surg.* 2011;27(8): 564-569.]

doi:10.3928/1081597X-20110607-01

Originally published in Journal of Refractive Surgery, *August 2011.*

Myopia and cataract are common disorders in the human population. Highly myopic eyes are more likely to develop cataract.[1] Cataract surgery has become a common, safe, and effective intervention performed worldwide.[2] However, surgery in eyes with long axial length is associated with increased risk of intra- and postoperative complications.[3]

Posterior capsular opacification is the most common surgically related cause of reduced vision after cataract surgery. Capsulorrhexis size, centration, and completely overlapping anterior capsule on the optic edge of the intraocular lens (IOL) affect the severity of this disorder. Although new IOL designs have diminished the incidence of posterior capsular opacification, a precise anterior capsulotomy is a crucial step in preventing the migration of lens epithelial cells.[4-6] Complete overlap helps prevent not only posterior capsular opacification but also results in better IOL centration and less myopic shift by maintaining the IOL in the proper position.[7,8]

In recent years, the most commonly applied technique during phacoemulsification is continuous curvilinear capsulorrhexis. Popularized by Gimbel and Neuhann,[9-11] it has several surgical and postoperative advantages, but special attention and surgical expertise are needed to complete it successfully. In highly myopic eyes, the larger size of the eye and pupillary diameter and optical distortion by the cornea may deceive surgeons to prepare a larger capsulorrhexis than intended.[12-14] This makes IOL malpositioning (eg, decentration, tilt, and luxation due to improper fixation in a larger capsular bag) more likely and may cause myopization and an increase in higher order aberrations.[15-17]

Nagy ZZ, ed. *Femtosecond Laser-Assisted Cataract Surgery: Facts and Results* (pp 87-92).

With the advent of femtosecond lasers in cataract surgery, a predictably sized, centered, and shaped anterior capsulotomy became possible through tissue reaction known as photodisruption.[18,19]

In a previous study, we demonstrated that laser capsulorrhexis in animal eyes is superior in precision and predictability to manual capsulorrhexis whereas strength (tear resistance) is the same.[19] The purpose of the current study is to evaluate the difference between standardized femtosecond laser capsulorrhexis and manual capsulorrhexis in both normal cataractous and highly myopic cataractous eyes.

Patients and Methods

Patients

In this study, femtosecond laser capsulotomies were carried out in 54 eyes of 53 patients and manual continuous curvilinear capsulorrhexis was performed in 57 eyes of 52 patients. All patients were examined 1 week after surgery. Each patient underwent complete ophthalmologic evaluation. Patients with previous ocular surgery, trauma, active ocular disease, poorly dilated pupils, or known zonular weakness were excluded from the study. Patient demographics are shown in Table 1.

Using computer randomization, patients and their right/left eyes were randomly selected for femtosecond and manual surgery.

Table 1

Demographic Data of Patients Undergoing Femtosecond Laser Capsulorrhexis and Manual Continuous Curvilinear Capsulorrhexis

Demographic	*FS Group*	*CCC Group*	*P Value**
No. of eyes (patients)	54 (53)	57 (52)	>.05
Mean age (y)	65±13	68±15	>.05
Sex (M:F)	15:39	17:40	>.05

FS = femtosecond, CCC = continuous curvilinear capsulorrhexis
**t test.*

Surgery

All surgeries were performed by the same surgeon (Z.Z.N.). Pupils were dilated with one drop of tropicamide 0.5% every 15 minutes for 45 minutes and topical anesthesia was achieved by the instillation of proparacaine HCl 0.5%.

In the laser capsulorrhexis group (FS group), surgery was started in a laser room outside the operating room, and a 4.5-mm capsulorrhexis was performed using the LenSx femtosecond laser system (LenSx Lasers Inc, Aliso Viejo, California). The eye was fixated with a curved applanator and the exact location of the lens and capsule was determined using optical coherence tomography built into the laser. The capsulotomy procedure was performed by scanning a cylindrical pattern starting at least 100 μm below the anterior capsule and ending at least 100 μm above the capsule. Proprietary energy and spot separation parameters, which had been optimized in previous studies, were used for all capsulotomies.

Following the laser procedure, all patients were brought into the operating room and standard phacoemulsification (Accurus; Alcon Laboratories Inc, Ft Worth, Texas) was performed. A 2.8-mm clear corneal incision was created, viscoelastic (Provisc, Alcon Laboratories Inc) was injected, and the cut capsule was removed with a capsulorrhexis forceps. In the manual capsulorrhexis group (CCC group), continuous curvilinear capsulorrhexis was performed with the aid of a cystotome and a capsulorrhexis forceps. The surgeon aimed for a 4.5-mm capsulorrhexis, but no guides were used during surgery. After hydrodissection, phacoemulsification of the nucleus and aspiration of the residual cortex were performed. A three-piece acrylic IOL was implanted in-the-bag in all eyes (MA60AC, Alcon Laboratories Inc) using the Monarch II injector and a C cartridge (Alcon Laboratories Inc). After IOL implantation, the viscoelastic material was removed from the anterior chamber and the capsular bag by irrigation/aspiration. All incisions were left sutureless. For the first 10 days postoperatively, all patients received a combination of antibiotic and steroid eye drops (Tobradex, Alcon Laboratories Inc).

Measurements

To document capsulotomies and IOL position, digital retroillumination photographs were taken 1 week after surgery with dilated pupils. Photos were imported into Adobe Photoshop CS4 Extended (Adobe Systems Inc, San Jose, California) to measure the area of the capsulorrhexis and its circularity. Circularity is a parameter used to determine the regularity of the shape of the capsulotomy according to the following formula: circularity=4Π (area/perimeter^2). Values of 1.0 indicate a perfect circle.

We also evaluated whether the capsulotomy showed circular overlap over the edge of the IOL optic or if there was only partial overlap. We did not evaluate the extent of the partial overlap, eg, 3 clock hours or 90°.

TABLE 2

COMPARISON OF LENS DECENTRATION PARAMETERS OF FEMTOSECOND LASER CAPSULORRHEXIS VS MANUAL CONTINUOUS CURVILINEAR CAPSULORRHEXIS

Parameter	Median±Quartile Range		P Value*
	FS Group	CCC Group	
Axial length (mm)	23.78±2.46	23.39±3.46	>.05
Refractive state (SE)	−0.75±7.1	−0.75±5.5	>.05
Area of capsulotomy (mm^2)	16.91±1.78	17.78±2.8	>.05
Circularity of capsulotomy	0.86±0.04	0.85±0.03	.032
Complete overlap (%)	89	72	.033
Incomplete overlap (%)	11	28	.033

FS = femtosecond, CCC = continuous curvilinear capsulorrhexis, SE = spherical equivalent refraction
**Mann-Whitney U test.*

Intraocular lens decentration was evaluated according to the method by Becker et al.[20] The previously described method was altered by changing the reference point to the center of the pupil because both the femtosecond and manual capsulotomies were aligned with the pupil center. Adobe Photoshop gives a vector (determined by its length and angle to the horizontal plane) between the pupil center and center of the IOL. The length of the vector shows the total decentration of the IOL in reference to the pupil. To eliminate the effect of mydriatic drops on changing the position of the pupil center, the same amount and type of mydriatic drops were used to dilate the pupils before surgery and before taking the photographs.[21] For evaluating the correlation between axial length and pupillary area, each patient's pupil area was also measured by Adobe Photoshop.

To eliminate the magnification effect of the cornea, the diameter of the implanted IOL (6 mm) was used as a scale to recalculate all of the above mentioned parameters.

Keratometry, axial length, and preoperative anterior chamber depth were measured with the Lenstar LS 900 (Haag-Streit AG, Koeniz, Switzerland). Refractive power of the cornea is influenced by both its anterior and posterior surface; however, to simplify clinical measurements, only the power of the anterior surface was measured.

Statistical Analyses

Statistical analyses were performed with SPSS 16.0 (SPSS Inc, Chicago, Illinois). Departure from normal distribution assumption was tested by the Shapiro-Wilks W test. Patient demographic data show mean and standard deviation due to normal distribution. Descriptive statistics show median and quartile range due to non-normal distribution of data. Correlations between parameters were tested with the Spearman rank correlation test. Statistical analysis was performed by comparing two samples at a time using the Student *t* test and Mann-Whitney U test, depending on the departure from normal distribution.

RESULTS

Patient and Capsulotomy Characteristics

No intra- or postoperative complications were noted. No statistically significant differences between the FS group and CCC group regarding age, sex distribution, axial length, refractive state, and area of capsulotomies were noted. However, circularity values in the FS group were significantly higher than in the CCC group, and the percentage of complete anterior capsule/IOL overlap was significantly higher in the FS group (Table 2).

Overlap Characteristics

The area of all capsulotomies proved to be smaller than the optical zone of the implanted IOL in all eyes. We found incomplete overlap in 28% (16/57 eyes) in the CCC group and 11% (6/54 eyes) in the FS group. The difference between groups was statistically significant (P=.033) (Table 2).

Anatomical Characteristics of Eyes and Associations With Capsulotomy Parameters

A statistically significant correlation was found between axial length and average keratometry values (R=−0.22, P=.018) and between axial length and preoperative anterior chamber depth (R=0.27, P=.007).

According to our data, a statistically significant correlation was also noted between axial length and area of pharmacologically dilated pupil (R=0.19, P=.049) (Fig 1).

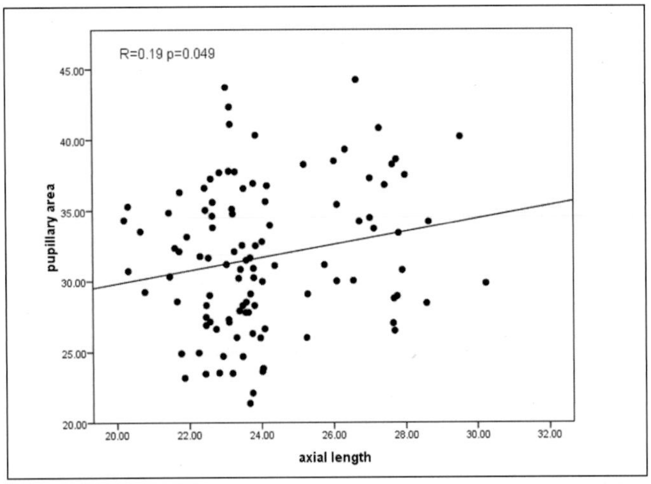

Figure 1. Correlation between axial length and area of dilated pupils (R=0.19; *P*=.049).

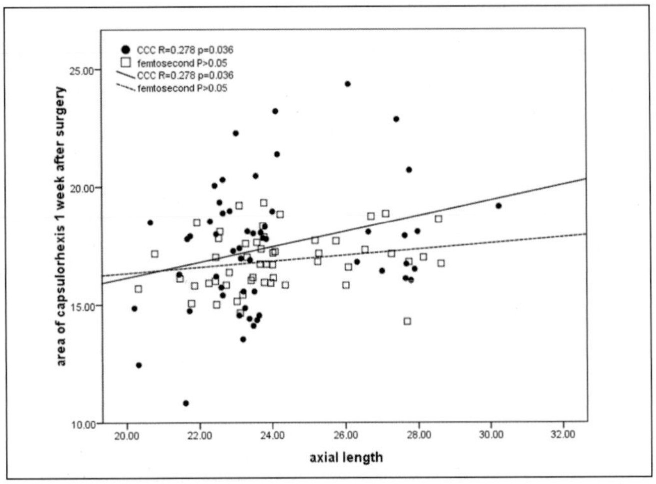

Figure 2. Correlation between axial length and area of capsulorrhexis 1 week after surgery. The correlation was significant in the manual capsulotomy group (CCC) (R=0.278, *P*=.036) but not in the laser capsulotomy group (femtosecond) (*P*>.05).

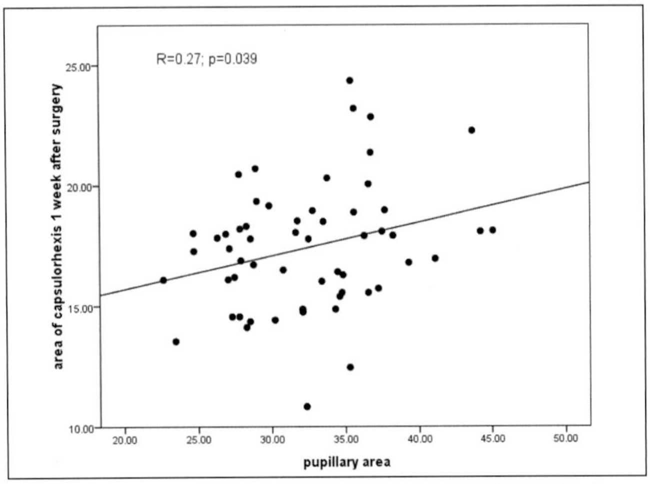

Figure 3. Correlation of pupillary area with area of capsulorrhexis 1 week after surgery in the manual capsulotomy group (R=0.27, *P*=.039).

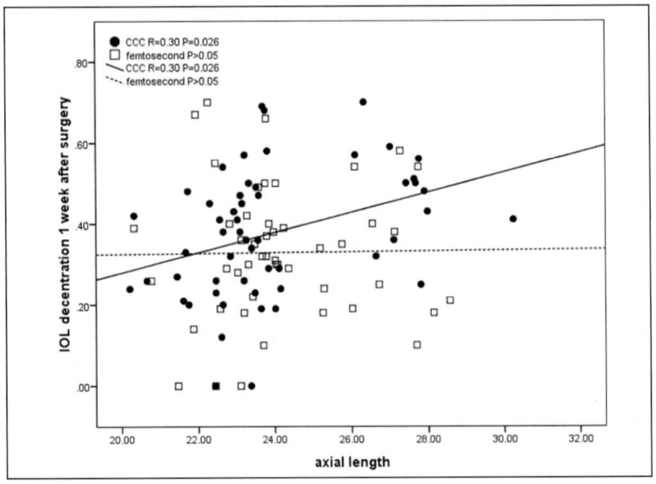

Figure 4. Correlation between axial length and intraocular lens decentration 1 week after surgery. The correlation was significant in the manual capsulotomy group (CCC) (R=0.30, *P*=.026) but not in the laser capsulotomy group (femtosecond) (*P*>.05).

Figure 2 shows significant correlations between axial length and area of capsulorrhexis in the CCC group (R=0.278, *P*=.036), but no statistically significant correlation was noted between these parameters in the FS group (*P*>.05). A statistically significant correlation between the average keratometry value of the cornea and the area of capsulorrhexis (R=−0.29, *P*=.033) in the CCC group was noted. No correlation was found between anterior chamber depth and capsulotomy area in either study group (*P*>.05).

As shown in Figure 3, the pupillary area correlated significantly with the area of capsulorrhexis in the CCC group (R=0.27, *P*=.039).

Values of IOL decentration showed a significant correlation with axial length in the CCC group (R=0.30, *P*=.026), but no statistically significant correlation was noted between IOL decentration and axial length in the FS group (*P*>.05) (Fig 4).

Discussion

The purpose of our study was to investigate the difference between a femtosecond laser capsulotomy and a manual continuous curvilinear capsulorrhexis during cataract surgery. We evaluated capsulotomy size, circularity, IOL centration, and IOL/capsulotomy overlap and correlated these findings to pupillary area, axial length, and average keratometry.

Special anatomical characteristics of myopic eyes make cataract surgery a challenge for experienced surgeons including the creation of a properly sized and centered capsulorrhexis and IOL implantation in the correct position.[14,22-25]

Our results are in accordance with previous reports of the association between axial length and average keratometry values and between axial length and preoperative anterior chamber depth.[22,23] Previous articles reported larger pupillary diameters in myopic eyes under mesopic conditions.[24,25] According to our data, a statistically significant correlation was also noted between axial length and area of pharmacologically dilated pupils (see Fig 1). The cornea magnifies the anterior capsule approximately 1.15 times.[26] This distortion effect varies according to individual anterior segment anatomy. There is no reliable reference marker to aid the surgeon in creating the correct size and shape of continuous curvilinear capsulorrhexis, unless an intraocular device is used. Most commonly, the pupil margin is used as a reference, despite large variation in pupil diameter. Figure 3 shows that even an experienced surgeon tends to prepare larger capsulotomies in eyes with larger pupils.

Another variable that introduces error in capsulotomy sizing is the magnification caused by the cornea. Figure 5 shows how the diameter of the capsulorrhexis varies depending on corneal magnification. Figure 5A represents a myopic eye and Figure 5B a hyperopic eye. The average keratometry value of a flatter myopic cornea seems to virtually compensate larger pupil diameters due to relatively smaller magnification effect. Our results confirm the previously reported fact that axial length is in inverse proportion to average keratometry.[22] According to our results, a statistically significant correlation exists between average keratometry and capsulorrhexis area 1 week after surgery. In addition, the optical effect of the anterior chamber depth on magnification should also be considered. However, we found no correlation between preoperative anterior chamber depth and area of capsulotomy 1 week after surgery. As a consequence of these effects, a manual capsulorrhexis is often larger in myopic eyes. Using a laser, these errors can be eliminated, which is shown by the lack of a correlation between capsulorrhexis and axial length in the laser group (see Fig 2).

Intraocular lens implantation in myopic eyes during conventional cataract surgery may lead to a higher risk of IOL decentration due to larger capsular bag and larger capsulorrhexis.[14] We did not find a correlation between IOL centration and axial length in the laser group, but one was found in the manual capsulotomy group (see Fig 4), which suggests that IOL centration is better after femtosecond laser capsulotomy. This is supported by our finding that an incomplete overlap between anterior capsule and IOL occurred more frequently in the manual capsulotomy group than in the laser group (Table 2).

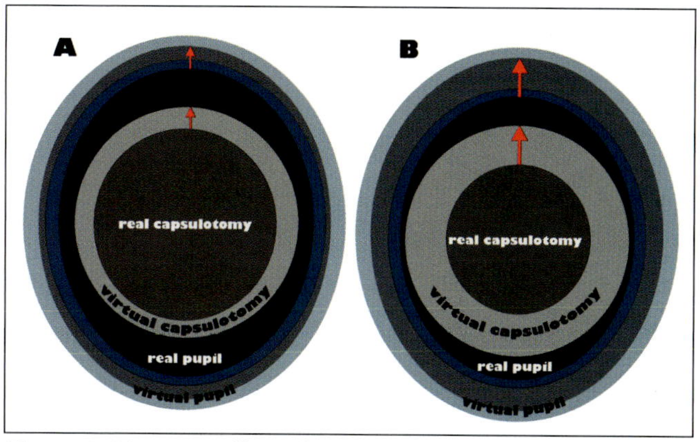

Figure 5. Distortion effect of **A)** myopic and **B)** hyperopic corneas. Red arrows show the magnification effect of the cornea depending on average keratometry values.

A decentered IOL with an incomplete anterior capsule overlap may cause myopization and, more importantly, a higher incidence of posterior capsule opacification due to an incomplete barrier effect; however, longer-follow up is needed to confirm these possibilities.

Our results show that capsulorrhexis performed with a femtosecond laser is more regularly shaped, does not correlate with pupil size and axial length, and results in a better IOL/capsule overlap and better IOL centration than manual capsulorrhexis.

Author Contributions

Study concept and design (Z.Z.N., K.K.); data collection (Z.Z.N., K.K., A.I.T., K.M., I.K.); analysis and interpretation of data (Z.Z.N., K.K., I.K., M.C.K.); drafting of the manuscript (Z.Z.N.); critical revision of the manuscript (K.K., A.I.T., K.M., I.K., M.C.K.); statistical expertise (Z.Z.N., K.K., K.M.); administrative, technical, or material support (Z.Z.N., A.I.T., M.C.K.); supervision (K.K., I.K.)

References

1. Younan C, Mitchell P, Cumming RG, Rochtchina E, Wang JJ. Myopia and incident cataract and cataract surgery: the blue mountains eye study. *Invest Ophthalmol Vis Sci.* 2002;43(12):3625-3632.
2. 2010 Comprehensive report on the global single-use ophthalmic surgical product market. Market Scope, LLC. August 2009. Market Scope website http://dev.market-scope.com/market_reports/2009/08/. Accessed August 19, 2009.
3. Li CY, Chen YC, See LC, Lin KK, Lee JS. Visual outcome after cataract surgery in extremely high axial myopia. *Ann Ophthalmol (Skokie).* 2007;39(1):27-35.

4. Ravalico G, Tognetto D, Palomba M, Busatto P, Baccara F. Capsulorhexis size and posterior capsule opacification. *J Cataract Refract Surg.* 1996;22(1):98-103.

5. Aykan U, Bilge AH, Karadayi K. The effect of capsulorhexis size on development of posterior capsule opacification: small (4.5 to 5.0 mm) versus large (6.0 to 7.0 mm). *Eur J Ophthalmol.* 2003;13(6):541-545.

6. Hollick EJ, Spalton DJ, Meacock WR. The effect of capsulorhexis size on posterior capsular opacification: one-year results of a randomized prospective trial. *Am J Ophthalmol.* 1999;128(3):271-279.

7. Smith SR, Daynes T, Hinckley M, Wallin TR, Olson RJ. The effect of lens edge design versus anterior capsule overlap on posterior capsule opacification. *Am J Ophthalmol.* 2004;138(4):521-526.

8. Cekiç O, Batman C. The relationship between capsulorhexis size and anterior chamber depth relation. *Ophthalmic Surg Lasers.* 1999;30(3):185-190. Erratum in: *Ophthalmic Surg Lasers.* 1999;30(9):714.

9. Neuhann T. Theory and surgical technic of capsulorhexis [German]. *Klin Monbl Augenheilkd.* 1987;190(6):542-545.

10. Gimbel HV, Neuhann T. Development, advantages, and methods of the continuous circular capsulorhexis technique. *J Cataract Refract Surg.* 1990;16(1):31-37.

11. Gimbel HV, Neuhann T. Continuous curvilinear capsulorhexis. *J Cataract Refract Surg.* 1991;17(1):110-111.

12. Tielsch JM, Legro MW, Cassard SD, et al. Risk factors for retinal detachment after cataract surgery. A population-based case-control study. *Ophthalmology.* 1996;103(10):1537-1545.

13. Subramaniam S, Tuft SJ. Early decentration of plate-haptic silicone intraocular lenses. *J Cataract Refract Surg.* 2001;27(2):330-332.

14. Vass C, Menapace R, Schmetterer K, Findl O, Rainer G, Steineck I. Prediction of pseudophakic capsular bag diameter based on biometric variables. *J Cataract Refract Surg.* 1999;25(10):1376-1381.

15. Taketani F, Matuura T, Yukawa E, Hara Y. Influence of intraocular lens tilt and decentration on wavefront aberrations. *J Cataract Refract Surg.* 2004;30(10):2158-2162.

16. Baumeister M, Bühren J, Kohnen T. Tilt and decentration of spherical and aspheric intraocular lenses: effect on higher-order aberrations. *J Cataract Refract Surg.* 2009;35(6):1006-1012.

17. Rohart C, Lemarinel B, Thanh HX, Gatinel D. Ocular aberrations after cataract surgery with hydrophobic and hydrophilic acrylic intraocular lenses: comparative study. *J Cataract Refract Surg.* 2006;32(7):1201-1205.

18. Krueger RR, Kuszak J, Lubatschowski H, Myers RI, Ripken T, Heisterkamp A. First safety study of femtosecond laser photodisruption in animal lenses: tissue morphology and cataractogenesis. *J Cataract Refract Surg.* 2005;31(12):2386-2394.

19. Nagy Z, Takacs A, Filkorn T, Sarayba M. Initial clinical evaluation of an intraocular femtosecond laser in cataract surgery. *J Refract Surg.* 2009;25(12):1053-1060.

20. Becker KA, Auffarth GU, Völcker HE. Measurement method for the determination of rotation and decentration of intraocular lenses [German]. *Ophthalmologe.* 2004;101(6):600-603.

21. Yang Y, Thompson K, Burns SA. Pupil location under mesopic, photopic, and pharmacologically dilated conditions. *Invest Ophthalmol Vis Sci.* 2002;43(7):2508-2512.

22. Sayegh FN. The correlation of corneal refractive power, axial length, and the refractive power of the emmetropizing intraocular lens in cataractous eyes. *Ger J Ophthalmol.* 1996;5(6):328-331.

23. Jivrajka R, Shammas MC, Boenzi T, Swearingen M, Shammas HJ. Variability of axial length, anterior chamber depth, and lens thickness in the cataractous eye. *J Cataract Refract Surg.* 2008;34(2):289-294.

24. Cakmak HB, Cagil N, Simavli H, Duzen B, Simsek S. Refractive error may influence mesopic pupil size. *Curr Eye Res.* 2010;35(2):130-136.

25. Camellin M, Gambino F, Casaro S. Measurement of the spatial shift of the pupil center. *J Cataract Refract Surg.* 2005;31(9):1719-1721.

26. Waltz KL, Rubin ML. Capsulorhexis and corneal magnification. *Arch Ophthalmol.* 1992;110(2):170.

Femtosecond Laser Capsulotomy and Manual Continuous Curvilinear Capsulorrhexis Parameters and Their Effects on Intraocular Lens Centration

Kinga Kránitz, MD; Agnes Takacs, MD; Kata Miháltz, MD; Illés Kovács, MD, PhD; Michael C. Knorz, MD; Zoltán Z. Nagy, MD, DSC

ABSTRACT

PURPOSE: To measure and compare sizing and positioning parameters of femtosecond laser capsulotomy with manual continuous curvilinear capsulorrhexis (CCC).

METHODS: Femtosecond capsulotomies (Alcon-LenSx Lasers Inc) and CCC were carried out in 20 eyes of 20 patients, respectively. Intraocular lens (IOL) decentration, circularity, vertical and horizontal diameters of capsulotomies, and capsule overlap were measured with Adobe Photoshop (Adobe Systems Inc) 1 week, 1 month, and 1 year after surgery. Between-group differences of parameters and predictors of IOL decentration were determined with repeated measures analysis of variance, chi-square test, and logistic regression analyses.

RESULTS: Vertical diameter of CCC was statistically significantly higher in the first week and month. Significantly higher values of capsule overlap over 1 year and circularity in the first week showed more regular femtosecond capsulotomies. Horizontal IOL decentration was statistically significantly higher in the CCC group over 1 year. A significant difference was noted between the two groups in dichotomized horizontal decentration values at 0.4 mm with chi-square test after 1 week and 1 year (P=.035 and P=.016, respectively). In univariable general estimating equation models, type of capsulorrhexis (P<.01) and capsule overlap (P=.002) were significant predictors of horizontal decentration. Vertical diameter showed significant correlation to the overlap in the CCC group (1 week: r=–0.91; 1 month: r=–0.76, P<.01; 1 year: r=–0.62, P<.01), whereas no significant correlation was noted in the femtosecond group (P>.05).

CONCLUSIONS: More precise capsulotomy sizing and centering can be achieved with femtosecond laser. Properly sized, shaped, and centered femtosecond laser capsulotomies resulted in better overlap parameters that help maintain proper positioning of the IOL. [*J Refract Surg.* 2011;27(8):558-563.]
doi:10.3928/1081597X-20110623-03

Originally published in Journal of Refractive Surgery, *August 2011.*

Creation of a precise anterior capsulorrhexis is one of the most important steps of cataract surgery. In recent years, the most commonly used technique during phacoemulsification is continuous curvilinear capsulorrhexis (CCC). Popularized by Gimbel and Neuhann,[1-3] CCC has several surgical and postoperative advantages but its completion takes special attention and surgical expertise. Obtaining a precise capsulorrhexis is essential to reach demanding refractive results because a properly sized and well-centered capsulorrhexis with a 360° overlapping capsular edge prevents optic decentration, tilt, myopic shift, posterior and anterior capsular opacification due to symmetric contractile forces of the capsular bag, and shrink wrap effect.[4-10] However, an eccentric or irregularly shaped capsulorrhexis with a diameter extending beyond the optic edge may lose these advantages.

Until now, capsulorrhexis has been a manual procedure. With the advent of femtosecond lasers in ophthalmic surgery, a predictably sized and centered anterior capsulotomy became possible through a laser–tissue interaction known as photodisruption.[11] Femtosecond lasers were initially developed for LASIK flap creation during corneal refractive surgery. Recently introduced laser technology enables surgeons to achieve efficient lens fragmentation or liquefaction and precise and reproducible creation of capsulotomies and corneal incisions during refractive cataract surgery.[11-14]

The purpose of this study was to measure and compare sizing and positioning parameters of the femtosecond laser capsulotomy with manual CCC during 1-year follow-up. We also studied the effects of these differences on IOL centration. To our knowledge, no such comparisons have been performed previously.

Nagy ZZ, ed. *Femtosecond Laser-Assisted Cataract Surgery: Facts and Results* (pp 93-98).

Patients and Methods

Femtosecond capsulotomies were carried out in 20 eyes of 20 patients and manual CCC was performed in 20 eyes of 20 patients undergoing cataract surgery with IOL implantation. Each patient underwent a complete ophthalmologic evaluation. Patients with previous ocular surgery, trauma, active ocular disease, poorly dilated pupils, or known zonular weakness were excluded from the study.

The study was conducted in compliance with the Declaration of Helsinki, as well as with applicable country and local requirements regarding ethics committee/institutional review boards and other statutes or regulations regarding protection of the rights and welfare of human subjects participating in biomedical research. A written informed consent was obtained prior to surgery from every patient.

Surgery

The surgical technique was standardized in each patient, except for the method of capsulorrhexis. All surgeries were performed by the same surgeon (Z.Z.N.).

After pupillary dilation (1 drop of tropicamide 0.5% every 15 minutes × 3) and instillation of topical anesthetics (proparacaine HCl 0.5%), the femtosecond laser (Alcon-LenSx Lasers Inc, Aliso Viejo, California) was docked to the eye using a curved contact lens to applanate the cornea. The location of the crystalline lens surface was determined with an integrated optical coherence tomography imaging system. A 4.5-mm diameter capsulotomy procedure was performed by scanning a cylindrical pattern starting at least 100 μm below the anterior capsule and ending at least 100 μm above the capsule. Proprietary energy and spot separation parameters, which had been optimized in previous studies, were used for all laser procedures.

Following the laser capsulotomy procedure, a 2.8-mm clear corneal incision was created with the laser. The cut capsule was removed with capsule forceps under a standard ophthalmic operating microscope. A 4.5-mm capsulorrhexis was attempted in the CCC group and was performed with the aid of a cystotome and capsulorrhexis forceps. After hydrodissection, phacoemulsification of the nucleus and aspiration of the residual cortex were performed using the Accurus phacoemulsification machine (Alcon Laboratories Inc, Ft Worth, Texas). All IOLs were folded and implanted in the capsular bag with the aid of an injection cartridge through the corneal wound. All IOLs were three-piece or one-piece spherical lenses of hydrophobic acrylic material. The haptics of the IOL were situated in the same position (at 3 and 9 o'clock). The IOL power was calculated using the SRK/T formula. After IOL implantation, the viscoelastic material was removed from the anterior chamber and capsular bag by irrigation/aspiration. No stromal hydration was needed. All incisions were left sutureless. No intra- or postoperative complications occurred. Within the first 10 days, all patients received a combination of antibiotic and steroid eye drops (dexamethasone and tobramycin).

Measurements

To document capsulotomies, digital retroillumination photographs were taken 1 week, 1 month, and 1 year after surgery. Photographs were imported into Adobe Photoshop (Adobe Systems Inc, San Jose, California) for measuring IOL decentration and the following capsulotomy parameters: vertical and horizontal diameter, circularity, and the shortest and longest distance between the edge of capsulorrhexis and the IOL optic edge (distance min, distance max) along an elongated radius of capsulorrhexis. The diameter of the implanted IOL was used as a scale to eliminate the magnification effect of the cornea (Fig 1).

Intraocular lens decentration was evaluated according to Becker et al.[15] The previously described method was altered by changing the reference point to the center of the pupil, because both the femtosecond capsulotomies and the manual procedures were aligned at the pupil center (Fig 2). To eliminate the effect of mydriatic drops on changing the position of the pupil center, the same amount and type of mydriatic drops were used to dilate patients' pupils before surgery and before taking the photographs.[16]

Adobe Photoshop gives a vector (determined by its length and angle to the horizontal plane) between the pupil center and center of the IOL. The length of the vector shows the total IOL decentration. Horizontal and vertical decentration were calculated using trigonometry analysis. To determine the magnitude of horizontal and vertical decentration without reference to nasal/temporal or up/down orientation, the absolute values of the above-mentioned parameters were counted.

Circularity is a parameter used for determining the regularity of capsulotomy shape according to the following formula: circularity = 4Π (area/perimeter^2). The quotient of the shortest and longest distance between the edge of the capsulorrhexis and the edge of the IOL optic was calculated to determine capsule–IOL overlap (overlap=distance min/distance max). Circularity and overlap values of 1.0 indicate a perfect circle and an absolute regularly overlapping anterior capsule on the optic of the implanted IOL, respectively.

Shifting of the visual axis from the pupil center was determined with a Lenstar biometer (Haag-Streit, Koeniz, Switzerland) in all eyes before and 1 year after cataract surgery.

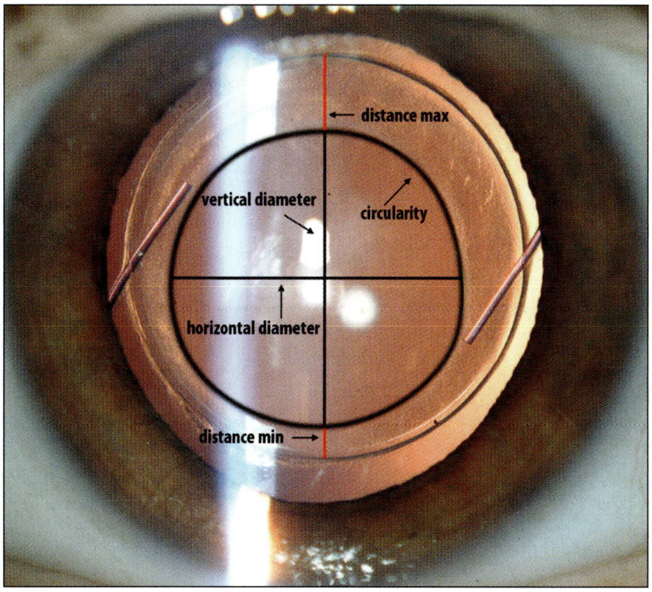

Figure 1. Parameters characteristic to the capsulorrhexis measured by Adobe Photoshop.

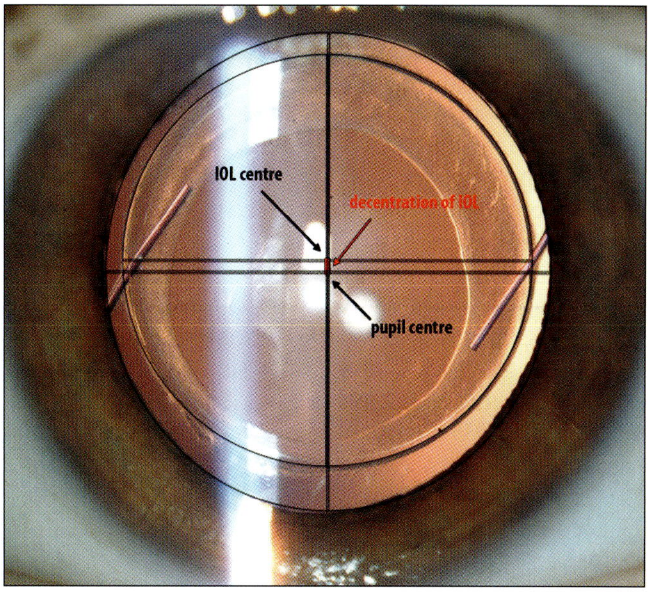

Figure 2. Decentration of the IOL from the pupil center.

Statistical Analyses

Statistical analyses were performed with SPSS 16.0 (SPSS Inc, Chicago, Illinois). Departure from normal distribution assumption was tested by the Shapiro-Wilks W test. Due to normality of data, descriptive statistics show mean and standard deviation.

Differences between the two groups of capsulorrhexis parameters were analyzed using repeated measures analysis of variance (ANOVA) test with Newman-Keuls test.

To determine predictors of IOL decentration, logistic regression analyses were performed via univariable general estimating equation (GEE) models treating data from eyes of patients in statistical analysis as repeated measures. This technique took into account the correlated nature of data from patients who contributed two eyes to the repeated measurements. We dichotomized decentration parameters at the level of 0.4 mm, as previous results showed that <0.4-mm decentration provides the best optical performance whereas >0.4 mm can worsen the visual outcome of aspheric and wavefront-corrected IOLs.[17]

Chi-square test of homogeneity was applied to compare the distribution of dichotomized horizontal decentration values at 0.4 mm between the two study groups.

Correlations between vertical diameter and overlap parameters were analyzed with Spearman rank correlation.

The significance level was set at $P<.05$ in all statistical analyses.

Results

No statistically significant differences were noted between the femtosecond (FS) and CCC groups in regards to age and gender distribution, refractive status, and axial length (Table 1).

Table 2 shows mean and standard deviation values of parameters characteristic to capsulotomies and IOL decentrations in the two study groups measured by Adobe Photoshop. Although capsulotomies were not perfectly round in the postoperative follow-up period in either the CCC or FS group, statistically significant differences were noted between the two groups at the given time point analyzed by repeated measures ANOVA. Vertical diameter was significantly higher 1 week and 1 month after surgery in the CCC group. Statistically significant differences were observed in the shortest and longest distance between the edge of the IOL optic and the edge of the capsulorrhexis 1 week and 1 month after surgery and in circularity 1 week after surgery. Significantly higher values of overlap and circularity showed more regular capsulotomies in the FS group. Horizontal decentration of the IOL was also significantly higher in the CCC group during the first year.

The type of capsulorrhexis was found to be a significant predictor of horizontal decentration in the univariable GEE model (odds ratio [OR]: 5.95, 95% confidence limit [CL]: 1.58-22.22, $P<.01$). When predictors of horizontal IOL decentration were explored, only capsulorrhexis overlap showed a significant effect ($P=.002$) among all capsulorrhexis parameters. Decentration was not influenced by type of implanted IOL according to a GEE model ($P>.05$). No statistically significant differences in total decentration or decentration in horizontal or vertical direction were noted between one-piece and three-piece IOLs according to repeated measurements ANOVA test with Newman-Keuls test ($P>.05$).

The ratios of <0.4 mm and >0.4 mm horizontal decentration values were 4/16, 3/17, and 5/15 eyes in the CCC group 1 week, 1 month, and 1 year after surgery, respectively. Horizontal decentration did not exceed 0.4 mm in any eye in the FS group (0/20 at all time points) (Table 3). Chi-square test of homogeneity was applied to compare the distribution of dichotomized horizontal decentration values at 0.4 mm between the two study groups. A statistically significant difference was found between groups at 1 week and 1 year postoperatively ($P=.035$ and .016, respectively). No statistically significant difference was noted between the FS and CCC group 1 month after surgery ($P>.05$).

According to Figures 3-5, vertical diameter demonstrated a statistically significant correlation to the overlap in the CCC group at all three time points (1 week: $r=-0.91$, $P<.01$; 1 month: $r=-0.76$, $P<.01$; and 1 year: $r=-0.62$, $P<.01$), whereas no significant correlation was noted between the two parameters in the FS group ($P>.05$).

No statistically significant difference was observed in shifting of the visual axis from the pupil center in either absolute value or in horizontal or vertical direction 1 year postoperatively between groups ($P>.05$).

TABLE 1

DEMOGRAPHICS OF PATIENTS WHO UNDERWENT MANUAL CONTINUOUS CURVILINEAR CAPSULORRHEXIS OR FEMTOSECOND LASER CAPSULOTOMY

Demographic	*Manual CCC*	*Femtosecond*	*P Value*
Age (y)	71.69±11.34 (52 to 84)	63.78±13.97 (28 to 86)	>.05
Gender (M:F)	6:14	5:15	>.05
MRSE (D)	−0.99±3.89 (−9.50 to 4.00)	−0.45±3.96 (−11.00 to 6.75)	>.05
Axial length (mm)	23.28±1.76 (20.32 to 27.76)	23.54±1.48 (20.32 to 26.55)	>.05

CCC = continuous curvilinear capsulorrhexis, MRSE = manifest refraction spherical equivalent
Note. Values presented as mean±standard deviation (range).

DISCUSSION

Cataract surgery techniques have undergone continued development since the introduction of phacoemulsification. However, with the advent of premium IOLs, an increasing need appeared for methods that ensure higher precision and predictability in cataract surgery. This is the first study to describe the better centration of IOLs 1 year after cataract surgery when capsulorrhexis was performed with a femtosecond laser.

A properly sized CCC provides several surgical advantages, and initial results with femtosecond laser showed higher precision of capsulorrhexis compared with manual techniques.[11]

Corresponding to previous results where we compared circularity of femtosecond capsulotomies and manually performed capsulorrhexis at 1 week, we observed more

TABLE 2

PARAMETERS OF CAPSULOTOMIES AND INTRAOCULAR DECENTRATIONS IN EYES THAT UNDERWENT CONTINUOUS CURVILINEAR CAPSULORRHEXIS OR FEMTOSECOND LASER CAPSULOTOMY

	1 Week		*1 Month*		*1 Year*	
Parameter	*CCC*	*Femtosecond*	*CCC*	*Femtosecond*	*CCC*	*Femtosecond*
Vertical diameter (mm)	4.79±0.36	4.51±0.11*	4.62±0.34	4.47±0.21*	4.67±0.42	4.54±0.22
Horizontal diameter (mm)	4.60±0.47	4.60±0.18	4.64±0.31	4.57±0.24	4.69±0.37	4.61±0.31
Circularity	0.83±0.02	0.86±0.01*	0.84±0.03	0.85±0.02	0.85±0.02	0.84±0.03
Distance min (mm)	0.17±0.21	0.42±0.16*	0.26±0.24	0.47±0.19*	0.12±0.18	0.46±0.16*
Distance max (mm)	1.09±0.21	0.95±0.17*	1.12±0.17	0.96±0.23*	1.09±0.14	1.00±0.24
Overlap	0.17±0.19	0.47±0.24*	0.24±0.23	0.53±0.25*	0.13±0.19	0.54±0.31*
Horizontal decentration (mm)	0.28±0.16	0.12±0.11*	0.26±0.14	0.13±0.09*	0.30±0.16	0.15±0.12*
Vertical decentration (mm)	0.18±0.14	0.23±0.17	0.19±0.13	0.19±0.19	0.20±0.10	0.22±0.10

CCC = continuous curvilinear capsulorrhexis
**P<.05 between groups at the given time point using repeated measures analysis of variance.*
Values presented as mean±standard deviation.

TABLE 3

DISTRIBUTION OF HORIZONTAL DECENTRATION VALUES >0.4 MM BETWEEN EYES THAT UNDERWENT MANUAL CONTINUOUS CURVILINEAR CAPSULORRHEXIS AND FEMTOSECOND LASER CAPSULOTOMY

Follow-up	*FS Group*	*CCC Group*	*P Value*
1 week	0/20	4/16	.035*
1 month	0/20	3/17	.072
1 year	0/20	5/15	.016*

FS = femtosecond laser, CCC = continuous curvilinear capsulorrhexis
**P<.05 between groups using Chi-square test.*

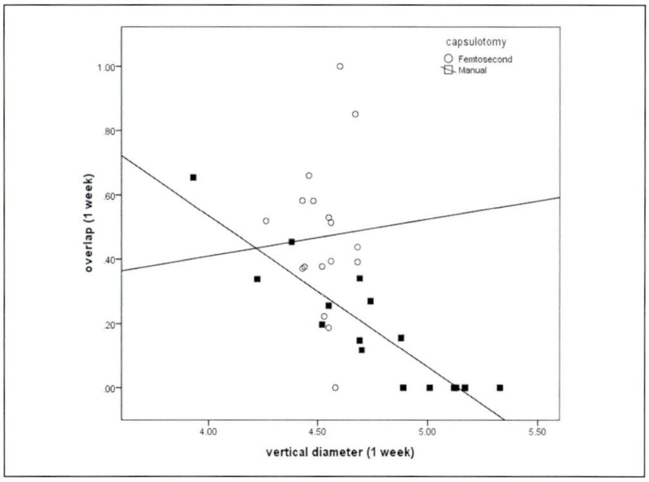

Figure 3. Correlation of vertical diameter to overlap 1 week after surgery. A statistically significant correlation was noted between the two parameters in the manual capsulorrhexis group (r=−0.91, *P*<−.01), but no correlation was found between these parameters in the femtosecond capsulotomy group (r=0.05, *P*>.05).

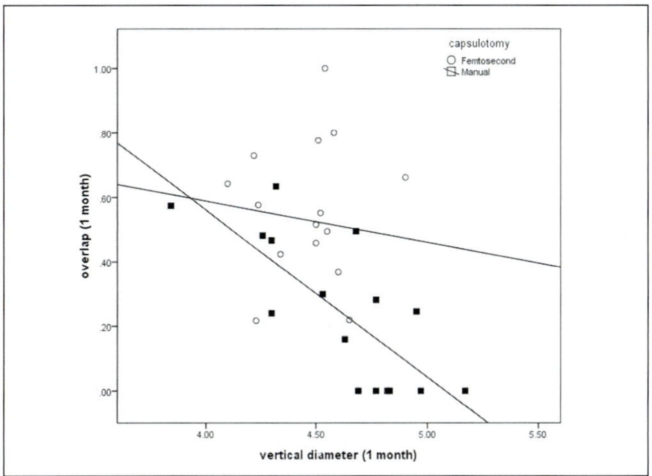

Figure 4. Correlation of vertical diameter to overlap 1 month after surgery. A statistically significant correlation was noted between the two parameters in the manual capsulorrhexis group (r=−0.76, *P*<.01), but no correlation was found between these parameters in the femtosecond capsulotomy group (r=−0.11, *P*>.05).

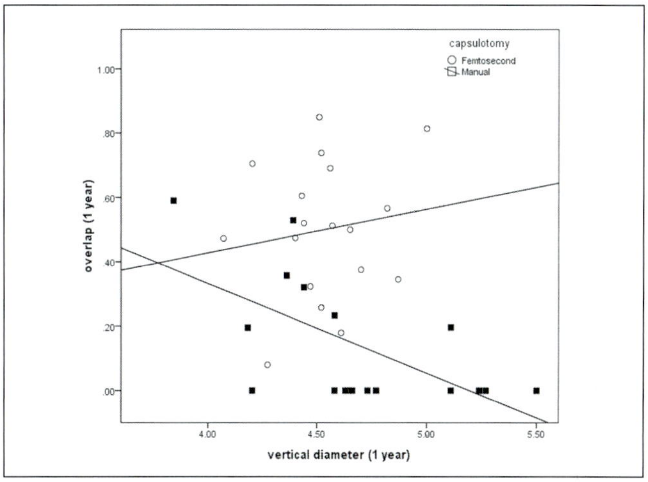

Figure 5. Correlation of vertical diameter to overlap 1 year after surgery. A statistically significant correlation was noted between the two parameters in the manual capsulorrhexis group (r=−0.62, *P*<−.01), but no correlation was found in the femtosecond capsulotomy group (r=0.14, *P*>.05).

regular shape in the FS group.[18] Difference in circularity between the two study groups can be explained by disproportion of vertical and horizontal diameter values in the CCC group. Properly sized, shaped, and centered femtosecond capsulotomies resulted in better overlap parameters during the first year. Worsening irregularity of manual capsulorrhexis through asymmetric contractile and vector forces aggravated the IOL centration over time. In our study, the length of vertical diameter correlated with the overlap of the anterior capsule in the manual capsulorrhexis group. Figures 3-5 demonstrate how higher values of this parameter are able to lead to irregular anterior capsule overlap. A 360° overlapping capsular edge is thought to be an important factor for standardizing refractive results by keeping the IOL in the desired center position. The overlap sets not only the horizontal–vertical but also the anteroposterior positioning of the IOL.[19]

In our study, we examined decentration of implanted IOLs according to a previous report from Becker et al.[15] Decentration >0.4 mm can deteriorate optical outcomes of accommodating and multifocal IOLs.[17] Our results show statistically higher horizontal decentration in the CCC group 1 week and 1 year after IOL implantation and a statistically significant difference in the distribution of dichotomized horizontal decentration values at 0.4 mm between the two study groups 1 week and 1 year after surgery. We found IOL decentration was six times more likely to occur when capsulorrhexis was performed manually. Moreover, it seems that "overlap" captures all characteristics of the capsulorrhexis shape. Among all capsulorrhexis parameters, only overlap showed significant effect on IOL horizontal decentration, representing the importance of precise sizing and centration of capsulotomy. During analysis of the centration results, we were able to statistically exclude the influence of implanted IOL type and larger capsular bag on IOL decentration because no statistically significant differences were found between the two study groups in preoperative refractive status or axial length. No differences in magnitude or direction of visual axis shifting from the pupil center were found between the two study groups that could influence the visual outcome of cataract surgery in relation to IOL decentration.

The limitation of our study is that we did not evaluate the anteroposterior position of the IOL. It would be interesting and important to examine whether the above described effect of regular femtosecond capsulotomies influences anteroposterior positioning and tilting of the IOL over time.

According to the results of our study, potential clinical advantages can be achieved during refractive cataract surgery through effective prevention of optic decentration with precisely controlled shape, size, and centration of capsulotomy with femtosecond laser. However, to present clinical relevance of more predictable postoperative IOL positioning, additional analyses are needed.

Author Contributions

Study concept and design (K.K., K.M., Z.Z.N.); data collection (K.K., A.T., I.K.); analysis and interpretation of data (K.K., I.K., M.C.K., Z.Z.N.); drafting of the manuscript (K.K., I.K.); critical revision of the manuscript (A.T., K.M., I.K., M.C.K., Z.Z.N.); statistical expertise (K.K., K.M.); administrative, technical, or material support (K.K.); supervision (Z.Z.N.)

References

1. Neuhann T. Theory and surgical technic of capsulorhexis [German]. *Klin Monatsbl Augenheilkd.* 1987;190(6):542-545.
2. Gimbel HV, Neuhann T. Development, advantages, and methods of the continuous circular capsulorhexis technique. *J Cataract Refract Surg.* 1990;16(1):31-37.
3. Gimbel HV, Neuhann T. Continuous curvilinear capsulorhexis. *J Cataract Refract Surg.* 1991;17(1):110-111.
4. Ravalico G, Tognetto D, Palomba M, Busatto P, Baccara F. Capsulorhexis size and posterior capsule opacification. *J Cataract Refract Surg.* 1996;22(1):98-103.
5. Aykan U, Bilge AH, Karadayi K. The effect of capsulorhexis size on development of posterior capsule opacification: small (4.5 to 5.0mm) versus large (6.0 to 7.0mm). *Eur J Ophthalmol.* 2003;13(6):541-545.
6. Hollick EJ, Spalton DJ, Meacock WR. The effect of capsulorhexis size on posterior capsular opacification: one-year results of a randomized prospective trial. *Am J Ophthalmol.* 1999;128(3):271-279.
7. Ram J, Pandey SK, Apple DJ, et al. Effect of in-the-bag intraocular lens fixation on the prevention of posterior capsule opacification. *J Cataract Refract Surg.* 2001;27(7):367-370.
8. Chang DF, Dewey S, Tipperman R, Wallace RB. Pearls for sizing the capsulorrhexis. *Cataract & Refractive Surgery Today Europe.* 2008;3(9):40-44.
9. Hayashi K, Hayashi H, Nakao F, Hayashi F. Anterior capsule contraction and intraocular lens decentration and tilt after hydrogel lens implantation. *Br J Ophthalmol.* 2001;85(11):1294-1297.
10. Hayashi H, Hayashi K, Nakao F, Hayashi F. Anterior capsule contraction and intraocular lens dislocation in eyes with pseudoexfoliation syndrome. *Br J Ophthalmol.* 1998;82(12):1429-1432.
11. Nagy Z, Takacs A, Filkorn T, Sarayba M. Initial clinical evaluation of an intraocular femtosecond laser in cataract surgery. *J Refract Surg.* 2009;25(12):1053-1060.
12. Ratkay-Traub I, Ferincz IE, Juhasz T, Kurtz RM, Krueger RR. First clinical results with the femtosecond neodymium-glass laser in refractive surgery. *J Refract Surg.* 2003;19(2):94-103.
13. Nordan LT, Slade SG, Baker RN, Suarez C, Juhasz T, Kurtz R. Femtosecond laser flap creation for laser in situ keratomileusis: six month follow-up of initial U.S. clinical series. *J Refract Surg.* 2003;19(1):8-14.
14. Tran DB, Sarayba MA, Bor Z, et al. Randomized prospective clinical study comparing induced aberrations with IntraLase and Hansatome flap creation in fellow eyes: potential impact on wavefront-guided laser in situ keratomileusis. *J Cataract Refract Surg.* 2005;31(1):97-105.
15. Becker KA, Auffarth GU, Völcker HE. Measurement method for the determination of rotation and decentration of intraocular lenses [German]. *Ophthalmologe.* 2004;101(6):600-603.
16. Yang Y, Thompson K, Burns SA. Pupil location under mesopic, photopic, and pharmacologically dilated conditions. *Invest Ophthalmol Vis Sci.* 2002;43(7):2508-2512.
17. Holladay JT, Piers PA, Koranyi G, van der Mooren M, Norrby NE. A new intraocular lens design to reduce spherical aberration of pseudophakic eyes. *J Refract Surg.* 2002;18(6):683-691.
18. Nagy ZZ, Kránitz K, Takacs AI, Mihaltz K, Kovacs I, Knorz MC. Comparison of IOL decentration parameters after femtosecond and manual capsulotomies. *J Refract Surg.* 2011;27(8):564-569.
19. Cekiç O, Batman C. The relationship between capsulorhexis size and anterior chamber depth relation. *Ophthalmic Surg Lasers.* 1999;30(3):185-190. Erratum in *Ophthalmic Surg Lasers.* 1999;30(9):714.

Intraocular Lens Tilt and Decentration Measured By Scheimpflug Camera Following Manual or Femtosecond Laser–created Continuous Circular Capsulotomy

Kinga Kránitz, MD; Kata Miháltz, MD; Gábor L. Sándor, MD; Agnes Takacs, MD; Michael C. Knorz, MD; Zoltán Z. Nagy, MD, DSC

ABSTRACT

PURPOSE: To compare intraocular lens (IOL) decentration and tilt following a circular capsulotomy created with a femtosecond laser (laser CCC) to a manually performed continuous curvilinear capsulorrhexis (manual CCC).

METHODS: In a prospective, randomized study, a laser CCC (Alcon LenSx Inc) was performed in 20 eyes from 20 patients and a manual CCC was performed in 25 eyes from 25 patients. Intraocular lens decentration and tilt were measured using a Scheimpflug camera (Pentacam, Oculus Optikgeräte GmbH) 1 year after surgery. Uncorrected (UDVA) and corrected distance visual acuity (CDVA) and manifest refraction were also determined postoperatively. Between-group differences of IOL decentration and tilt as well as the correlation between IOL decentration and postoperative refractive changes and between IOL tilt and visual acuity were analyzed.

RESULTS: Horizontal and vertical tilt were significantly higher in the manual CCC group (P=.007 and P<.001, respectively). Lenses implanted after manual CCC showed greater horizontal and total decentration (P=.034 and P=.022, respectively). Significant differences were found in the homogeneity of dichotomized IOL vertical tilt and both horizontal and total decentration distribution (P=.008, P=.036, and P=.017, respectively). Total IOL decentration showed a significant correlation with changes in manifest refraction values between 1 month and 1 year after surgery (R=0.33, P=.032). A significant correlation was noted between IOL vertical tilt and CDVA (R^2=0.17, β=−0.41, 95% confidence limit: −0.69 to −0.13, P=.005).

CONCLUSIONS: Continuous curvilinear capsulorrhexis created with a femtosecond laser resulted in a more stable refractive result and less IOL tilt and decentration than manual CCC. [*J Refract Surg*. 2012;28(4):259-263.]
doi:10.3928/1081597X-20120309-01

Originally published in Journal of Refractive Surgery, *April 2012.*

Microincisional cataract surgery by phacoemulsification and implantation of an artificial intraocular lens (IOL) has become a safe and effective intervention.[1] Due to new surgical techniques and IOL designs, surgically induced astigmatism and complications such as posterior capsular opacification are rare.[2-4] Continuous curvilinear capsulorrhexis (CCC) is one of the most important steps of cataract surgery. Obtaining a "perfect" CCC is important to maintain IOL centration and prevent IOL tilt. An eccentric or irregularly shaped capsulorrhexis with a diameter extending beyond the optic edge loses these advantages.[5-11] Tilt and decentration of an IOL can induce changes in postoperative refraction and decrease image quality due to induced higher order ocular aberrations.[12,13]

With the advent of femtosecond lasers in ophthalmic surgery, a properly sized and centered CCC became possible through a laser–tissue interaction known as photodisruption.[14,15] A reproducibly sized, shaped, and centered femtosecond laser CCC was shown to result in better overlap between capsulorrhexis edge and IOL, which helps maintain proper positioning of the IOL.[16,17]

The effect of IOL tilt and decentration depends greatly on the actual combination of these positioning parameters in an eye. Several laboratory tests have been performed to identify the maximum decentration and tilt that does not impair the visual outcome of aspheric IOLs. Holladay et al[18] calculated the critical amount of decentration to be 0.4 mm and tilt of 5°. Piers et al[19] calculated a greater range of decentration and tilt (0.8 mm and 10°, respectively).

Intraocular lens tilt and decentration can be measured by several methods, such as retroillumination photographs, Purkinje imaging systems, or with a Scheimpflug camera. A Scheimpflug camera provides images of the anterior chamber

Nagy ZZ, ed. *Femtosecond Laser-Assisted Cataract Surgery: Facts and Results* (pp 99-103).

of the eye. Initial Scheimpflug images suffered from geometrical distortion. However, in new systems, images are corrected using custom algorithms, which provide high reproducibility for this device in the measurement of IOL tilt and decetration.[20-22]

We evaluated the use of an intraocular femtosecond laser in performing capsulotomies of the anterior lens capsule. The purpose of this study was to evaluate the effects of laser capsulotomy on centration and anteroposterior displacement of implanted IOLs and to compare results with those achieved with manually performed CCC.

PATIENTS AND METHODS

Patient Population

In a prospective, randomized study, a laser CCC (Alcon LenSx Inc, Aliso Viejo, California) was performed in 20 eyes from 20 patients and a manual CCC was performed in 25 eyes from 25 patients undergoing cataract surgery with IOL implantation (Table 1). Each patient had undergone a complete ophthalmologic evaluation. Patients with previous ocular surgery, trauma, active ocular disease, poorly dilated pupils, or known zonular weakness were excluded from the study. Randomization was done using computer-generated tables (Microsoft Excel; Microsoft Corp, Redmond, Washington).

The study was conducted in compliance with the Declaration of Helsinki, as well as with applicable country and local requirements regarding ethics committee/ institutional review boards and other statutes or regulations regarding protection of the rights and welfare of human subjects participating in biomedical research. A written informed consent was obtained prior to surgery from every patient.

Surgical Technique

The surgical technique was standardized in each patient, except for the method of capsulorrhexis. All surgeries were performed by the same surgeon (Z.Z.N.). After pupillary dilation (1 drop of tropicamide 0.5% every 15 minutes ×3) and instillation of topical anesthetics (proparacaine HCl 0.5%), the laser was docked to the eye using a curved contact lens to applanate the cornea. The location of the crystalline lens surface was determined with an integrated optical coherence tomography (OCT, Alcon LenSx Inc) imaging system. A 4.5-mm diameter capsulotomy procedure was performed by scanning a cylindrical pattern starting at least 100 μm below the anterior capsule and ending at least 100 μm above the capsule. The capsulotomy was centered on the dilated pupil. Proprietary energy and spot separation parameters, which had been optimized in previous studies, were used for all laser procedures. A 4.5-mm capsulorrhexis, also centered on the dilated pupil, was attempted in the manual CCC group and performed with the aid of a cystotome and capsulorrhexis forceps. A marker was not used. Incisions were done with a disposable keratome (Alcon Laboratories Inc, Ft Worth, Texas) in both groups. After hydrodissection, phacoemulsification of the nucleus and aspiration of the residual cortex was performed using the Accurus phacoemulsification machine (Alcon Laboratories Inc).

All IOLs were folded and implanted in the capsular bag with the aid of an injection cartridge through the corneal wound. Intraocular lenses were all one-piece (SA60AT, Alcon Laboratories Inc) of hydrophobic acrylic material. Lens haptics were placed in the same position (at 3 and 9 o'clock). Intraocular lens power was calculated using the SRK-T formula. After IOL implantation, the viscoelastic material was removed from the anterior chamber and capsular bag by irrigation/aspiration. All incisions were left sutureless. No intra- or postoperative complications occurred. During the first 10 days, all patients received a combination of antibiotic and steroid eye drops (dexamethasone and tobramycin).

Measurements

A Scheimpflug imaging system (Pentacam; Oculus Optikgeräte GmbH, Wetzlar, Germany) was used to evaluate IOL tilt and decentration. Lens decentration and tilt were measured according to de Castro et al[21] as follows: IOL decentration is obtained from the distance between the IOL center and pupillary axis. Positive horizontal coordinates stand for nasal in the right eye and temporal in the left eye. Positive vertical coordinates stand for superior decentrations, and negative for inferior ones. By eliminating positive and negative signs, the magnitude of horizontal and vertical decentration could be determined without reference to nasal/temporal and superior/inferior orientation, respectively. Total decentration, determined by trigonometry analysis, shows the magnitude of the result vector of horizontal and vertical decentration. Regarding IOL tilt, positive tilt around the x-axis indicates that the superior edge of the IOL is moved forward, and vice versa for negative tilt. Positive tilt around the y-axis shows, in the right eye, nasal tilt and indicates that the nasal edge of the IOL is moved backward and vice versa for a negative tilt around the y-axis in right eyes. A positive tilt around the y-axis stands for temporal tilt (nasal edge of the IOL moves forward) in left eyes. By eliminating positive and negative signs, the magnitude of horizontal and vertical tilt could be determined without reference to any orientation.

TABLE 1

AGE AND GENDER DISTRIBUTION AND AXIAL LENGTH IN EYES THAT UNDERWENT FEMTOSECOND LASER AND MANUAL CONTINUOUS CURVILINEAR CAPSULORRHEXIS

	Manual CCC	*Laser CCC*	*P Value**
Age (y)	68.24±10.77	63.55±13.65	>.05
Gender (M:F)	2:23	5:15	>.05
Axial length (mm)	23.92±1.99	23.72±1.99	>.05

CCC = continuous curvilinear capsulorrhexis
**t test for independent samples.*

Postoperative manifest refraction was determined 1 week, 1 month, and 1 year after cataract surgery, and shift in postoperative refraction was calculated.

Statistical Analyses

Statistical analyses were performed with SPSS 16.0 (SPSS Inc, Chicago, Illinois). Departure from normal distribution assumption was tested by the Shapiro-Wilks W test. Due to normality of data, descriptive statistics, visual acuity, and IOL positioning parameters show mean and standard deviation. Differences between the two study groups in visual acuity and IOL tilt and decentration values were tested with *t* test for independent samples.

The chi-square test of homogeneity was applied to compare the distribution of dichotomized tilt and decentration values of 5° and 0.4 mm, respectively, between the study groups. Due to non-normal distribution of values representing spherical equivalent changes postoperatively, correlation between IOL total decentration and spherical equivalent changes was analyzed with Spearman rank correlation. Linear regression analysis was performed to determine correlation between the absolute value of IOL vertical tilt and distance visual acuity using coefficient of determination R^2, regression coefficient β, and the corresponding *P* value. Significance level was set at $P<.05$ in all statistical analyses. Power calculation analysis was also performed, which showed 88% statistical power of our statistical analysis.

RESULTS

No statistically significant differences were noted in age, gender distribution, or axial length between the laser CCC and manual CCC groups (Table 1).

Table 2 shows no significant differences were noted between the two groups in regards to UDVA at any postoperative time point. However, CDVA proved to be significantly better in the laser CCC group 1 month and 1 year after surgery.

TABLE 2

UNCORRECTED AND CORRECTED DISTANCE VISUAL ACUITY IN EYES THAT UNDERWENT FEMTOSECOND LASER AND MANUAL CONTINUOUS CURVILINEAR CAPSULORRHEXIS

	Manual CCC	*Laser CCC*	*P Value*
UDVA (decimal)			
1 week	0.51±0.29	0.59±0.23	>.05
1 month	0.61±0.28	0.69±0.19	>.05
1 year	0.60±0.25	0.63±0.23	>.05
CDVA (decimal)			
1 week	0.77±0.25	0.89±0.17	>.05
1 month	0.84±0.16	0.94±0.11	.031*
1 year	0.92±0.09	0.97±0.06	.038*

CCC = continuous curvilinear capsulorrhexis, UDVA = uncorrected distance visual acuity, CDVA = corrected distance visual acuity
**P<.05 between groups using t test for independent samples.*

Significant differences in centration and tilt were noted between the study groups. Vertical and horizontal tilt was significantly higher in the manual CCC group than in the laser CCC group. Horizontal and total decentration was significantly higher in the manual CCC group as well (Table 3).

Applying the chi-square test of homogeneity to compare the distribution of dichotomized tilt and decentration values (at 5° and 0.4 mm, respectively) between the study groups, a significant difference was found in vertical tilt and horizontal and total decentration (Table 4). A significant correlation was also noted between the absolute value of total decentration and the absolute value of changes in spherical manifest refraction between 1 month and 1 year postoperatively (R=0.33, *P*=.032; Fig). Manifest refraction changes in spherical or cylindrical values did not show a correlation with IOL tilt parameters (*P*>.05).

Linear regression analysis showed significant correlation between IOL vertical tilt and CDVA ($R^2=0.17$, $\beta=-0.41$, 95% confidence limit: −0.69 to −0.13, *P*=.005).

DISCUSSION

In our experience, femtosecond laser capsulotomies are accurate, round, and reproducible, with accurate diameters, whereas manual capsulorrhexis can be irregular in shape and difficult to control in centration.[15-17] A properly sized and centered anterior capsulotomy causes a circular overlap of the IOL optic rim by the anterior capsule and can maintain the correct position of the

TABLE 3

INTRAOCULAR LENS POSITIONING PARAMETERS IN EYES THAT UNDERWENT FEMTOSECOND LASER AND MANUAL CONTINUOUS CURVILINEAR CAPSULORRHEXIS

Parameter	*Manual CCC*	*Laser CCC*	*P Value*
Horizontal tilt (°)	2.75±1.67	1.53±1.08	.007*
Vertical tilt (°)	4.34±2.40	2.15±1.41	<.001*
Horizontal decentration (µm)	270.83±190.85	164.25±113.78	.034*
Vertical decentration (µm)	148.40±101.59	131.00±124.72	>.05
Total decentration (µm)	334.91±169.67	230.27±111.54	.022*

CCC = continuous curvilinear capsulorrhexis
**P<.05 between groups using t test for independent samples.*

TABLE 4

DISTRIBUTION OF INTRAOCULAR LENS TILT >5° AND DECENTRATION VALUES >0.4 MM IN EYES THAT UNDERWENT FEMTOSECOND LASER AND MANUAL CONTINUOUS CURVILINEAR CAPSULORRHEXIS

	Manual CCC	*Laser CCC*	*P Value*
Horizontal tilt (°)	1/25	0/20	>.05
Vertical tilt (°)	10/25	0/20	.008*
Horizontal decentration (mm)	6/25	0/20	.036*
Vertical decentration (mm)	1/25	0/20	>.05
Total decentration (mm)	8/25	0/20	.017*

**P<.05 between groups using chi-square test.*

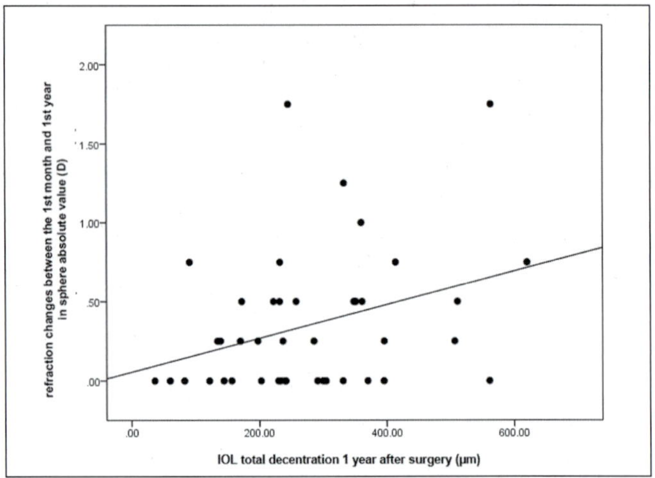

Figure. Correlation between the absolute value of intraocular lens total decentration and the absolute value of changes in manifest refraction spherical equivalent between the first postoperative month and year. Spearman-rank correlation: R=0.33; *P*=.032.

implanted IOL.[16,17] The crystalline lens in young phakic eyes is not perfectly centered and free of tilt. However, comparing the amount and direction of lens decentration and tilt measured by Mester et al[23] and misalignments of IOLs implanted after CCC, malpositions in pseudophakic eyes are more significant.

The ultimate limitation of the potential use of a customized IOL is precision in its positioning. Intraocular lens misalignments worsen visual quality and change the planned postoperative refraction due to induced astigmatism, myopic or hyperopic shift, higher order aberrations, reflections, and halos.[12,24,25]

In our study, we found significant differences in both tilt and decentration between the laser CCC and manual CCC groups 1 year after cataract surgery. The magnitude of both horizontal and vertical tilt was significantly higher in the manual CCC group. More than 5° of tilt can deteriorate visual outcomes of IOLs. Our results show a statistically significant difference in the distribution of dichotomized vertical tilt of ≥5° between the study groups (Table 4). Intraocular lenses in the manual CCC group showed higher horizontal and total decentration than in the laser CCC group. These outcomes correlate well with our previous results.[16] Deviations from the optical axis and pupil center might affect the refractive outcome of IOLs. The effect of IOL tilt and decentration on the final refractive power depends greatly on the actual combination of tilt and decentration in an individual eye. According to our results, IOL decentration influenced the stability of the postoperative manifest refraction. In our study, we found significantly better CDVA, associated with lower vertical tilt, in the laser CCC group. Correlation between these parameters shows that tilt of the IOL from the right anteroposterior position worsens visual quality, supposedly because of induced higher order aberrations that cannot be corrected with spectacles.[25]

A significant difference in axial length was not found between the study groups, which means that a possible difference in capsular bag size is not a likely reason for the larger decentrations observed in the manual CCC group.

In this study, we were able to demonstrate that the use of a femtosecond laser to create an anterior curvilinear capsulotomy results in less IOL decentration and tilt and better CDVA than the use of a manual CCC.

In an ongoing study, we plan to determine how different diameters of femtosecond laser capsulotomies influence postoperative visual performance of premium IOLs by maintaining the optic in the correct position. In the future, unique femtosecond laser caspulotomy diameters will be defined for IOLs with different optical diameters and principles of operation to ensure more standardized surgical procedures.

Author Contributions

Study concept and design (K.K., K.M., Z.Z.N.); data collection (K.M., G.L.S., A.T.); analysis and interpretation of data (K.K., M.C.K.); drafting the manuscript (K.K., Z.Z.N.); critical revision of the manuscript (K.M., G.L.S., A.T., M.C.K.); statistical expertise (K.K.); administrative, technical, or material support (G.L.S., A.T.); supervision (K.M., Z.Z.N.)

References

1. 2009 comprehensive report on the global single-use ophthalmic surgical product market. *Market Scope.* August 2009.
2. Paul T, Braga-Mele R. Bimanual microincisional phacoemulsification: the future of cataract surgery? *Curr Opin Ophthalmol.* 2005;16(1):2-7.
3. Auffarth GU, Rabsilber TM, Kohnen T, Holzer MP. Design and optical principles of multifocal lenses [German]. *Ophthalmologe.* 2008;105(6):522-526.
4. Riederle F, Buchwald HJ, Preissinger C, Lang GK. Refractive aspects of modern cataract surgery [German]. *Klin Monbl Augenheilkd.* 2006;223(12):943-951.
5. Ravalico G, Tognetto D, Palomba M, Busatto P, Baccara F. Capsulorhexis size and posterior capsule opacification. *J Cataract Refract Surg.* 1996;22(1):98-103.
6. Aykan U, Bilge AH, Karadayi K, Akin T. The effect of capsulorhexis size on development of posterior capsule opacification: small (4.5 to 5.0 mm) versus large (6.0 to 7.0 mm). *Eur J Ophthalmol.* 2003;13(6):541-545.
7. Hollick EJ, Spalton DJ, Meacock WR. The effect of capsulorhexis size on posterior capsular opacification: one-year results of a randomized prospective trial. *Am J Ophthalmol.* 1999;128(3):271-279.
8. Ram J, Pandey SK, Apple DJ, et al. Effect of in-the-bag intraocular lens fixation on the prevention of posterior capsule opacification. *J Cataract Refract Surg.* 2001;27(7):1039-1046.
9. Chang DF, Dewey S, Tipperman R, Wallace RB. Pearls for sizing the capsulorrhexis. *Cataract & Refractive Surgery Today Europe.* 2008;3(9):40-44.
10. Hayashi K, Hayashi H, Nakao F, Hayashi F. Anterior capsule contraction and intraocular lens decentration and tilt after hydrogel lens implantation. *Br J Ophthalmol.* 2001;85(11):1294-1297.
11. Hayashi H, Hayashi K, Nakao F, Hayashi F. Anterior capsule contraction and intraocular lens dislocation in eyes with pseudoexfoliation syndrome. *Br J Ophthalmol.* 1998;82(12):1429-1432.
12. Baumeister M, Bühren J, Kohnen T. Tilt and decentration of spherical and aspheric intraocular lenses: effect on higher-order aberrations. *J Cataract Refract Surg.* 2009;35(6):1006-1012.
13. Auran JD, Koester CJ, Donn A. In vivo measurement of posterior chamber intraocular lens decentration and tilt. *Arch Ophthalmol.* 1990;108(1):75-79.
14. Krueger RR, Kuszak J, Lubatschowski H, Myers RI, Ripken T, Heisterkamp A. First safety study of femtosecond laser photodisruption in animal lenses: tissue morphology and cataractogenesis. *J Cataract Refract Surg.* 2005;31(12):2386-2394.
15. Nagy Z, Takacs A, Filkorn T, Sarayba M. Initial clinical evaluation of an intraocular femtosecond laser in cataract surgery. *J Refract Surg.* 2009;25(12):1053-1060.
16. Nagy ZZ, Kránitz K, Takacs AI, Miháltz K, Kovács I, Knorz MC. Comparison of intraocular lens decentration parameters after femtosecond and manual capsulotomies. *J Refract Surg.* 2011;27(8):564-569.
17. Kránitz K, Takacs A, Miháltz K, Kovács I, Knorz MC, Nagy ZZ. Femtosecond laser capsulotomy and manual continuous curvilinear capsulorrhexis parameters and their effects on intraocular lens centration. *J Refract Surg.* 2011;27(8):558-563.
18. Holladay JT, Piers PA, Koranyi G, van der Mooren M, Norrby NE. A new intraocular lens design to reduce spherical aberration of pseudophakic eyes. *J Refract Surg.* 2002;18(6):683-691.
19. Piers PA, Weeber HA, Artal P, Norrby S. Theoretical comparison of aberration-correcting customized and aspheric intraocular lenses. *J Refract Surg.* 2007;23(4):374-384.
20. Becker KA, Auffarth GU, Völcker HE. Measurement method for the determination of rotation and decentration of intraocular lenses [German]. *Ophthalmologe.* 2004;101(6):600-603.
21. de Castro A, Rosales P, Marcos S. Tilt and decentration of intraocular lenses in vivo from Purkinje and Scheimpflug imaging. Validation study. *J Cataract Refract Surg.* 2007;33(3):418-429.
22. Rosales P, De Castro A, Jiménez-Alfaro I, Marcos S. Intraocular lens alignment from Purkinje and Scheimpflug imaging. *Clin Exp Optom.* 2010;93(6):400-408.
23. Mester U, Sauer T, Kaymak H. Decentration and tilt of a single-piece aspheric intraocular lens compared with the lens position in young phakic eyes. *J Cataract Refract Surg.* 2009;35(3):485-490.
24. Eppig T, Scholz K, Löffler A, Messner A, Langenbucher A. Effect of decentration and tilt on the image quality of aspheric intraocular lens designs in a model eye. *J Cataract Refract Surg.* 2009;35(6):1091-1100.
25. Mihaltz K, Knorz MC, Alió JL, et al. Internal aberrations and optical quality after femtosecond laser anterior capsulotomy in cataract surgery. *J Refract Surg.* 2011;27(10):711-716.

Comparison of Long-term Visual Outcome and IOL Position With a Single-optic Accommodating IOL After 5.5- or 6.0-mm Femtosecond Laser Capsulotomy

Andrea Szigeti, MD; Kinga Kránitz, MD; Agnes I. Takacs, MD; Kata Mihältz, MD; Michael C. Knorz, MD; Zoltan Z. Nagy, MD, DSC

ABSTRACT

PURPOSE: To evaluate the long-term visual outcome and intraocular (IOL) position parameters with a single-optic accommodating IOL after 5.5- or 6.0-mm femtosecond laser capsulotomy.

METHODS: This prospective, randomized, pilot study comprised 17 eyes from 11 patients (7 men) with a mean age of 65.82±10.64 years (range: 51 to 79 years). All patients received a Crystalens AT-50AO (Bausch & Lomb) accommodating IOL after femtosecond laser refractive cataract surgery using either a 5.5-mm capsulotomy (5.5-mm group; 9 eyes) or 6.0-mm capsulotomy (6.0-mm group; 8 eyes). Near and distance visual acuities, manifest refraction spherical equivalent (MRSE), and IOL tilt and decentration were evaluated 1 year postoperatively.

RESULTS: No significant differences were noted between groups for postoperative uncorrected distance visual acuity, uncorrected near visual acuity, distance-corrected near visual acuity, and MRSE. Vertical and horizontal tilt were significantly higher in the 6.0-mm group than in the 5.5-mm group (P=.014 and P=.015, respectively). No significant difference was observed between groups regarding IOL decentration.

CONCLUSIONS: A 5.5-mm capsulotomy created with a femtosecond laser is associated with less IOL tilt and therefore may be superior to a 6.0-mm capsulotomy when implanting a single-optic accommodating IOL. [*J Refract Surg*. 2012;28(9):609-613.]

doi:10.3928/1081597X-20120815-04

Originally published in Journal of Refractive Surgery, *September 2012.*

Implantation of accommodating intraocular lenses (IOLs) is an option to treat presbyopia. Accommodating IOLs were designed to avoid optical side effects of multifocal IOLs, eg, decreased contrast sensitivity,[1,2] glare disability, and halos.[3,4]

The mechanism of action of accommodating IOLs remains controversial.[5] The recommended capsulorrhexis size for a single-optic accommodating IOL is 5.5 to 6.0 mm.[6] Until the introduction of femtosecond laser refractive cataract surgery,[7-11] the only way to perform a capsulorrhexis was via a manual procedure. In previous studies using femtosecond laser refractive cataract surgery,[10,11] a precisely sized and centered femtosecond laser capsulorrhexis proved to maintain centration of monofocal IOLs in a stable postoperative position.

The aim of this prospective pilot study was to evaluate long-term outcomes of a single-optic accommodating IOL after femtosecond laser refractive cataract surgery, comparing two different capsulotomy diameters.

PATIENTS AND METHODS

This prospective, randomized, pilot study included 17 eyes from 11 patients (7 men, 4 women) with a mean age of 65.82±10.64 years (range: 51 to 79 years). All patients had a thorough discussion with the surgeon about the risks, benefits, and alternatives of the treatment. The study adhered to the tenets of the Declaration of Helsinki and was approved by the local ethics committee. Inclusion criteria were senile cataract and age 50 years or older. Patients with diabetes, glaucoma, uveitis,

The authors thank Béla Csákány, MD, for preparing the biometries.

Nagy ZZ, ed. *Femtosecond Laser-Assisted Cataract Surgery: Facts and Results* (pp 105-109).

TABLE 1

PREOPERATIVE CHARACTERISTICS OF PATIENTS WHO UNDERWENT 5.5- OR 6.0-MM CAPSULOTOMY

Parameter	Mean±Standard Deviation (Range)		P Value*
	5.5-mm Group	6.0-mm Group	
Eyes (n)	9	8	
Age (y)	65.4±10.03 (53 to 78)	66.25±11.98 (51 to 79)	.743
MRSE (D)	0.22±0.96 (−1.50 to +1.50)	0.094±1.49 (−2.00 to +2.00)	.834
Corneal astigmatism (D)	0.64±0.22 (0.43 to 1.00)	0.53±0.33 (0.08 to 0.97)	.448
Mean K (D)	42.27±0.71 (41.47 to 43.59)	42.52±1.11 (41.07 to 44.45)	.625
UDVA (decimal)	0.13±0.05 (0.05 to 0.2)	0.14±0.07 (0.05 to 0.25)	.744
CDVA (decimal)	0.21±0.06 (0.1 to 0.3)	0.19±0.07 (0.1 to 0.3)	.569
Axial length (mm)	23.05±1.08 (21.51 to 24.4)	23.67±0.60 (22.95 to 24.49)	.329
IOL power (D)	22.57±1.92 (20.50 to 25.50)	21.13±0.99 (20.00 to 23.00)	.126

MRSE = manifest refraction spherical equivalent, K = keratometry, UDVA = uncorrected distance visual acuity, CDVA = corrected distance visual acuity, IOL = intraocular lens
**Independent t test.*

previous ocular surgery and trauma, retinal diseases, anterior segment pathology (iris atrophy, synechiae, incomplete or damaged zonules, aniridia), non-dilating pupil, a difference between steep and flat keratometry (K) cylinder >1.00 diopter (D), and axial length <19.0 mm or >25.0 mm were excluded from the study.

Eyes were divided into two groups by computer-generated randomization tables. In 9 eyes, a 5.5-mm capsulotomy was performed (5.5-mm group), and in 8 eyes a 6.0-mm capsulotomy (6.0-mm group) was performed. Table 1 shows the preoperative characteristics in both groups. No statistically significant differences were present between groups in age, visual acuity (uncorrected and corrected), manifest refraction spherical equivalent (MRSE), K, corneal astigmatism, axial length, or power of the implanted IOL.

Preoperative Assessment

Baseline preoperative examination included uncorrected distance visual acuity (UDVA) and corrected distance visual acuity (CDVA) measurements using a Snellen chart, MRSE, intraocular pressure by Goldmann applanation tonometry, slit-lamp evaluation, and funduscopy after pupil dilation.

Intraocular Lens and Power Calculation

A Crystalens AT-50AO (Bausch & Lomb, Rochester, New York) accommodating IOL was implanted in all eyes, which has a biconvex aspheric 5.0-mm single-optic design from Biosil with a refractive index of 1.4301 and a total diameter of 11.5. Optical biometry was performed in all eyes (IOLMaster; Carl Zeiss Meditec, Jena, Germany). Keratometry was measured using the Len-Star LS 900 (Haag-Streit International, Koeniz, Switzerland). The SRK/T formula with an A-constant of 119.1 was used for IOL power calculations for eyes with axial lengths measuring ≥22.01 mm. The Holladay II formula was used for eyes with axial lengths measuring ≤22.0 mm and for eyes with K flatter than 42.00 D independent of axial length. The target was emmetropia in all cases.

Surgical Technique

The same surgeon (Z.Z.N.) performed all cataract extractions and IOL implantations using topical anesthesia (oxybuprocain). Pupils were dilated with one drop of tropicamide 0.5% every 15 minutes for 45 minutes preoperatively.

Surgery was started in a laser room outside the operating room, and a 5.5-mm (5.5-mm group) or 6.0-mm (6.0-mm group) capsulotomy was performed using the LenSx femtosecond laser system (Alcon LenSx Inc, Aliso Viejo, California). The eye was fixated with a curved patient interface and the exact location of the lens and capsule were determined using optical coherence tomography built into the laser. The capsulotomy procedure was performed by scanning a circular pattern starting at least 100 μm below the anterior capsule and ending at least 100 μm above the capsule. Proprietary energy and spot separation parameters, which had been optimized in previous studies, were used for all capsulotomies.

Following the laser procedure, all patients were brought into the operating room and standard phacoemulsification (Infiniti; Alcon Laboratories Inc, Ft Worth, Texas) was performed. A 2.8-mm clear corneal incision was created with a disposable keratome, viscoelastic material (Provisc, Alcon Laboratories Inc) was injected, and the cut capsule was removed with a capsulorrhexis forceps. After hydrodissection, phacoemulsification of the nucleus and aspiration of the residual cortex were performed. The accommodating IOL was implanted in the intact capsular bag. After IOL implantation, the viscoelastic material was removed from the anterior chamber and capsular bag by irrigation and aspiration. All incisions were left sutureless. Immediately after hydration of the corneal incision, one drop of atropine 1% was instilled. One day postoperatively, one drop of atropine 1% was instilled to completely relax the ciliary muscle for the first 7 days so the accommodating IOL would remain firmly in contact with the posterior capsule. Patients were instructed to instill one drop of dexamethasone 0.1%–tobramycin 0.3% (Tobradex, Alcon Laboratories Inc) five times daily for 1 week and four times daily for the following week.

Postoperative Assessment

On the first postoperative day, patients had slit-lamp examination with dilated pupil to check the position of the accommodating IOL optic. Examinations at 1 week and 1, 3, 6, and 12 months after surgery were the same as preoperatively.

Uncorrected near visual acuity (UNVA) was measured using a Rosenbaum-Jaeger reading chart at 35 cm 12 months postoperatively; the chart was directly illuminated by a lamp with a 60-W bulb. Distance-corrected near visual acuity (DCNVA) was measured similarly to eliminate potential pseudoaccommodative effects of residual myopia and corneal cylinder. Uncorrected distance visual acuity, CDVA, UNVA, and DCNVA readings were converted to decimal notation for statistical analysis.

A Scheimpflug imaging system (Pentacam; Oculus Optikgeräte GmbH, Wetzlar, Germany) was used to evaluate IOL tilt and decentration 12 months postoperatively according to de Castro et al[12] as follows: IOL decentration is obtained from the distance between the IOL center and pupillary axis. Positive horizontal coordinates stand for nasal in the right eye and temporal in the left eye. Positive vertical coordinates stand for superior decentrations, and negative for inferior decentrations. By eliminating positive and negative signs, the magnitude of horizontal and vertical decentration could be determined without reference to nasal/temporal and superior/inferior orientation, respectively. Regarding IOL tilt, positive tilt around the x-axis indicates that the superior edge of the IOL is moved forward and vice versa for negative tilt. Positive tilt around the y-axis means, in the right eye, nasal tilt and indicates that the nasal edge of the IOL is moved backward and vice versa for a negative tilt around the y-axis in right eyes. A positive tilt around the y-axis stands for temporal tilt (nasal edge of the IOL moves forward) in left eyes. By eliminating positive and negative signs, the magnitude of horizontal and vertical tilt could be determined without reference to any orientation. The same examiner (K.K.) obtained the tilt measurements.

Statistical Analysis

Statistical analysis of the results was performed using SPSS for Windows software (version 9.0; SPSS Inc, Chicago, Illinois). Departure from normal distribution assumption was tested by the Shapiro-Wilks W test. In the case of normal distribution, data were presented as mean ± standard deviation, whereas median ± interquartile range was used if data showed non-normal distribution. For comparison of pre- and postoperative data, paired *t* test or Wilcoxon rank sum test was used, and for analyzing between-group differences unpaired *t* test or Mann-Whitney test was used.

To evaluate clinical significance between groups regarding tilt and decentration parameters, the Chi-square test of homogeneity was applied to compare the distribution of dichotomized tilt and decentration values at the level of 5° and 0.4 mm, respectively.[13]

The significance level was set at $P<.05$ in all statistical analyses.

RESULTS

No intraoperative complications or abnormal postoperative inflammations occurred. Mild corneal edema was found in four eyes on the first postoperative day, which resolved by the end of the first week. No cases of posterior capsule opacification occurred during the study period. All patients presented for 1-year follow-up.

Mean corneal astigmatism (difference between steep and flat K readings) was 0.64 ± 0.22 D preoperatively and 0.78 ± 0.20 D 12 months postoperatively in the 5.5-mm group and 0.53 ± 0.33 D preoperatively and 0.84 ± 0.32 D 12 months postoperatively in the 6.0-mm group. The difference between pre- and postoperative corneal astigmatism was not statistically significant in either group (5.5-mm group, P=.851; 6.0-mm group, P=.058; paired *t* test).

Visual and Refractive Outcomes

Table 2 shows the mean UDVA, UNVA, and DCNVA in decimal notation and MRSE in the study groups. One year after surgery, 7 (77.8%) eyes in the 5.5-mm group and 4 (50%) eyes in the 6.0-mm group had UDVA of 20/25 (0.8) or better 12 months postoperatively. Uncorrected near

TABLE 2

12-MONTH POSTOPERATIVE DATA OF EYES THAT UNDERWENT 5.5-MM OR 6.0-MM CAPSULOTOMY*

Parameter	*5.5-mm Group*	*6.0-mm Group*	*P Value†*
Eyes (n)	9	8	
MRSE (D)	−0.52±0.44 (−1.00 to 0.25)	−0.61±0.70 (−1.87 to 0.50)	.774
Corneal astigmatism (D)	0.78±0.20 (0.51 to 1.00)	0.84±0.32 (0.40 to 1.21)	.723
Mean K (D)	42.52±0.89 (41.27 to 44.25)	43.41±0.95 (42.05 to 44.65)	.101
UDVA (decimal)	0.8±0.2 (0.7 to 1.0)	0.75±0.38 (0.6 to 1.0)	.399‡
UNVA (decimal)	0.63±0.21 (0.32 to 1)	0.60±0.22 (0.32 to 1.0)	.750
DCNVA (decimal)	0.63±0.3 (0.4 to 0.8)	0.57±0.23 (0.32 to 0.63)	.488‡

MRSE = manifest refraction spherical equivalent, K = keratometry, UDVA = uncorrected distance visual acuity, UNVA = uncorrected near visual acuity, DCNVA = distance-corrected near visual acuity
**Normal distribution data are presented as mean±standard deviation (range). Non-normal distribution data are presented as median±interquartile range.*
†Independent t test.
‡Mann-Whitney test.

TABLE 3

TILT AND DECENTRATION PARAMETERS OF EYES THAT UNDERWENT 5.5-MM OR 6.0-MM CAPSULOTOMY

	Mean±SD (Range)		
Parameter	*5.5-mm Group*	*6.0-mm Group*	*P Value**
Tilt (°)			
Vertical	1.42±0.81 (0.49 to 2.99)	4.29±2.52 (1.45 to 8.77)	.014
Horizontal	1.62±0.85 (0.36 to 2.55)	4.77±2.62 (1.77 to 8.14)	.015
Decentration (mm)			
Vertical	0.083±0.079 (0.000 to 0.200)	0.086±0.095 (0.010 to 0.280)	.976
Horizontal	0.136±0.109 (0.010 to 0.340)	0.193±0.141 (0.010 to 0.350)	.414

**Independent t test.*

TABLE 4

DISTRIBUTION OF DICHOTOMIZED TILT VALUES AT 5.0° IN EYES THAT UNDERWENT 5.5-MM OR 6.0-MM CAPSULOTOMY

Parameter	*5.5-mm Group*	*6.0-mm Group*	*P Value**
Vertical tilt	0:9	2:8	.156
Horizontal tilt	0:9	3:8	.089

**Chi-square test.*

visual acuity was J3 (0.5) or better in 8 (88.9%) eyes in the 5.5-mm group and 6 (75.0%) eyes in the 6.0-mm group. The difference between groups was not statistically significant (*P*=.75; independent *t* test). Median DCNVA was J3 in both groups postoperatively. Distance-corrected near visual acuity was J3 or better in 77.7% of eyes (7/9) in the 5.5-mm group and 75.0% of eyes (6/8) in the 6.0-mm group. The difference between groups was not statistically significant (*P*=.48; Mann-Whitney test). No statistically significant difference was noted between groups in MRSE preoperatively (*P*=.834, independent *t* test) and 1 year postoperatively (*P*=.14, Mann-Whitney test).

Accommodating IOL Tilt and Decentration Parameters

Table 3 shows the mean horizontal and vertical accommodating IOL tilt and decentration parameters. Both vertical and horizontal tilt parameters were statistically significantly higher in the 6.0-mm group. No statistically significant difference was noted between groups in any decentration parameter. None of the implanted IOLs showed a decentration >0.4 mm.

In the 6.0-mm group, >5° vertical and horizontal tilt was measured in 2 (25%) and 3 (37.5%) eyes, respectively. In the 5.5-mm group, none of the eyes showed IOL tilt >5°. No significant difference was noted in the distribution of dichotomized tilt values at 5° between groups (Table 4).

DISCUSSION

To our knowledge, this is the first pilot study to report single-optic accommodating IOL implantation after femtosecond laser capsulotomy and to evaluate accommodating IOL tilt and decentration taking into consideration capsulorrhexis size. Accommodating IOLs[5] were developed with the aim of providing accommodative capability and functional near vision and independence from spectacles after cataract extraction without the compromises of a multifocal IOL.[1-4] For the implantation of a 5.0-mm diameter single-optic accommodating IOL, the capsulorrhexis should be central, circular, and between 5.5 and 6 mm in diameter.[6] A large or eccentric capsulorrhexis increases the risk of IOL dislocation.[10,11]

The introduction of femtosecond laser refractive cataract surgery provides the means to perform more precise, accurate, reproducible, and stronger capsulotomies than those created with the conventional manual technique.[7-11,14] A properly sized, shaped, and centered femtosecond laser capsulotomy resulted in better IOL centration and less tilt when compared to a manual capsulotomy.[9-11] Kránitz et al[11] reported six-times higher odds for IOL decentration when the capsulorrhexis was performed manually compared to a femtosecond laser capsulotomy.

Until now there has been no clear evidence in the published literature regarding whether a 5.5- or 6.0-mm capsulorrhexis is the most suitable for a 5.0-mm diameter single-optic accommodating IOL (Crystalens AT-50AO). We therefore compared both diameters in this prospective study. We found no significant difference between the two study groups regarding postoperative UDVA, UNVA, and DCNVA. We also did not find a difference in IOL decentration between the 5.5-mm and 6.0-mm groups, and none of the implanted IOLs exceeded 0.4 mm of decentration. Altmann[15] warned that the advantage of an aspheric IOL can be lost in the case of decentration >0.5 mm. Holladay et al[16] indicated that the performance of aspheric IOLs is worse compared to spherical IOLs when decentration is >0.4 mm.

When evaluating the anteroposterior position of the accommodating IOLs, we found significantly higher horizontal and vertical tilt in the 6.0-mm group, and two (25%) IOLs exceeded 5.0° of vertical tilt and three (37.5%) IOLs exceeded 5° of horizontal tilt in the 6.0-mm group, whereas no IOL exceeded 5° in the 5.5-mm group. Guyton et al[13] reported that IOL tilt >5° can impair visual quality. Other authors[17,18] demonstrated a significant correlation between IOL tilt and ocular coma-like aberrations, and the quality of the retinal image improves by reducing IOL tilt.

Limitations of our study include the small number of eyes evaluated and the potential bias introduced by including both eyes of some patients.

Our results indicate that a 5.5-mm capsulotomy created with an intraocular femtosecond laser causes less IOL tilt than a 6.0-mm capsulotomy and may therefore be superior when implanting a single-optic accommodating IOL.

Author Contributions

Study concept and design (A.S., Z.Z.N.); data collection (A.S., K.K., A.I.T., Z.Z.N.); analysis and interpretation of data (A.S., K.K., K.M., M.C.K.); drafting of the manuscript (A.S.); critical revision of the manuscript (K.K., A.I.T., K.M., M.C.K., Z.Z.N.); statistical expertise (A.S.); administrative, technical, or material support (A.S.); supervision (K.K., A.I.T., Z.Z.N.)

References

1. Kamlesh M, Dadeya S, Kaushik S. Contrast sensitivity and depth of focus with aspheric multifocal versus conventional monofocal intraocular lens. *Can J Ophthalmol.* 2001;36(4):197-201.
2. Montés-Micó R, Alió JL. Distance and near contrast sensitivity function after multifocal intraocular lens implantation. *J Cataract Refract Surg.* 2003;29(4):703-711.
3. Pieh S, Lackner B, Hanselmayer G, et al. Halo size under distance and near conditions in refractive multifocal intraocular lenses. *Br J Ophthalmol.* 2001;85(7):816-821.
4. Allen ED, Burton RL, Webber SK, et al. Comparison of a diffractive bifocal and a monofocal intraocular lens. *J Cataract Refract Surg.* 1996;22(4):446-451.
5. Sheppard AL, Bashir A, Wolffsohn JS, Davies LN. Accommodating intraocular lenses: a review of design concepts, usage and assessment methods. *Clin Exp Optom.* 2010;93(9):441-452.
6. Chang DF. *Mastering Refractive IOLs: The Art and Science.* Thorofare, NJ: SLACK Inc; 2008.
7. Nagy Z, Takacs A, Filkorn T, Sarayba M. Initial clinical evaluation of an intraocular femtosecond laser in cataract surgery. *J Refract Surg.* 2009;25(12):1053-1060.
8. Nagy ZZ, Kránitz K, Takacs A, Filkorn T, Gergely R, Knorz MC. Intraocular femtosecond laser use in traumatic cataracts following penetrating and blunt trauma. *J Refract Surg.* 2012;28(2):151-153.
9. Mihàltz K, Knorz MC, Alió JL, et al. Internal aberrations and optical quality after femtosecond laser anterior capsulotomy in cataract surgery. *J Refract Surg.* 2011;27(10):711-716.
10. Nagy ZZ, Kránitz K, Takacs AI, Mihàltz K, Kovács I, Knorz MC. Comparison of intraocular lens decentration parameters after femtosecond and manual capsulotomies. *J Refract Surg.* 2011;27(8):564-569.
11. Kránitz K, Takacs AI, Mihàltz K, Kovács I, Knorz MC, Nagy ZZ. Femtosecond laser capsulotomy and manual continuous curvilinear capsulorrhexis parameters and their effects on intraocular lens centration. *J Refract Surg.* 2011;27(8):558-563.
12. de Castro A, Rosales P, Marcos S. Tilt and decentration of intraocular lenses in vivo from Purkinje and Scheimpflug imaging. Validation study. *J Cataract Refract Surg.* 2007;33(3):418-429.
13. Guyton DL, Uozato H, Wisnicki HJ. Rapid determination of intraocular lens tilt and decentration through the undilated pupil. *Ophthalmology.* 1990;97(10):1259-1264.
14. Friedman NJ, Palanker DV, Schuele G, et al. Femtosecond laser capsulotomy. *J Cataract Refract Surg.* 2011;37(7):1189-1198.
15. Altmann GE. Wavefront-customized intraocular lenses. *Curr Opin Ophthalmol.* 2004;15(4):358-364.
16. Holladay JT, Piers PA, Koranyi G, van der Mooren M, Norrby NE. A new intraocular lens design to reduce spherical aberration of pseudophakic eyes. *J Refract Surg.* 2002;18(6):683-691.
17. Taketani F, Matuura T, Yukawa E, Hara Y. Influence of intraocular lens tilt and decentration on wavefront aberrations. *J Cataract Refract Surg.* 2004;30(10):2158-2162.
18. Oshika T, Kawana K, Hiraoka T, Kaji Y, Kiuchi T. Ocular higher-order wavefront aberration caused by major tilting of intraocular lens. *Am J Ophthalmol.* 2005;140(4):744-746.

Internal Aberrations and Optical Quality After Femtosecond Laser Anterior Capsulotomy in Cataract Surgery

Kata Miháltz, MD; Michael C. Knorz, MD; Jorge L. Alió, MD, PhD; Ágnes I. Takács, MD; Kinga Kránitz, MD; Illés Kovács, MD, PhD; Zoltán Z. Nagy, MD, DSc

ABSTRACT

PURPOSE: To compare ocular and internal aberrations after femtosecond laser anterior capsulotomy and continuous curvilinear capsulorrhexis in cataract surgery.

METHODS: In this prospective study, anterior capsulotomy was performed during cataract surgery with an intraocular femtosecond (FS) laser (Alcon LenSx Inc) in 48 eyes. As a control group, continuous curvilinear capsulorrhexis (CCC) was performed in 51 eyes. Wavefront aberrometry, corneal topography, and objective visual quality were measured using the OPD-Scan (NIDEK Co Ltd). Vertical and horizontal tilt, coma, and visual quality metrics were evaluated separately to determine whether the source of aberrations was ocular or internal. Main outcome measures included postoperative residual refraction, uncorrected and corrected visual acuities, ocular and internal aberrations, Strehl ratio, and modulation transfer function (MTF).

RESULTS: No statistically significant differences were noted between the FS and CCC groups, respectively, in postoperative sphere (−0.60±1.50 vs −0.50±1.40 diopters [D]), postoperative cylinder (1.30±1.01 vs 1.10±1.10 D), uncorrected distance visual acuity (0.86±0.15 vs 0.88±0.08), or corrected distance visual acuity (0.97±0.08 vs 0.97±0.06). The FS group had significantly lower values of intraocular vertical tilt (−0.05±0.36 vs 0.27±0.57) and coma (−0.003±0.11 vs 0.1±0.15), and significantly higher Strehl ratios (0.02±0.02 vs 0.01±0.01) and MTF values at all measured cycles per degree, compared to the CCC group.

CONCLUSIONS: Capsulotomy performed with an intraocular FS laser induced significantly less internal aberrations measured by the NIDEK OPD-Scan aberrometer compared to eyes that underwent CCC, which may result in better optical quality after the procedure.
[*J Refract Surg*. 2011;27(10):711-716.]
doi:10.3928/1081597X-20110913-01

Originally published in Journal of Refractive Surgery, *October 2011.*

Performing a precise anterior capsulorrhexis is crucial in cataract surgery. A capsulorrhexis with a 360° overlapping capsular edge prevents optic decentration, tilt, myopic shift, posterior and anterior capsular opacification due to symmetric contractile forces of the capsular bag, and shrink wrap effect.[1-6] In earlier reports from our research group, we have demonstrated higher precision capsulorrhexis creation and reduced lens decentration with the intraocular femtosecond laser.[7,8] This technology also has the potential to reduce the risk of capsular tear and intraoperative complications during cataract surgery and reduced phacoemulsification power.[9]

Optical quality is a subjective entity and can currently only be described indirectly by objective metrics, such as wavefront error measurements, and visual quality metrics or functional data, such as visual acuity and contrast sensitivity.[10-13] Wavefront analysis isolates the effect of lower order aberrations (defocus, astigmatism) and higher order aberrations, as well as the contribution of individual aberrations on optical quality. Strehl ratio, point spread function (PSF), and modulation transfer function (MTF) are parameters of the quality of an optical system including a human eye. The PSF of an optical system is the intensity distribution of light from a point source projected onto the retina and indicates the extent of blurring of the retinal image. Modulation transfer function is defined as the amplitude of the image contrast divided by the amplitude of the object contrast and is a function of spatial frequency, which could describe the reduction in contrast of sine wave stimuli by the optical medium. Modulation transfer function can be measured by directly imaging the PSF on the retinal surface or by calculating from wavefront aberrations.[14,15]

Nagy ZZ, ed. *Femtosecond Laser Assisted Cataract Surgery: Facts and Results* (pp 111-116).

The purpose of this study was to evaluate optical and visual effects of capsulorrhexis performed by an intraocular femtosecond laser during cataract surgery compared to manually performed continuous curvilinear capsulorrhexis (CCC).

PATIENTS AND METHODS

Patient Population

Femtosecond capsulotomies were performed in 48 eyes of 43 patients with cataract for IOL implantation (FS group). Continuous curvilinear capsulorrhexis by forceps was performed on 51 eyes of 38 patients, which served as a control group (CCC group). All surgeries were performed by the same surgeon (Z.Z.N.). For comparison of postoperative results, all patients were examined 6 months after surgery. Each patient underwent a complete ophthalmological evaluation. Patients with previous ocular surgery, trauma, active ocular disease, poorly dilated pupils, or known zonular weakness were excluded from the study.

The study was conducted in compliance with the Declaration of Helsinki, as well as with applicable country and local requirements regarding ethics committee/institutional review boards, informed consent, and other statutes or regulations regarding protection of the rights and welfare of human subjects participating in biomedical research.

Surgery

The surgical technique was standardized in each patient, except for the method of capsulorrhexis.

After pupillary dilation (one drop of tropicamide 0.5% every 15 minutes × 3) and instillation of topical anesthesia (proparacaine HCl 0.5%), the following procedures were performed by the femtosecond laser system: the LenSx laser system (Alcon LenSx Inc, Aliso Viejo, California) uses a curved patient interface to applanate the cornea. The location of the crystalline lens surface is determined following applanation using proprietary optical methodology. A 4.5-mm diameter capsulotomy procedure was performed by scanning a cylindrical pattern starting at least 100 μm below the anterior capsule and ending at least 100 μm above the capsule. Proprietary energy and spot separation parameters, which had been optimized in previous studies, were used for all laser procedures.

Following the laser procedure, a 2.8-mm biplanar clear corneal incision was created with a trapezoid knife and the cut capsule was removed with a rhexis forceps under a standard ophthalmic operating microscope. The clear corneal incision was always placed at the 11-o'clock position; the side-port incision was created with a 15° steel blade at the 1-o'clock position. Corneal incision and side-port were created with the same technique in the CCC group as well. For manual capsulorrhexis procedures, a 4.5-mm diameter round corneal marker was initially used to aid the surgeon in creating the correct size and shape capsulorrhexis. Continuous curvilinear capsulorrhexis was performed with the aid of a cystotome and capsular forceps. After hydrodissection, phacoemulsification of the nucleus and aspiration of the residual cortex were performed using the Accurus (Alcon Laboratories Inc, Ft Worth, Texas) phacoemulsification machine.

All intraocular lenses (IOL) were folded and implanted in the capsular bag with the aid of an injection cartridge; the haptics were placed at the 3- and 9-o'clock positions. In all eyes in the FS and CCC groups, AcrySof MA60AC three-piece acrylic spherical IOLs (Alcon Laboratories Inc) were implanted. The IOL power was calculated using the SRK/T formula. After IOL implantation, the viscoelastic material was removed from the anterior chamber and capsular bag by irrigation/aspiration. Stromal hydration of the paracentesis and main incision ended the procedure. All incisions were left sutureless. No intra- or postoperative complications occurred. Within the first month, all patients received a combination of antibiotic and steroid eye drops (dexamethasone and tobramycin).

Aberrometry Measurements

Total, corneal, and internal optical aberrations were measured using the NIDEK OPD-Scan II (NIDEK Co Ltd, Gamagori, Japan). This device measures the autorefraction, keratometry, photopic and mesopic pupil diameters, corneal topography, and wavefront aberrations simultaneously on the same axis. All wavefront aberrations were calculated and plotted with respect to the corneal vertex. The corneal topography was measured using Placido-disk technology, and the ocular wavefront was measured using the principle of skiascopic phase difference.[16,17] Wavefront measurements were performed in a dark room and were standardized to a 4.5-mm pupil. No dilating drop was used to assess the aberration profile of the natural view normally experienced by the patient. We chose to perform aberrometry measurements without applying mydriatic drops as we believe that results of a natural aberrometry profile are more representative for optical performances of the eye than results of a 6- or 7-mm dilated pupil. In the eye, wavefront errors typically increase with pupil size, but also a smaller aperture causes greater diffraction.[14,15,18] Total, corneal, and internal wavefront aberrations

TABLE 1

DEMOGRAPHICS OF PATIENTS WHO UNDERWENT MANUAL CONTINUOUS CURVILINEAR CAPSULORRHEXIS OR FEMTOSECOND LASER CAPSULOTOMY

	Mean±Standard Deviation		
Demographic	CCC Group (n=51)	FS Group (n=48)	P Value*
Age (y)	70.7±14.3	75.0±10.4	>.05
Sex (M:F)	7:31	9:34	>.05
Spherical refractive error (D)	−0.50±1.40	−0.60±1.50	>.05
Cylindrical refractive error (D)	1.10±1.10	1.30±1.01	>.05

CCC = continuous curvilinear capsulorrhexis, FS = femtosecond
**Unpaired t test.*

were reconstructed using a 6th order Zernike polynomial decomposition. Visual quality was described by uncorrected (UDVA) and corrected distance visual acuity (CDVA), and by MTF and Strehl ratio. Images of PSF were depicted to demonstrate characteristic image degradation in the two groups. Point spread function is represented by a figure displaying how a point is reproduced on the retina by the eye's optical system. Strehl ratio was used to compare image quality metrics in the two groups. The Strehl ratio is defined as the ratio between the PSF of an eye and the PSF of that eye when optical quality is limited only by diffraction. It is a number between 0 and 1. The OPD-Scan provides the MTF curves from 0 to 60 cycles per degree (cpd), obtained from aberrations for the 4.5-mm optical zone. The spatial frequencies selected as landmarks were 5, 10, 15, 20, 25, 30, 35, 40, 45, 50, 55, and 60 cpd.

Statistical Analyses

Statistical analyses were performed with SPSS 16.0 (SPSS Inc, Chicago, Illinois). Departure from normal distribution assumption was tested by the Shapiro-Wilks W test. Due to normality of data, descriptive statistics show mean and standard deviation. Statistical analysis was performed by comparing two samples at a time using the Student *t* test for analysis of mean visual and refractive values and intraocular optical quality parameters in both study groups. To determine predictors of Strehl ratio, multiple regression analysis was performed. Among all tested models, the best fitting model was used,[19] and model fit was assessed by pseudo r^2 as goodness-of-fit statistics.

TABLE 2

OCULAR, CORNEAL, AND INTERNAL ABERROMETRY PARAMETERS 6 MONTHS AFTER SURGERY IN EYES THAT UNDERWENT CONTINUOUS CURVILINEAR CAPSULORRHEXIS OR FEMTOSECOND LASER CAPSULOTOMY

	Mean±Standard Deviation		
Parameter	CCC Group (n=51)	FS Group (n=48)	P Value*
Ocular			
Vertical tilt	0.09±0.44	−0.08±0.35	>.05
Horizontal tilt	0.10±0.49	0.16±0.39	>.05
Vertical coma	0.04±0.19	−0.02±0.16	>.05
Horizontal coma	−0.01±0.16	0.02±0.14	>.05
Corneal			
Vertical tilt	−0.11±0.49	−0.06±0.38	>.05
Horizontal tilt	−0.05±0.41	−0.04±0.32	>.05
Vertical coma	−0.04±0.17	−0.04±0.11	>.05
Horizontal coma	−0.03±0.11	−0.02±0.12	>.05
Internal			
Vertical tilt	0.27±0.57	−0.05±0.36	.006
Horizontal tilt	0.15±0.59	0.16±0.63	>.05
Vertical coma	0.10±0.15	0.003±0.11	.006
Horizontal coma	0.03±0.18	0.06±0.11	>.05

CCC = continuous curvilinear capsulorrhexis, FS = femtosecond
**Unpaired t test.*

RESULTS

Patient Characteristics

All patients were evaluated 6 months after surgery. Table 1 shows the patient demographic data and postoperative refractive error values. No statistically significant differences were noted in any variable.

Zernike Polynomials

The FS group had significantly lower values of intraocular vertical tilt (Z_1^{-1}) and coma (Z_3^{-1}) aberrations compared with the CCC group (*P*=.006) (Table 2). No statistically significant differences were noted in any ocular, corneal, or other internal aberrations between the two groups. Linear regression analysis showed a strong correlation (*P*<.001, r=0.73) between internal vertical coma and internal vertical tilt in both groups (Fig 1).

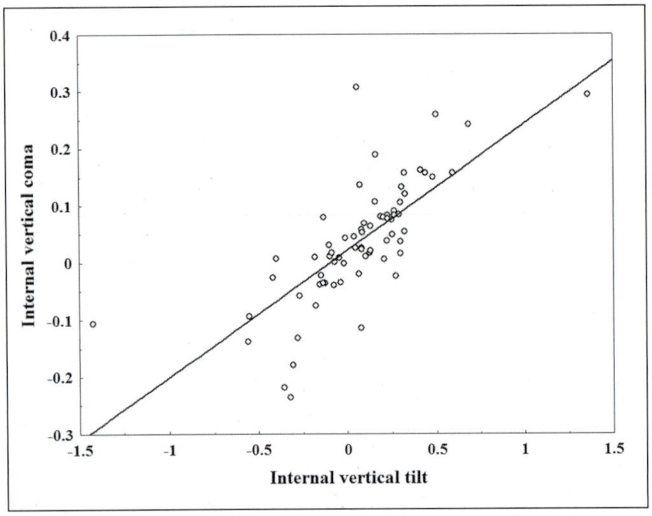

Figure 1. Linear regression for internal vertical tilt and coma. Correlation is significant ($P<.001$), r=0.73.

Image Quality

Although no significant difference in UDVA or CDVA could be detected between groups, the FS group had a statistically significantly higher Strehl ratio. The MTF value was also significantly increased in the FS group at all studied cpds; the differences were statistically significant ($P<.05$) for all values (Table 3).

To determine predictors of Strehl ratio, multivariable regression analysis was performed. In this model, Zernike terms that showed significant differences between groups and the most important confounders (lower order aberrations) were included. The model was fitted not only to test the additive effects of data but also included interaction terms. This model showed that after adjustment for lower order aberrations (astigmatism and defocus), the amount of internal vertical tilt had significant influence on Strehl ratio with a significant interaction between vertical tilt and coma (Table 4).

Figure 2 demonstrates PSF images of two patients, representative of the two study groups, whose visual performance, measured by Strehl ratio, was closest to the average value of the given group. The PSF plot of the CCC eye shows more astigmatic and coma-like degradation of the retinal image (see Fig 2B). On the contrary, PSF of the FS eye is smaller and round (see Fig 2A). On average, FS eyes had higher MTF performance than CCC eyes across all spatial frequencies (Fig 3).

Table 3

Visual Quality Characteristics in Eyes That Underwent Continuous Curvilinear Capsulorrhexis or Femtosecond Laser Capsulotomy

Characteristic	*CCC Group (n=51)*	*FS Group (n=48)*	P Value*
UDVA	0.88±0.08	0.86±0.15	>.05
CDVA	0.97±0.06	0.97±0.08	>.05
Strehl ratio	0.01±0.007	0.02±0.024	.001
MTF (cpd)			
5	0.25±0.15	0.32±0.19	.04
10	0.10±0.06	0.17±0.12	.001
15	0.07±0.04	0.11±0.08	.001
20	0.05±0.04	0.08±0.07	.008
25	0.04±0.03	0.06±0.06	.003
30	0.03±0.02	0.05±0.05	.002
35	0.02±0.02	0.04±0.04	.006
40	0.02±0.02	0.04±0.04	.003
45	0.02±0.01	0.03±0.03	.005
50	0.02±0.01	0.03±0.03	.002
55	0.01±0.01	0.03±0.02	.002
60	0.01±0.01	0.02±0.02	.006

CCC = continuous curvilinear capsulorrhexis, FS = femtosecond, UDVA = uncorrected distance visual acuity, CDVA = corrected distance visual acuity, MTF = modulation transfer function, cpd = cycles per degree
**Unpaired t test.*

Discussion

Although no significant difference could be demonstrated in any ocular aberrations, the FS group had a statistically significant reduction in intraocular vertical tilt and coma aberrations. A statistically significant increase in Strehl ratio and MTF values at all studied cpds could be detected in the FS group as well, suggesting a better image quality in these patients. Aside from vertical tilt and coma, FS group or CCC group was also a significant predictor of Strehl ratio, confirming our hypothesis, that the type of surgery has a significant effect on the visual outcome of cataract surgery. During analysis of OPD-Scan tilt, coma, and Strehl ratio results, we excluded the influence of implanted IOL type on optical aberrations and visual quality metrics. As all implanted IOLs were of spherical design, their influence on ocular spherical aberration was equal and therefore not analyzed separately.

Tilt is a prismatic error that is not a true optical aberration because it does not induce distortion of the image, rather a shift in its position. Coma aberration is a higher order aberration, which may occur either due to the incident wavefront being tilted or decentered with respect to the optical surface. It may originate from the axial misalignment of optical surfaces.[13,20-22] Comatic

TABLE 4

REGRESSION BETA COEFFICIENTS FOR SIGNIFICANT PREDICTORS OF STREHL RATIO AFTER ADJUSTMENT FOR ASTIGMATISM AND DEFOCUS IN MULTIPLE REGRESSION MODELING

Parameters	β	95% CL	P Value
Internal vertical tilt	0.38	0.03-0.72	<.05
Interaction of internal vertical tilt and coma	1.55	0.67-2.42	<.05

CL = confidence limit

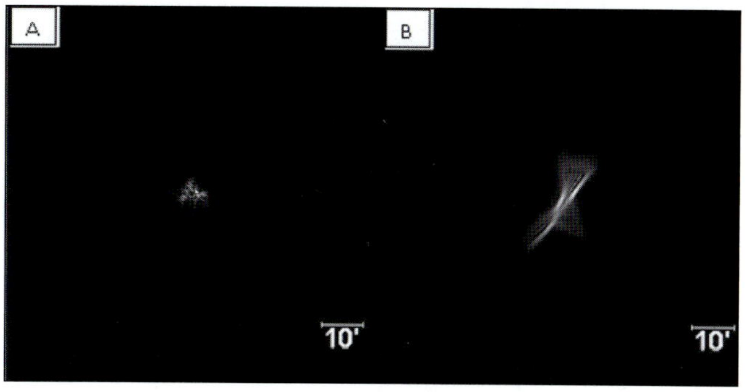

Figure 2. Representative point spread function images in the **A)** femtosecond laser and **B)** manual continuous curvilinear capsulorrhexis (control) groups.

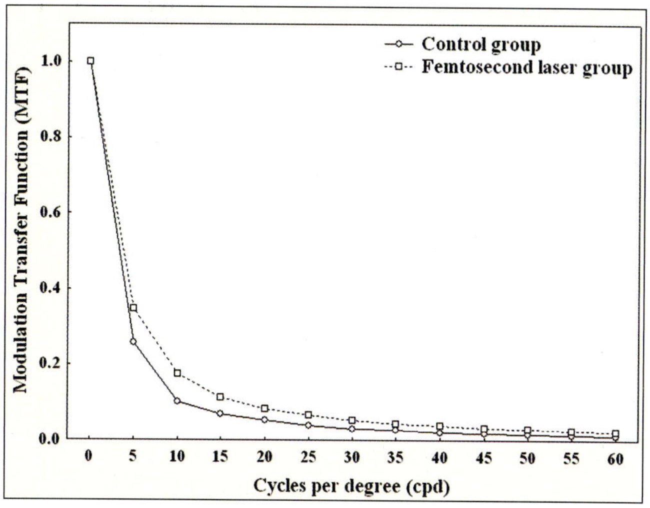

Figure 3. Modulation transfer function (MTF) in the **A)** femtosecond laser and **B)** manual continuous curvilinear capsulorrhexis (control) groups representing the average of MTF values in the sagittal and meridional directions at different spatial frequencies.

wavefront deviation forms a blurred spot image with a comet-shaped tail, similar to the PSF image demonstrated in Figure 2B. As demonstrated by Applegate et al,[23] when combined, Zernike modes can interact. A decentration of an aberration mode induces aberration of another order. For example, the translation of spherical aberration generates coma. With an increasing amount of decentration, an increasing amount of coma is introduced.[24,25] Thibos et al[26] demonstrated an existing positive correlation between modes of the same frequency, eg, between vertical coma and vertical tilt. Our results also prove a strong positive correlation between vertical tilt and coma, which according to previous theories, is due to the decentration of the IOL.

Femtosecond lasers represent an important technological advance in ophthalmic surgery. Combined with computer-controlled optical delivery systems, femtosecond lasers can produce precise surgical incisions without collateral damage to surrounding tissues.[27,28] A potential benefit of this new technology is that it will provide a better capsulotomy prior to implantation of aspheric or multifocal IOLs.[7-9] A tilted or decentered multifocal IOL or an IOL with a negative spherical aberration can induce higher asymmetrical aberrations; thus, the desired effect on the optical quality could be impaired by IOL displacement.[29,30]

In the present study, femtosecond laser capsulotomy resulted in decreased internal tilt and coma aberrations; however, internal aberrations may originate not only from the lens, but also from the posterior surface of the cornea. The separation of these different sources is not possible with the OPD-Scan. Dubbelman et al[31,32] have isolated aberrations resulting from the posterior corneal surface from those of the anterior corneal surface with the use of a Scheimpflug camera. They found a strong relationship between anterior and posterior corneal surface asphericity. They stated that the posterior corneal surface compensates approximately 3.5% of the coma of the anterior surface and that for the coma aberration of the whole eye, only the anterior corneal surface and crystalline lens play a role.[31,32] According to these findings, we can conclude that the decreased internal aberrations measured in the current study are resultant of the better IOL position due to better sizing of the capsulorrhexis performed by the femtosecond laser.

AUTHOR CONTRIBUTIONS

Study concept and design (K.M., J.L.A.); data collection (K.M., J.L.A., K.K., I.K.); analysis and interpretation of data (K.M., M.C.K., J.L.A., A.T., I.K., Z.Z.N.); drafting of the manuscript (K.M., I.K.); critical revision of the manuscript (K.M., M.C.K., J.L.A., A.T., K.K., I.K., Z.Z.N.); statistical expertise (I.K.); obtained funding (J.L.A., Z.Z.N.); administrative, technical, or material support (J.L.A., A.T., K.K.); supervision (J.L.A., Z.Z.N.)

References

1. Dick HB, Pena-Aceves A, Manns A, Krummenauer F. New technology for sizing the continuous curvilinear capsulorhexis: prospective trial. *J Cataract Refract Surg.* 2008;34(7):1136-1144.
2. Tan JC. Capsulotomy. *Curr Opin Ophthalmol.* 2001;12(1):82-85.
3. Ravalico G, Tognetto D, Palomba M, Busatto P, Baccara F. Capsulorhexis size and posterior capsule opacification. *J Cataract Refract Surg.* 1996;22(1):98-103.
4. Aykan U, Bilge AH, Karadayi K. The effect of capsulorhexis size on development of posterior capsule opacification: small (4.5 to 5.0 mm) versus large (6.0 to 7.0 mm). *Eur J Ophthalmol.* 2003;13(6):541-545.
5. Hollick EJ, Spalton DJ, Meacock WR. The effect of capsulorhexis size on posterior capsular opacification: one-year results of a randomized prospective trial. *Am J Ophthalmol.* 1999;128(3):271-279.
6. Krueger RR, Kuszak J, Lubatschowski H, Myers RI, Ripken T, Heisterkamp A. First safety study of femtosecond laser photodisruption in animal lenses: tissue morphology and cataractogenesis. *J Cataract Refract Surg.* 2005;31(12):2386-2394.
7. Kránitz K, Takacs A, Mihåltz K, Kovács I, Knorz MC, Nagy ZZ. Femtosecond laser capsulotomy and manual continuous curvilinear capsulorrhexis parameters and their effects on intraocular lens centration. *J Refract Surg.* 2011;27(8):558-563.
8. Nagy ZZ, Kránitz K, Takacs AI, Mihåltz K, Kovács I, Knorz MC. Comparison of intraocular lens decentration parameters after femtosecond and manual capsulotomies. *J Refract Surg.* 2011;27(8):564-569.
9. Nagy Z, Takacs A, Filkorn T, Sarayba M. Initial clinical evaluation of an intraocular femtosecond laser in cataract surgery. *J Refract Surg.* 2009;25(12):1053-1060.
10. Baumeister M, Bühren J, Kohnen T. Tilt and decentration of spherical and aspheric intraocular lenses: effect on higher-order aberrations. *J Cataract Refract Surg.* 2009;35(6):1006-1012.
11. Mester U, Sauer T, Kaymak H. Decentration and tilt of a single-piece aspheric intraocular lens compared with the lens position in young phakic eyes. *J Cataract Refract Surg.* 2009;35(3):485-490.
12. Pieh S, Fiala W, Malz A, Stork W. In vitro strehl ratios with spherical, aberration-free, average, and customized spherical aberration-correcting intraocular lenses. *Invest Ophthalmol Vis Sci.* 2009;50(3):1264-1270.
13. Rohart C, Lemarinel B, Thanh HX, Gatinel D. Ocular aberrations after cataract surgery with hydrophobic and hydrophilic acrylic intraocular lenses: comparative study. *J Cataract Refract Surg.* 2006;32(7):1201-1205.
14. Liang J, Grimm B, Goelz S, Bille JF. Objective measurement of wave aberrations of the human eye with the use of the Hartmann–Shack wave front sensor. *J Opt Soc Am A.* 1994;11(7):1949-1957.
15. Walsh G, Charman WN, Howland HC. Objective technique for the determination of monochromatic aberrations of the eye. *J Opt Soc Am A.* 1984;1(9):987-992.
16. Gatinel D, Hoang-Xuan T. Objective assessment of the quality of vision before and after repositioning of a dislocated iris-fixated aphakic anterior chamber lens. *J Refract Surg.* 2007;23(9 Suppl):S1005-S1010.
17. Levy J, Lifshitz T, Klemperer I, et al. The effect of Nd:YAG laser posterior capsulotomy on ocular wave front aberrations. *Can J Ophthalmol.* 2009;44(5):529-533.
18. Tutt R, Bradley A, Begley C, Thibos LN. Optical and visual impact of tear break-up in human eyes. *Invest Ophthalmol Vis Sci.* 2000;41(13):4117-4123.
19. Lu M, Tilley BC; NINDS t-PA Stroke Trial Study Group. Use of odds ratio or relative risk to measure a treatment effect in clinical trials with multiple correlated binary outcomes: data from the NINDS t-PA stroke trial. *Stat Med.* 2001;20(13):1891-1901.
20. Taketani F, Matuura T, Yukawa E, Hara Y. Influence of intraocular lens tilt and decentration on wavefront aberrations. *J Cataract Refract Surg.* 2004;30(10):2158-2162.
21. Korynta J, Bok J, Cendelin J, Michalova K. Computer modeling of visual impairment caused by intraocular lens misalignment. *J Cataract Refract Surg.* 1999;25(1):100-105.
22. Dai GM. Ocular wavefront presentation. In: *Wavefront Optics for Vision Correction.* Bellingham, WA: SPIE; 2008:33-96.
23. Applegate RA, Marsack JD, Ramos R, Sarver EJ. Interaction between aberrations to improve or reduce visual performance. *J Cataract Refract Surg.* 2003;29(8):1487-1495.
24. Mihåltz K, Kránitz K, Kovács I, Takács, Németh J, Nagy ZZ. Shifting of the line of sight in keratoconus measured by a Hartmann-Shack sensor. *Ophthalmology.* 2010;117(1):41-48.
25. Guirao A, Williams DR. Effect of rotation and translation on the expected benefit of an ideal method to correct the eye's higher-order aberrations. *J Opt Soc Am A Opt Image Sci Vis.* 2001;18(5):1003-1015.
26. Thibos LN, Hong X, Bradley A, Cheng X. Statistical variation of aberration structure and image quality in a normal population of healthy eyes. *J Opt Soc Am A Opt Image Sci Vis.* 2002;19(1):2329-2348.
27. Soong HK, Malta JB. Femtosecond lasers in ophthalmology. *Am J Ophthalmol.* 2009;147(2):189-197.
28. Chung SH, Mazur E. Surgical applications of femtosecond lasers. *J Biophotonics.* 2009;2(10):557-572.
29. Kohnen T, Klaproth OK, Bühren J. Effect of intraocular lens asphericity on quality of vision after cataract removal: an intraindividual comparison. *Ophthalmology.* 2009;116(9):1697-1706.
30. Holladay JT, Piers PA, Koranyi G, et al. A new intraocular lens design to reduce spherical aberration of pseudophakic eyes. *J Refract Surg.* 2002;18(6):683-691.
31. Dubbelman M, Weeber HA, van der Heijde RG, Völker-Dieben HJ. Radius and asphericity of the posterior corneal surface determined by corrected Scheimpflug photography. *Acta Ophthalmol Scand.* 2002;80(4):379-383.
32. Dubbelman M, Sicam VA, van der Heijde RG. The contribution of the posterior surface to the coma aberration of the human cornea. *J Vis.* 2007;7(7):10.1-8.

Comparison of IOL Power Calculation and Refractive Outcome After Laser Refractive Cataract Surgery With a Femtosecond Laser Versus Conventional Phacoemulsification

Tamás Filkorn, MD; Illés Kovács, MD, PhD; Ágnes Takács, MD; Éva Horváth, MD; Michael C. Knorz, MD; Zoltán Z. Nagy, MD, DSC

Abstract

PURPOSE: To compare intraocular lens (IOL) power calculation and refractive outcome between patients who underwent laser refractive cataract surgery with a femtosecond laser and those with conventional cataract surgery.

METHODS: In this prospective study, 77 eyes from 77 patients underwent laser refractive cataract surgery (laser group; Alcon LenSx femtosecond laser), and conventional cataract surgery with phacoemulsification was performed in 57 eyes from 57 patients (conventional group). Biometry was done with optical low coherence reflectometry (Lenstar LS900, Haag-Streit AG), and IOL calculation was performed with third-generation IOL formulas (SRK/T, Hoffer Q, and Holladay). The refractive outcome was analyzed using the mean absolute error (MAE; difference between predicted and achieved postoperative spherical equivalent refraction), and multivariable regression analysis was performed to compare the two groups.

RESULTS: No significant differences were found between age, axial length, keratometry, and preoperative corrected visual acuity in the laser and conventional groups ($P>.05$; Mann-Whitney U test). At least 6 weeks after surgery, MAE was significantly lower in the laser group (0.38 ± 0.28 diopters [D]) than in the conventional group (0.50 ± 0.38 D) ($P=.04$). The difference was the greatest in short (axial length <22.0 mm, 0.43 ± 0.41 vs 0.63 ± 0.48) and long (axial length >26.0 mm, 0.33 ± 0.24 vs 0.63 ± 0.42) eyes.

CONCLUSIONS: Laser refractive cataract surgery with a femtosecond laser resulted in a significantly better predictability of IOL power calculation than conventional phacoemulsification surgery. This difference is possibly due to a more precise capsulorrhexis, resulting in a more stable IOL position. [*J Refract Surg*. 2012;28(8):540-544.]
doi:10.3928/1081597X-20120703-04

Originally published in Journal of Refractive Surgery, *August 2012.*

Laser refractive cataract surgery with an intraocular femtosecond laser became available recently to create controlled incisions through photodisruption in eye tissue.[1] Initial clinical results of our group demonstrated a more predictable capsulorrhexis and reduced effective phacoemulsification energy compared to conventional surgery in porcine and human eyes.[2] With the use of aberration-correcting or multifocal intraocular lenses (IOLs), there is a higher expectation to achieve a precise refractive outcome after cataract surgery. With the increasing use of optical biometry, the error in IOL power calculation is less likely due to imprecise axial length measurement but remains affected by the variability of the effective lens position after surgery.[3,4] Intraocular lens tilt, decentration, and anteroposterior movement contribute to variations in effective lens position and are, among other reasons, caused by variations in capsulotomy size, shape, and position. The use of an intraocular femtosecond laser to perform the capsulorrhexis was shown to result in higher predictability of the capsulotomy,[5,6] which may result in better refractive outcomes. We therefore compared IOL power calculation and refractive outcome in laser refractive cataract surgery and conventional phacoemulsification using optical biometry and three third-generation IOL calculation formulas.

Patients and Methods

Patients

In this prospective study, 77 eyes from 77 patients underwent laser refractive cataract surgery with an intraocular

Nagy ZZ, ed. *Femtosecond Laser-Assisted Cataract Surgery: Facts and Results* (pp 117-121).

femtosecond laser (Alcon LenSx, Ft Worth, Texas) (laser group), and conventional cataract surgery with phacoemulsification was performed on 57 eyes from 57 patients (conventional group). Table 1 shows the preoperative demographics; no significant differences were noted between groups regarding these parameters (P>.05; Mann-Whitney U test). Patients were randomly assigned to each group using a computer randomization chart. Exclusion criteria were previous ocular surgery, corneal diseases such as keratoconus, known zonular weakness, corneal astigmatism >3.00 diopters (D), anterior capsule tear, posterior capsule rupture, severe macular disease, and amblyopia. Every patient underwent a complete ophthalmologic evaluation, which included uncorrected (UDVA) and corrected distance visual acuity (CDVA), applanation tonometry, slit-lamp microscopy, and funduscopy.

The study was conducted in compliance with the Declaration of Helsinki, as well as with applicable country and local requirements regarding ethical committee/institutional review board, informed consent, and other statutes or regulations regarding protection of the rights and welfare of human subjects participating in biomedical research.

TABLE 1

PREOPERATIVE PATIENT DEMOGRAPHICS: FEMTOSECOND LASER AND CONVENTIONAL PHACOEMULSIFICATION*

	Mean±SD (Range)	
Parameter	***Laser Group (n=77)***	***Conventional Group (n=57)***
Age (y)	65.18±12.6 (23 to 88)	64.37±12.37 (23 to 86)
Axial length (mm)	23.93±2.62 (20.12 to 34.33)	24.07±2.28 (20.66 to 31.5)
Average K (D)	43.53±1.53 (39.67 to 47.56)	43.13±1.64 (39.89 to 47.45)
SE (D)	−1.62±5.55 (−23.00 to +7.75)	−1.37±5.27 (−18.00 to +8.50)
CDVA (logMAR)	0.45±0.29 (0 to 1.3)	0.37±0.26 (0 to 1.22)

SD = standard deviation, K = keratometry, SE = spherical equivalent, CDVA = corrected distance visual acuity
**No statistically significant differences were found between groups (Mann-Whitney U test).*

Surgery

Patients in the conventional group had uneventful cataract surgery with a 2.75-mm clear corneal incision at 120°, a side-port at 60°, manual continuous curvilinear capsulorrhexis (CCC) with an attempted diameter of 4.5 mm, phacoemulsification (Accurus; Alcon Laboratories Inc, Ft Worth, Texas) with the same technique (chop), and IOL implantation in the capsular bag.

Patients in the laser group underwent a laser procedure prior to the phacoemulsification surgery. All laser procedures were performed using the Alcon LenSx laser system. After pupillary dilation and instillation of topical or retrobulbar anesthesia, a curved applanator with a suction ring was applied. A 2.75-mm clear corneal laser incision at 120° and a 1.2-mm side-port at 60° were placed in all eyes. The capsulorrhexis was centered to the dilated pupil with a diameter of 4.5 mm and followed with a cross-shaped nucleus fragmentation with a diameter of 4.5 mm, extending 500 μm above the posterior capsule to 300 μm below the anterior capsule. Proprietary energy and spot separation parameters, which had been optimized in previous studies,[2] were used for all laser procedures. Loss of suction or capsular tag did not occur in any case in this study sample. Neither astigmatic keratotomy nor limbal relaxing incisions were performed. After the laser procedure, the corneal incisions were opened using a blunt spatula, viscoelastic material was injected (Provisc, Alcon Laboratories Inc), and the anterior capsule was removed with forceps. The nucleus fragments were removed using phacoemulsification, followed by irrigation-aspiration and implantation of an IOL in the bag.

Several IOLs were used in the course of this study (Alcon AcrySof MA30AC, n=37; MA60AC, n=23; SA60AT, n=8; Bausch & Lomb [Rochester, New York] LI60AO, n=43; Oculentis [Preisvergleich, Germany] L-302-1, n=16; and Medicontur [Zsámbék, Hungary] 690AB, n=7). The average power of the implanted IOLs was 20.34±5.92 D (range: −2.00 to +32.00 D). All operations were performed by the same surgeon (Z.Z.N.).

IOL Calculation

All patients had axial length and keratometry measurements by low coherence optical reflectometry (Lenstar LS900; Haag-Streit AG, Koeniz, Switzerland) before surgery. All three available third-generation IOL formulas (SRK/T, Hoffer Q, and Holladay 1) and optimized IOL constants were used for IOL calculation. To determine which formula to use, patients were divided into four subgroups. The Hoffer Q was used for short eyes (axial length <22.0 mm; n=20 [10 laser group and 10 conventional group]), the average of the three formulas for medium eyes (axial length 22.00 to 24.49 mm; n=81 [51 laser group and 30 conventional group]), the Holladay 1 for medium long eyes (axial length 24.50 to 25.99 mm; n=11 [4 laser group and 7 conventional group]), and the SRK/T for long eyes (axial length >26.0 mm, n=22 [12 laser group and 10 conventional

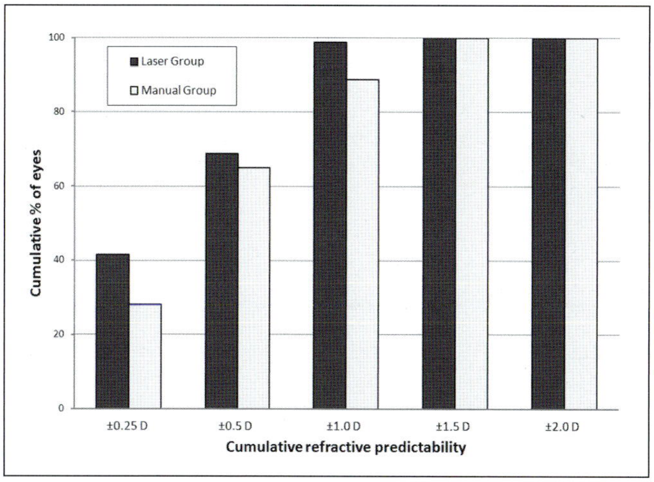

Figure 1. Cumulative refractive predictability of the eyes in the laser and conventional (manual) groups.

TABLE 2

POSTOPERATIVE OUTCOMES: FEMTOSECOND LASER AND CONVENTIONAL PHACOEMULSIFICATION

	Mean±SD (Range)	
Parameter	***Laser Group (n=77)***	***Conventional Group (n=57)***
MRSE (D)*	−0.50±1.06 (−5.00 to +1.25)	−0.58±1.28 (−4.125 to +2.125)
CDVA (logMAR)*	0.03±0.06 (0 to 0.26)	0.02±0.04 (0 to 0.22)
MAE (D)	0.38±0.28 (0 to 1.09)	0.50±0.38 (0 to 1.48)
ME (D)*	−0.03±0.47 (−1.09 to +0.97)	0.07±063 (−1.40 to +1.48)
Avg K (D)*	43.59±1.50 (39.88 to 46.97)	43.22±1.62 (39.98 to 47.58)
Follow-up (wk)*	9.72±2.82 (6 to 12)	9.67±2.66 (6 to 12)

SD = standard deviation, MRSE = manifest refraction spherical equivalent, CDVA = corrected distance visual acuity, MAE = mean absolute error, ME = mean error, K = keratometry
**No statistically significant differences were found between groups (Mann-Whitney U test).*

group]), as recommended in our national biometry protocol.

Postoperative refraction and CDVA were measured 6 to 12 weeks after surgery. Patients with CDVA 20/40 or worse were excluded (one patient in each group) to avoid errors in manifest refraction.

Mean absolute error (MAE) was calculated as the difference of the postoperative manifest refraction (spherical equivalent) and the predicted postoperative target refraction and used to analyze the accuracy of the power IOL calculation.

The MAE was calculated for all eyes to compare the two groups depending on the different IOL calculation formulas in all axial length subgroups. The percentage of eyes within ±0.25, ±0.50, ±1.00, ±1.50, and ±2.00 D of MAE was also determined.

Statistical Analysis

Statistical analyses were performed with SPSS 15.0 software (SPSS Inc, Chicago, Illinois). The Mann-Whitney U test was used for between-group comparisons of age and axial length. $P<.05$ was considered statistically significant. Correlation between MAE and axial length was tested using linear and nonlinear regression analysis. Multivariable regression analysis was performed to determine the effect of the type of surgery on postoperative refractive error after adjusting for the effect of axial length and IOL type. Akaike's Information Criterion was used to find the best fitting model.[7]

RESULTS

Table 2 presents the postoperative data. Comparing refractive predictability, 41.6% of eyes were within ±0.25 D of target refraction in the laser group compared to 28.1% of eyes in the conventional group; 68.8% and 64.9% were within ±0.50 D, respectively; and 98.7% and 87.7% were within ±1.00 D, respectively. All eyes were within ±1.50 D in both groups (Fig 1).

Using the IOL power calculation formulas described above, the MAE was 0.38±0.28 D for all eyes in the laser group and 0.50±0.38 D for all eyes in the conventional group. The correlation between axial length and MAE in the two groups is shown in Figure 2. Significant cubic correlation was found in the conventional group ($r=0.14$, $P=.011$), whereas no correlation was found in the laser group ($P>.05$).

In multivariable modeling, the type of surgery showed significant effect on the postoperative MAE after adjusting for the effect of axial length and IOL type ($P=.04$). In the laser group, the MAE was lower than in the conventional group, with an average difference of 0.12 D. The IOL type had no effect on postoperative refractive error ($P=.19$) in the multivariable regression analysis. Differences were largest in short (axial length <22.0 mm; MAE=0.43±0.41 vs 0.63±0.48) and long eyes (axial length >26.0 mm; MAE=0.33±0.24 vs 0.63±0.42), both in favor of the laser group.

Analyzing the mean error (ME), no significant difference was noted between groups (−0.03±0.47 vs 0.07±0.63, $P>.05$ [Mann-Whitney U test]). No correlation was found between ME and axial length in the laser group (*P*=.41). In the conventional group, a weak but significant correlation (r=−0.29, *P*=.03) was present, in which more myopic errors were found in eyes with long axial length.

Discussion

Cataract surgery is also refractive surgery and the use of modern aberration-correcting or multifocal or accommodating IOLs requires a high degree of refractive predictability. Optical biometry reduces the error in axial length measurements, but calculation errors are still caused by variations in effective lens position.[4] Despite precise calculation of the effective lens position, the real IOL position and refractive effect depend on other factors, such as lens thickness, refraction, and age.[8] Our IOL calculation results are in agreement with previously published large studies using ultrasound[9] and laser interferometry[10] for IOL calculation.

We found a subtle but significant difference (0.12 D) in postoperative IOL power calculation error and better refractive outcomes after laser refractive cataract surgery with an intraocular femtosecond laser than after conventional phacoemulsification cataract surgery, when evaluated in multivariate analysis. The difference between IOL power calculation errors was highest in short (0.20 D) and long (0.30 D) eyes. Presumably, the higher the IOL power (short eyes), the higher the refractive change due to IOL displacement.[11] Moreover, it was previously shown that IOL tilt, decentration, and anteroposterior movement are greater in long eyes.[6] In previous studies, we measured and compared sizing and positioning parameters of femtosecond laser capsulotomy with manual continuous curvilinear capsulorrhexis.[5] We found that more precise capsulotomy sizing, circularity, and centering can be achieved with a femtosecond laser. Properly sized, shaped, and centered femtosecond laser capsulotomies resulted in better overlap parameters. More consistent capsulorrhexis may explain smaller variations in IOL position, effecting the refractive outcome.[5,6]

Intraocular lens misalignment is a well-known factor that can induce changes in postoperative refraction.[11-15] Several studies used different methods for IOL power calculation, but did not differ in conclusions. Intraocular lens decentration and tilt induce myopic shift and oblique astigmatism, cause lateral shift of focus, and the resulting refractive error depends on the amount of decentration and tilt. Longitudinal IOL position errors are the principal component of visual outcome, whereas alignment errors have minor but significant effects on postoperative refraction.[14] Some authors used

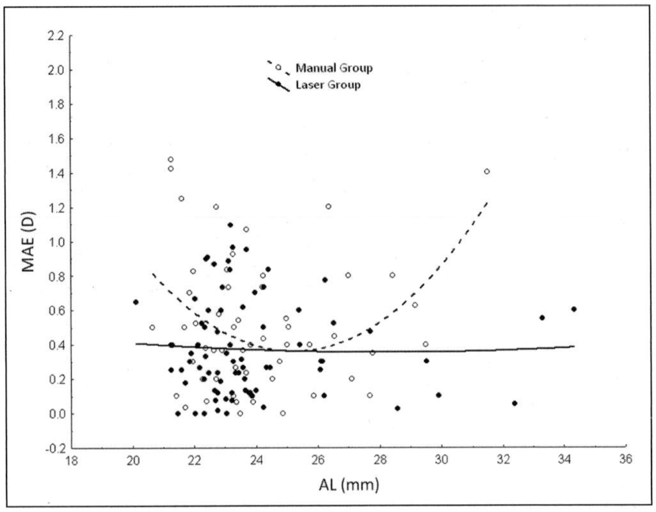

Figure 2. Correlation between axial length (AL) (Lenstar LS900) and mean absolute error (MAE) following laser refractive cataract surgery with a femtosecond laser (laser group) and conventional phacoemulsification (manual group).

a computer program to model the visual impairment caused by IOL misalignment.[16] Aberration-free IOLs were proven to be less sensitive to decentration and tilt than aberration-correcting IOLs.[17] The type and shape of the capsulorrhexis has a major effect on IOL position. Conventional CCC was shown to be safer and less likely to be associated with anterior capsular tears than a can opener or linear capsulotomy,[18] and showed less IOL decentration and tilt.[19-21] Even with an intact CCC, asymmetric capsular shrinkage, which is affected by capsulotomy shape, increases IOL decentration.[22] Furthermore, the size of the capsulotomy and the area and regularity of anterior capsule–IOL overlap influence the IOL position.[23]

In previous studies, our research group established that the decentration and tilt of an IOL can be significantly decreased when the capsulorrhexis is performed with a femtosecond laser as compared to the standard conventional technique.[5,6] In this study, we found that the use of an intraocular femtosecond laser resulted in significantly lower IOL power calculation errors as expressed by a smaller MAE than in manual capsulorrhexis. The more predictable size, shape, and position of a femtosecond laser–created capsulorrhexis may contribute to minimized IOL misalignment, decentration, and tilt and therefore results in a smaller variability of the precalculated effective lens position. A limitation of our study is that several different IOL types were used; however, statistical analysis did not show a correlation based on IOL type.

AUTHOR CONTRIBUTIONS

Study concept and design (T.F., Z.Z.N.); data collection (T.F., A.T., E.H.); analysis and interpretation of data (T.F., I.K., M.C.K.); drafting of the manuscript (T.F.); critical revision of the manuscript (I.K., A.T., E.H., M.C.K., Z.Z.N.); statistical expertise (T.F., I.K.); administrative, technical, or material support (Z.Z.N.); supervision (I.K., Z.Z.N.)

REFERENCES

1. Krueger RR, Kuszak J, Lubatschowski H, Myers RI, Ripken T, Heisterkamp A. First safety study of femtosecond laser photodisruption in animal lenses: tissue morphology and cataractogenesis. *J Cataract Refract Surg.* 2005;31(12):2386-2394.
2. Nagy Z, Takacs A, Filkorn T, Sarayba M. Initial clinical evaluation of an intraocular femtosecond laser in cataract surgery. *J Refract Surg.* 2009;25(12):1053-1060.
3. Olsen T. Sources of error in intraocular lens power calculation. *J Cataract Refract Surg.* 1992;18(2):125-129.
4. Norrby S. Sources of error in intraocular lens power calculation. *J Cataract Refract Surg.* 2008;34(3):368-376.
5. Kránitz K, Takacs A, Miháltz K, Kovács I, Knorz MC, Nagy ZZ. Femtosecond laser capsulotomy and manual continuous curvilinear capsulorrhexis parameters and their effects on intraocular lens centration. *J Refract Surg.* 2011;27(8):558-563.
6. Nagy ZZ, Kránitz K, Takacs AI, Miháltz K, Kovács I, Knorz MC. Comparison of intraocular lens decentration parameters after femtosecond and manual capsulotomies. *J Refract Surg.* 2011;27(8):564-569.
7. Akaike H. A new look at the statistical model identification. *IEEE Transactions on Automatic Control.* 1974;19(6):716-723.
8. Olsen T. Prediction of the effective postoperative (intraocular lens) anterior chamber depth. *J Cataract Refract Surg.* 2006;32(3):419-424.
9. Gale RP, Saha N, Johnston RL. National Biometry Audit II. *Eye (Lond).* 2006;20(1):25-28.
10. Aristodemou P, Knox Cartwright NE, Sparrow JM, Johnston RL. Formula choice: Hoffer Q, Holladay 1, or SRK/T and refractive outcomes in 8108 eyes after cataract surgery with biometry by partial coherence interferometry. *J Cataract Refract Surg.* 2011;37(1):63-71.
11. Lakshminarayanan V, Enoch JM, Raasch T, Crawford B, Nygaard RW. Refractive changes induced by intraocular lens tilt and longitudinal displacement. *Arch Ophthalmol.* 1986;104(1):90-92.
12. Atchison DA. Refractive errors induced by displacement of intraocular lenses within the pseudophakic eye. *Optom Vis Sci.* 1989;66(3):146-152.
13. Erickson P. Effects of intraocular lens position errors on postoperative refractive error. *J Cataract Refract Surg.* 1990;16(3):305-311.
14. Kozaki J, Tanihara H, Yasuda A, Nagata M. Tilt and decentration of the implanted posterior chamber intraocular lens. *J Cataract Refract Surg.* 1991;17(5):592-595.
15. Korynta J, Bok J, Cendelin J. Changes in refraction induced by change in intraocular lens position. *J Refract Corneal Surg.* 1994;10(5):556-564.
16. Korynta J, Bok J, Cendelin J, Michalova K. Computer modeling of visual impairment caused by intraocular lens misalignment. *J Cataract Refract Surg.* 1999;25(1):100-105.
17. Eppig T, Scholz K, Löffler A, Messner A, Langenbucher A. Effect of decentration and tilt on the image quality of aspheric intraocular lens designs in a model eye. *J Cataract Refract Surg.* 2009;35(6):1091-1100.
18. Assia EI, Apple DJ, Barden A, Tsai JC, Castaneda VE, Hoggatt JS. An experimental study comparing various anterior capsulectomy techniques. *Arch Ophthalmol.* 1991;109(5):642-647.
19. Caballero A, López MC, Losada M, Pérez Flores D, Salinas M. Long-term decentration of intraocular lenses implanted with envelope capsulotomy and continuous curvilinear capsulotomy: a comparative study. *J Cataract Refract Surg.* 1995;21(3):287-292.
20. Akkin C, Ozler SA, Mentes J. Tilt and decentration of bag-fixated intraocular lenses: a comparative study between capsulorhexis and envelope techniques. *Doc Ophthalmol.* 1994;87(3):199-209.
21. Oner FH, Durak I, Soylev M, Ergin M. Long-term results of various anterior capsulotomies and radial tears on intraocular lens centration. *Ophthalmic Surg Lasers.* 2001;32(2):118-123.
22. Ohmi S. Decentration associated with asymmetric capsular shrinkage and intraocular lens size. *J Cataract Refract Surg.* 1993;19(5):640-643.
23. Nanavaty MA, Raj SM, Vasavada VA, Vasavada VA, Vasavada AR. Anterior capsule cover and axial movement of intraocular lens. *Eye (Lond).* 2008;22(8):1015-1023.

The Effect of Femtosecond Laser Capsulotomy on the Development of Posterior Capsule Opacification

Illés Kovács, MD, PhD; Kinga Kránitz, MD; Gábor L. Sándor, MD; Michael C. Knorz, MD; Eric D. Donnenfeld, MD, FACS; Rudy M. Nuijts, MD, PhD; Zoltán Z. Nagy, MD, DSC

Abstract

PURPOSE: To evaluate and compare the effects of femtosecond laser-assisted anterior capsulotomy and manual anterior capsulorhexis on posterior capsule opacification (PCO) development.

METHODS: Femtosecond laser-assisted anterior capsulotomy was performed in 40 eyes of 40 patients (FS group) and manual anterior capsulorhexis was performed in 39 eyes of 39 patients (CCC group). An AcrySof one-piece hydrophobic acrylic intraocular lens (Alcon Laboratories, Inc., Fort Worth, TX) was implanted in all eyes. The PCO level was measured using Open-Access Systematic Capsule Assessment (OSCA) software 18 to 26 months after surgery. Postoperative intraocular lens position (ie, tilt and decentration) was measured using Scheimpflug images (Pentacam; Oculus Optikgeräte GmbH, Wetzlar, Germany).

RESULTS: There was no statistically significant difference in age, axial length, and follow-up time between the two groups ($P > .05$). Vertical tilt, horizontal and total decentration of intraocular lenses, and PCO proved to be significantly higher in the CCC group ($P = .03$, .04, .03, and .01, respectively). After adjusting for axial length and follow-up time, manual anterior capsulorhexis was found to be a significant predictor of higher PCO scores in the multivariable regression model (β: 0.33; 95% CI: 0.01 to 0.65; $P = .04$). Vertical tilt affected PCO scores after adjusting for axial length and follow-up time (β: 0.07; 95% CI: 0.01 to 0.12; $P = .02$). No capsulotomies were performed during follow-up in either group.

CONCLUSIONS: Femtosecond laser-assisted anterior capsulotomy proved to be a safe procedure for postoperative PCO rates. Due to better intraocular lens position, femtosecond laser-assisted anterior capsulotomy resulted in slightly decreased PCO scores; however, evaluating its clinical significance requires further studies.

[*J Refract Surg.* 2014;30(3):154-158.]

Originally published in Journal of Refractive Surgery, *March 2014.*

Posterior capsule opacification (PCO) is currently the most common postoperative complication and is caused by migration and proliferation of lens epithelial cells that remain in the capsular bag.[1,2] Creating a precise anterior capsulorhexis is essential to avoid PCO because a 360° overlapping capsular edge prevents optic decentration and tilt due to symmetric contractile forces of the capsular bag and shrink-wrap effect.[3] However, an eccentric or irregularly shaped capsulorhexis extending beyond the optic edge of the intraocular lens may result in malpositioned intraocular lens with incomplete anterior capsule overlap, which in turn may result in higher incidence of PCO through migration of retained lens epithelial cells because of an incomplete barrier.[4,5] Until recently, capsulorhexis has been a manual procedure. However, femtosecond laser technology enables surgeons to create precise and reproducible capsulotomies.[6]

In our previous studies, properly sized, shaped, and centered femtosecond laser-assisted anterior capsulotomy resulted in better overlap parameters compared to manual anterior capsulorhexis during the postoperative first year. A 360° overlapping capsular edge was thought to be important for standardizing refractive results by keeping the intraocular lens in the desired center position and preventing tilt.[5,7]

The purpose of this study was to evaluate the effects of femtosecond laser-assisted anterior capsulotomy and manual anterior capsulorhexis on PCO development in the intermediate term.

doi:10.3928/1081597X-20140217-01

Nagy ZZ, ed. *Femtosecond Laser-Assisted Cataract Surgery: Facts and Results* (pp 123-127).

Patients and Methods

Patient Population

In this study, PCO levels were retrospectively evaluated in 79 eyes of 79 patients at the Department of Ophthalmology at Semmelweis University, Budapest, Hungary. All patients from a previous prospective, randomized study on femtosecond laser surgery with a minimum follow-up time of 18 months were identified in our database and their data were processed for further statistical analyses. Femtosecond laser-assisted anterior capsulotomy (creating a 4.9-mm anterior capsulotomy) was performed in 40 eyes of 40 patients (FS group). At the same time, 39 eyes of 39 patients receiving manual anterior capsulorhexis with attempted 4.9-mm capsulotomy served as controls (CCC group). In all cases, an AcrySof hydrophobic acrylic, one-piece intraocular lens (Alcon Laboratories, Inc., Fort Worth, TX) with a 6-mm optic was implanted in the capsular bag.

All patients had undergone preoperative ophthalmologic evaluations. Patients with previous ocular surgery, trauma, active ocular disease (eg, pseudoexfoliation syndrome and uveitis), poorly dilated pupils, or known zonular weakness were excluded. The study was conducted in compliance with the Declaration of Helsinki, applicable country and local requirements regarding ethics committees and institutional review boards, and other statutes or regulations regarding protection of the rights and welfare of human subjects participating in biomedical research. Written, informed consent was obtained from participants before surgery.

Surgical Technique

Axial length measurements were performed using the Lenstar LS 900 optical biometer (Haag-Streit AG, Koeniz, Switzerland). The surgical technique was standardized in all patients, except for capsulorhexis. All surgeries were performed by the same surgeon. After pupillary dilation (1 drop of tropicamide 0.5% every 15 minutes [3 times]) and instillation of topical anesthetic (proparacaine hydrochloride 0.5%), the laser (LenSx; Alcon Laboratories, Inc.) was docked to the eyes using a curved contact lens to applanate the cornea. The location of the crystalline lens surface was found with an integrated optical coherence tomography imaging system. A 4.9-mm diameter capsulotomy was performed by scanning a cylindrical pattern starting at least 300 μm below the anterior capsule and ending at least 300 μm above the anterior capsule. The capsulotomy was centered on the dilated pupil. Proprietary energy and spot separation parameters (optimized in previous studies) were used. A 4.9-mm manual anterior capsulorhexis (centered on the dilated pupil) was attempted in the CCC group and performed with a cystotome and forceps; a capsulorhexis marker was not used. In both groups, corneal incisions were made with a disposable keratome (Alcon Laboratories, Inc.). After hydrodissection, standard phacoemulsification of the nucleus and aspiration of the residual cortex were performed using the Infinity Vision System (Alcon Laboratories, Inc.) in both groups.

In all cases, one-piece hydrophobic acrylic intraocular lenses were folded and implanted in the capsular bag with injection cartridges through the corneal wounds. Intraocular lens power was calculated using the SRK-T formula. After intraocular lens implantation, viscoelastic material was removed from the anterior chamber and capsular bag by irrigation or aspiration. All corneal incisions were left sutureless. No intraoperative or postoperative complications occurred. During the first postoperative 10 days, patients received a combination of dexamethasone 0.1% and tobramycin 0.3% drops four times a day.

PCO Analysis

Digital retroillumination photographs were taken under maximal pupil dilation (focusing the camera on the posterior capsule) 18 to 26 months postoperatively and imported to an open-access software platform for masked, objective PCO evaluation.[8] Two images (showing various angles) of one eye were used to identify and remove light reflections. During PCO evaluation, OSCA used location-sensitive, entropy-based texture analysis to calculate PCO scores. Validation analyses of this method showed PCO scores correlate with contrast sensitivity and visual acuity (two factors significantly affected by PCO), thus providing an objective, valid, and reliable method of PCO quantification. The range of possible OSCA scores is 0 (no PCO) to approximately 15 (practical expected maximum). Typical OSCA values were approximately 0.5 for images with very little or no PCO. OSCA values for patients warranting laser capsulotomy were approximately 4 to 5.[8]

Evaluation of Postoperative Intraocular Lens Position

A Scheimpflug imaging system (Pentacam; Oculus Optikgeräte GmbH, Wetzlar, Germany) was used to evaluate intraocular lens tilt and decentration 12 months postoperatively. Decentration and tilt were measured according to de Castro et al.[9] as follows. Intraocular lens decentration is obtained from the distance between the intraocular lens center and pupillary axis. Positive horizontal coordinates represent nasal in the right eye and temporal in the left eye. Positive vertical coordinates represent superior decentrations and negative vertical coordinates represent inferior decentrations. Using ab-

TABLE 1
DESCRIPTIVE STATISTICS OF THE TWO GROUPS

Variable	FS Group (n = 40) Mean	FS Group (n = 40) SD	CCC Group (n = 39) Mean	CCC Group (n = 39) SD	P
Age (y)	65.50	12.94	68.95	10.84	.37
Gender (female:male)	28:12		29:10		.67[a]
Axial length (mm)	23.25	1.48	23.82	1.93	.31
Follow-up (months)	22.37	4.36	21.74	5.46	.30
Horizontal tilt (degrees)	2.01	2.24	2.24	1.36	.69
Vertical tilt (degrees)	3.50	2.13	5.10	2.23	.03
Vertical decentration (μm)	106.32	114.66	158.50	101.27	.14
Horizontal decentration (μm)	154.74	126.24	260.50	187.07	.05
Total decentration (μm)	212.01	126.62	320.54	172.07	.03
PCO level (OSCA score)	0.58	0.30	0.84	0.52	.01

FS = femtosecond laser-assisted capsulotomy; CCC = manual capsulorhexis; SD = standard deviation; PCO = posterior capsule opacification; OSCA = Open-Access Systematic Capsule Assessment (Osca, Inc., Carson, CA)
[a]Chi-square test.

solute values, the magnitude of horizontal and vertical decentrations is determined without reference to nasal or temporal and superior or inferior orientations. Total decentration (determined by trigonometry analysis) shows the magnitude of the resulting vector of horizontal and vertical decentrations. For intraocular lens tilt, positive vertical tilt around the horizontal axis indicates the superior edge has moved forward, whereas negative vertical tilt means it moved backward. Positive horizontal tilt around the vertical axis in the right eye indicates the nasal edge of the intraocular lens moved backward and positive horizontal tilt in the left eye shows it moved forward. Negative horizontal tilt values correspond to similar temporal edge movements. By expressing tilt as absolute values, magnitudes of horizontal and vertical tilt are determined without reference to orientation.

Statistical Analysis

Statistical analyses were performed using SPSS version 16.0 (SPSS, Inc., Chicago, IL). A *P* value less than .05 was considered significant. Departure from normal distribution assumption was tested by the Shapiro-Wilks *W* test. Due to normality of data, descriptive statistics show mean and standard deviation. The Student's *t* test for independent samples was used to compare FS group and CCC group data. To determine the effect of multiple predictors on PCO, multivariable regression analyses were performed via generalized estimating equation models by adding axial length and follow-up time as covariates to adjust for their effects on PCO development. Generalized estimating equation models were used to show possible dependencies between predictor variables, therefore providing reasonable estimates of regression coefficients and standard errors.

RESULTS

Age, gender, and axial length were not statistically significantly different between the two groups (**Table 1**).

In all cases, a 360° overlapping anterior capsulorhexis was created. However, there were statistically significant postoperative differences in both decentration and tilt values between the two groups. Significantly higher vertical intraocular lens tilt was measured in the CCC group (**Table 1**). There were also higher horizontal and total decentration values in the CCC group than in the FS group (**Table 1**). PCO levels were significantly lower in the FS group (0.58 ± 0.30) compared to the CCC group (0.84 ± 0.52) ($P = .01$) (**Table 1**). No capsulotomies were performed during follow-up.

After adjusting for axial length and follow-up time, manual anterior capsulorhexis was found to be a significant predictor for PCO development in the multivariable regression model (β: 0.33; 95% CI: 0.01 to 0.65; $P = .04$). Neither axial length nor follow-up time were significant PCO predictors in this model ($P > .05$ for both parameters). Among postoperative intraocular lens position parameters, only vertical tilt showed significant correlation with PCO levels in both groups (FS: r = 0.58, $P < .001$; CCC: r = 0.35, $P = .03$) (**Figure 1**). Similarly, in multivariable modeling, vertical tilt was a significant predictor of postoperative PCO after adjusting for the effect of axial length, follow-up time, and capsulorhexis type (β: 0.07; 95% CI: 0.01 to 0.12; $P = .02$).

Discussion

PCO is the most frequent long-term complication following phacoemulsification with intraocular lens implantation.[1] Although Nd:YAG laser capsulotomy is effective treatment for PCO, increased intraocular pressure, cystoid macular edema, and retinal detachment are known complications.[10]

Design and diameter of intraocular optics, intraocular lens material, edge profile, and optic–haptic junction influence PCO development. Moreover, implantation of an intraocular lens in the capsular bag with complete anterior capsular overlap has significant, preventative effects on PCO development.[5,11-13]

Creating a properly sized and centered anterior capsulorhexis to achieve complete anterior capsular overlap is often challenging, but surgery has become more standardized with the advent of femtosecond lasers. According to our previous results, femtosecond laser-assisted anterior capsulotomies are round and reproducible with accurate diameters, whereas manual anterior capsulorhexes can be irregular in shape and it is difficult to control centration.[6] A properly sized and centered anterior capsulotomy results in complete, circular overlap, maintaining the correct postoperative position of the implanted intraocular lens.[4,7] In this study, we found statistically significant differences between the FS and CCC groups for intraocular lens positioning parameters. Postoperative vertical tilt and horizontal and total decentrations proved to be significantly higher in the CCC group compared to the FS group, confirming our previously published results.

According to multivariable statistical analyses, capsulorhexis type was found to be an independent, significant predictor of PCO after adjusting for the effects of axial length and follow-up time (which were already described as predictors of PCO).[1,14] After adjusting for axial length and follow-up time, manual anterior capsulorhexis increased PCO scores by 33% compared to femtosecond laser-assisted anterior capsulotomy in our series. Neither axial length nor follow-up time proved to be significant PCO predictors. There was a statistically significant, positive correlation between vertical tilt and PCO severity. According to multivariable modeling, after adjusting for the effects of axial length, follow-up time, and capsulorhexis type (laser-assisted or manual) every 1° of intraocular lens tilt resulted in a 7% increase in PCO scores. These results support the barrier principle in PCO prevention that is based on symmetric contractile forces of a 360° overlapping anterior capsular edge pushing the intraocular lens optic to the posterior capsule, leading to continuous circular contact between them, and creating an effective barrier to migrating lens epithelial cells. In our study, a 360° overlapping anterior capsulorhexis was created in both groups and there was no difference in irrigation and aspiration techniques or time.

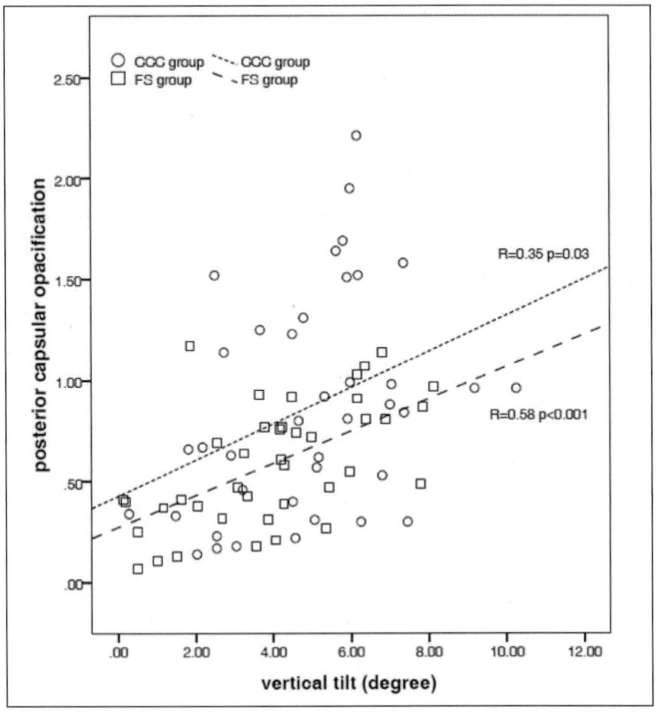

Figure 1. Significant correlation between vertical intraocular lens tilt and posterior capsular opacification in the femtosecond laser-assisted capsulotomy (FS) group (r = 0.58; $P < .001$) and manual anterior capsulorhexis (CCC) group (r = 0.35; $P = .03$).

According to our previous results, more accurate capsulotomies are performed with femtosecond lasers than manually in eyes with emmetropia or high mypopia.[15] When performing a capsulotomy for eyes with high myopia, it is important to provide perfect overlap and a continuous, circular barrier for lens epithelial cells to prevent PCO because laser capsulotomy has an increased risk for retinal detachment in eyes with longer axial length.[16]

Our results suggest a centered and accurate anterior capsulotomy may have an additive role to intraocular lens edge design and hydrophobic intraocular lens material for PCO prevention. In this study, no capsulotomies were required because of severe PCO and femtosecond laser-assisted anterior capsulotomy proved to be a safe procedure that did not increase PCO scores. In fact, we observed a slight decrease in PCO formation, which is a supplemental advantage of this method. Further studies are needed in patient groups at increased risk for PCO development to assess the clinical significance of these results.

Author Contributions

Study concept and design (EDD, IK, KK, ZZN); data collection (ZZN, GLS); analysis and interpretation of data (MCK, IK, KK, RMN); drafting of the manuscript (IK); critical revision of the manuscript (EDD, MCK, KK, ZZN, RMN, GLS); statistical expertise (IK); administrative, technical, or material support (ZZN); supervision (EDD, IK, KK, ZZN)

References

1. Schaumberg DA, Dana MR, Christen WG, Glynn RJ. A systematic overview of the incidence of posterior capsule opacification. *Ophthalmology*.1998;105:1213-1221.
2. Nishi O, Nishi K, Sakanishi K. Inhibition of migrating lens epithelial cells at the capsular bend created by the rectangular optic edge of a posterior chamber intraocular lens. *Ophthalmic Surg Lasers*. 1998;29:587-594.
3. Ravalico G, Tognetto D, Palomba M, Busatto P, Baccara F. Capsulorhexis size and posterior capsule opacification. *J Cataract Refract Surg*. 1996;22:98-103.
4. Kránitz K, Miháltz K, Sándor GL, Takacs A, Knorz MC, Nagy ZZ. Intraocular lens tilt and decentration measured by Scheimpflug camera following manual or femtosecond laser created continuous circular capsulotomy. *J Refract Surg*. 2012;28:259-263.
5. Smith SR, Daynes T, Hinckley M, Wallin TR, Olson RJ. The effect of lens edge design versus anterior capsule overlap on posterior capsule opacification. *Am J Ophthalmol*. 2004;138:521-526.
6. Nagy Z, Takacs A, Filkorn T, Sarayba M. Initial clinical evaluation of an intraocular femtosecond laser in cataract surgery. *J Refract Surg*. 2009;25:1053-1060.
7. Kránitz K, Takacs A, Miháltz K, Kovács I, Knorz MC, Nagy ZZ. Femtosecond laser capsulotomy and manual continuous curvilinear capsulorrhexis parameters and their effects on intraocular lens centration. *J Refract Surg*. 2011;27:558-563.
8. Aslam TM, Patton N, Rose CJ. OSCA: a comprehensive open-access system of analysis of posterior capsular opacification. *BMC Ophthalmol*. 2006;6:30.
9. de Castro A, Rosales P, Marcos S. Tilt and decentration of intraocular lenses in vivo from Purkinje and Scheimpflug imaging. Validation study. *J Cataract Refract Surg*. 2007;33:418-429.
10. Burq MA, Taqui AM. Frequency of retinal detachment and other complications after neodymium:YAG laser capsulotomy. *J Pak Med Assoc*. 2008;58:550-552.
11. Hollick EJ, Spalton DJ, Ursell PG, et al. The effect of PMMA, silicone, and polyacrylic lenses on posterior capsule opacification 3 years after surgery. *Ophthalmology*. 1998;106:49-54.
12. Schmidbauer JM, Escobar-Gomez M, Apple DJ, Peng Q, Arthur SN, Vargas LG. Effect of haptic angulation on posterior capsule opacification in modern foldable lenses with a square, truncated optic edge. *J Cataract Refract Surg*. 2002;28:1251-1255.
13. Meacock WR, Spalton DJ, Boyce JF, Jose RM. Effect of optic size on posterior capsule opacification: 5.5mm versus 6.0mm AcrySof intraocular lenses. *J Cataract Refract Surg*. 2001;27:1194-1198.
14. Zhao Y, Li J, Lu W, et al. Capsular adhesion to intraocular lens in highly myopic eyes evaluated in vivo using ultralong-scan depth optical coherence tomography. *Am J Ophthalmol*. 2013;155:484-491.
15. Nagy ZZ, Kránitz K, Takacs AI, Miháltz K, Kovács I, Knorz MC. Comparison of intraocular lens decentration parameters after femtosecond and manual capsulotomies. *J Refract Surg*. 2011;27:564-569.
16. Dardenne MU, Gerten GJ, Kokkas K, Kermani O. Retrospective study of retinal detachment following neodymium: YAG laser posterior capsulotomy. *J Cataract Refract Surg*. 1989;15:676-680.

Effect of Femtosecond Laser Cataract Surgery on the Macula

Mónika Ecsedy, MD; Kata Miháltz, MD; Illés Kovács, MD, PhD; Ágnes Takács, MD; Tamás Filkorn, MD; Zoltán Z. Nagy, MD, DSc

Abstract

PURPOSE: To compare the effect of conventional and femtosecond laser–assisted (Alcon LenSx Inc) phacoemulsification on the macula using optical coherence tomography (OCT).

METHODS: Twenty eyes of 20 patients underwent uneventful cataract surgery in both study groups: femtosecond laser–assisted (laser group) and conventional phacoemulsification (control group). Macular thickness and volume were evaluated by OCT preoperatively and 1 week and 1 month postoperatively. Primary outcomes were OCT retinal thickness in 3 macular areas and total macular volume at 1 week and 1 month postoperative. Secondary outcomes were changes in retinal thickness at 1 week and 1 month postoperatively, with respect to preoperative retinal thickness values and effective phacoemulsification time.

RESULTS: Multivariable modeling of the effect of surgery on postoperative macular thickness showed significantly lower macular thickness in the inner retinal ring in the laser group after adjusting for age and preoperative thickness across the time course (P=.002). In the control group, the inner macular ring was significantly thicker at 1 week (mean: 21.68 μm; 95% confidence limit [CL]: 11.93-31.44 μm, P<.001). After 1 month, this difference decreased to a mean of 17.56 μm (95% CL: −3.21-38.32 μm, P=.09) and became marginally significant.

CONCLUSIONS: Results of this study suggest that femtosecond laser–assisted cataract extraction does not differ in postoperative macular thickness as compared with standard ultrasound phacoemulsification.
[*J Refract Surg*. 2011;27(10):717-722.]
doi:10.3928/1081597X-20110825-01

Originally published in Journal of Refractive Surgery, *October 2011.*

Initial results of our study group with an intraocular femtosecond laser (LenSx laser system; Alcon LenSx Inc, Aliso Viejo, California) used during phacoemulsification have demonstrated higher precision and safety of capsulorrhexis and reduced phacoemulsification power in porcine and human eyes as compared to traditional techniques.[1]

During the femtosecond laser procedure, a suction ring is applied to avoid eye movements and laser misdirection, exerting pressure on the pars plana region at the limbus. Previous experimental and clinical studies demonstrated that the application of the suction ring causes short but considerable fluctuations (up to 40 mmHg in the LenSx technique) in intraocular pressure,[2] which can induce several changes in ocular structure—from the deterioration of goblet cells of the conjunctiva up to the retina.[3] During application of microkeratome suction in LASIK, a decrease in the lens thickness and an increase of the vitreous distance have been described, suggesting anterior traction on the posterior segment.[4] These alterations can cause posterior hyaloid detachment, transient choroidal circulation abnormalities,[5,6] macular hemorrhage,[7] and optic atrophy.[8]

On the other hand, phacoemulsification itself may induce postoperative macular edema owing to its traumatic effect. Clinical cystoid macular edema is one of the most common complications, with a prevalence of 0.1% to 12.0%.[9,10] Furthermore, studies using angiographic assessment have shown an incidence of subclinical perifoveal leakage up to 19% after cataract surgery.[11,12] Recent studies using optical coherence tomography (OCT) also demonstrated that uncomplicated phacoemulsification is followed by increase of the parafoveal retinal thickness, foveal volume, and volume of the entire macula.[13-16]

Nagy ZZ, ed. *Femtosecond Laser-Assisted Cataract Surgery: Facts and Results* (pp 129-134).

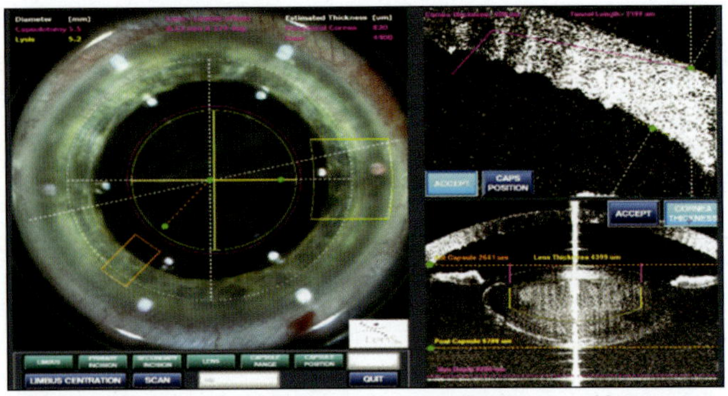

Figure 1. Photograph of the intraoperative femtosecond laser monitor and real-time optical coherence tomography scan. The corneal incision, capsulorrhexis, and lens fragmentation can be visualized.

The purpose of this study was to evaluate effects of femtosecond laser–assisted cataract surgery on macular thickness to that of traditional phacoemulsification using OCT measurements.

PATIENTS AND METHODS

Patients

In this prospective study, femtosecond laser–assisted phacoemulsification with the LenSx laser system was carried out in 20 eyes from 20 patients with cataract (laser group). Traditional phacoemulsification was performed on 20 eyes from 20 additional patients with cataract (control group). Patients with previous ocular surgery, trauma, other ocular disease, and known macular alteration (patients with diabetic retinopathy or age-related macular degeneration) were excluded from the study.

The study was conducted in compliance with the Declaration of Helsinki, as well as with applicable country and local requirements regarding ethics committee/institutional review boards, informed consent, and other statutes or regulations regarding protection of the rights and welfare of human subjects participating in biomedical research.

Surgery

All surgeries were performed by the same surgeon (Z.Z.N.) using the Accurus (Alcon Laboratories Inc, Ft Worth, Texas) phacoemulsification machine.

After pupillary dilation and instillation of topical anesthetics or retrobulbar anesthesia, the following procedures were performed by the femtosecond laser system. The LenSx laser system uses a curved contact lens to applanate the cornea. The location of the crystalline lens surface is determined following applanation using OCT. A 4.5-mm diameter capsulotomy procedure was performed by scanning a cylindrical pattern starting at least 100 μm below the anterior capsule and ending at least 200 μm above the capsule. For lens fragmentation, a cross pattern was used to fragment the crystalline lens into four quadrants. The laser created a self-sealing biplanar corneal incision (2.8 mm) and a side-port incision (1.0 mm). Proprietary energy and spot separation parameters (lens fragmentation: 11-μJ spot and layer separation 8/6 μm; capsulotomy 13 μJ; and primary and secondary corneal incision 6-μJ spot separation 6 μm and layer separation 3 μm), which had been optimized in previous studies, were used (Fig 1).

After femtolaser pretreatment, the patient was brought to the main operating room. The self-sealing corneal incisions were opened by a blunt spatula, and the anterior chamber was filled with viscoelastic material. The 4.5-mm diameter capsulotomy was identified with a cystotome and the capsule as a whole was pulled out of the eye with rhexis forceps, followed by hydrodissection. The lens was divided into four quadrants with the aid of a chopper without using any phaco energy. The four lens quadrants were removed with traditional phacoemulsification technique. Surgery concluded with cortex removal and implantation of a one-piece, hydrophobic, acrylic, posterior chamber lens and the viscoelastic material was completely removed by irrigation-aspiration. In the laser group, no hydration of the corneal wound was necessary because of the self-sealing nature of the wound. In the traditional phacoemulsification (control) group, the divide and conquer technique was used for lens fragmentation.

No intra- or postoperative complications occurred during any procedure. Within the first 10 days, all patients used a combination of antibiotic and steroid eye drops (tobramycin and dexamethasone, Tobradex; Alcon Laboratories Inc) five times daily. Nonsteriodal anti-inflammatory drugs were not used.

OCT Measurements

Optical coherence tomography measurements (Stratus OCT3; Carl Zeiss Meditec, Dublin, California) were performed 2 hours before surgery and postoperatively at 1 week and 1 month. Macular measurements were performed using the Early Treatment of Diabetic Retinopathy Study (ETDRS) macular mapping protocol, which consists of six individual line scans regularly arranged in a radial pattern with a scan length of 6 mm. Scans were performed using a default axial length (24.46 mm) and refractive error (right eye) for consistency with usual clinical practice. The scans were accepted if free of artifacts, and complete cross-sectional images were seen for all individual line scans. Retinal thickness was automatically determined by the instrument software as the distance between the internal limiting membrane and retinal pigment epithelium. Measurements were provided for three concentric regions. The central disc (foveal region) was a region with a radius of 0.5 mm (CSMT), and the inner and outer rings had outer radii of 1.5 and 3 mm, respectively, and were divided into four quadrants. Average retinal thickness was provided for each of the nine regions, and total macular volume (TMV) was calculated by the software automatically from these data. Foveal thickness (FT) was measured by the software at the cutting point of the six individual line scans. The average retinal thicknesses of the four inner (inner macular ring AT) and the four outer segments (outer macular ring AT) were also calculated.

Statistical Analysis

Statistical analyses were performed with SPSS 15.0 software (SPSS Inc, Chicago, Illinois). Data are expressed as median with the corresponding interquartile range (IQR). For group comparisons, the Mann-Whitney U test was used. A *P* value <.05 was considered statistically significant.

Multivariable regression analysis was performed to determine predictors of postoperative macular thickness 1 week and 1 month after surgery. Age and preoperative macular thickness values were incorporated as covariates into this repeated measures regression model to adjust for their effects on postoperative results. The effect of surgery on the foveal region thickness (CSMT and FT), inner and outer macular rings, and TMV was tested. The relationship between effective phaco time and retinal thickness changes were also evaluated. Effective phaco time was calculated by multiplying the total phaco time with the percentage of the power used. In the multivariable analyses, variables were kept in the models if they were associated with a *P* value <.05 and the overall fit of the model improved.

Results

Patient Characteristics

The laser group comprised 12 (60%) women and 8 (40%) men with a mean age of 58.85±15.27 years (range: 23 to 75 years). The control group comprised 15 (75%) women and 5 (25%) men with a mean age of 66.85±11.77 years (range: 52 to 84 years). There were no significant differences between the two groups regarding age (*P*=.53), refractive error (*P*=.95), axial length (*P*=.12), and effective phaco time (*P*=.94) (Table 1).

Functional Results

In the laser group, median corrected distance visual acuity (CDVA) was 0.32±0.24 logMAR preoperatively and 0.16±0.27 logMAR at 1 week and 0.08±0.19 logMAR at 1 month after surgery. In the control group, median CDVA was 0.39±0.28 logMAR preoperatively and 0.08±0.16 logMAR 1 week and 0.02±0.06 logMAR 1 month postoperatively.

Table 1

Comparison of Eyes That Underwent Conventional or Femtosecond Laser-Assisted Phacoemulsification

Demographic	Median (IQR) Laser Group	Median (IQR) Control Group	P Value
Age (y)	64 (53.5 to 69.5)	66 (59 to 74.5)	.18
SE (D)	0.25 (−3.50 to 2.00)	0.25 (−2.75 to 2.75)	.95
AL (mm)	22.66 (22.01 to 23.84)	23.81 (22.42 to 24.77)	.12
Phaco time (s)	0.08 (0.03 to 0.12)	0.08 (0.03 to 0.15)	.94

IQR = interquartile range, SE = spherical equivalent refraction, AL = axial length

OCT Parameters

Pre- and postoperative retinal thickness parameters in the laser and control groups are summarized in Table 2.

Although differences between the two groups in terms of macular thickness parameters did not achieve statistical significance, multivariable modeling of the effect of surgery on postoperative macular thickness showed significantly lower macular thickness in the inner retinal ring in the laser group after adjusting for age and preoperative thickness across the time course (*P*=.002). In the control group, the inner macular ring was significantly thicker at 1 week (mean: 21.68 µm; 95% confidence limit [CL]: 11.93-31.44, *P*<.001). After 1 month this difference decreased to a mean of 17.56 µm (95% CL: −3.21-38.32, *P*=.09) and became marginally significant (Table 3). Type of surgery showed no statistically significant effect on total macular volume, foveal thickness, and outer macular ring average thickness 1 week and 1 month postoperatively (*P*>.05, Table 2).

Figure 2 shows the tendency of postoperative inner macular ring thickness in the two groups after adjusting for age and preoperative thickness. Macular thickness increased in the control group (mean: 287.76 µm; 95% CL: 282.32-293.20; *P*<.001) but not in the laser group (mean: 268.38 µm; 95% CL: 253.10-273.67; *P*>.05) 1 week after surgery compared to the baseline average (mean: 273.3 µm). At 1 month, mean thickness of the inner macular ring was increased in the laser

TABLE 2

RETINAL THICKNESS VALUES PREOPERATIVELY, 1 WEEK, AND 1 MONTH AFTER CONVENTIONAL AND FEMTOSECOND LASER–ASSISTED PHACOEMULSIFICATION MEASURED BY OPTICAL COHERENCE TOMOGRAPHY

Time/Parameter	Median (IQR) Laser Group	Median (IQR) Control Group	P Value
Preoperative			
TMV	6.93 (6.44 to 7.14)	6.66 (6.3 to 7.2)	.63
FT	169.5 (144.0 to 205.5)	174.5 (160.0 to 199.0)	.46
CSMT	210.0 (186.0 to 239.0)	211.5 (195.0 to 226.5)	.80
Inner macular ring AT	280.0 (263.1 to 291.5)	259.75 (252.8 to 283.8)	.12
Outer macular ring AT	238.25 (229.5 to 253.5)	238.0 (219.8 to 247.3)	.40
1 week			
TMV	6.99 (6.63 to 7.33)	6.91 (6.61 to 7.34)	.84
FT	172.0 (155.0 to 200.0)	195.5 (172.0 to 212.0)	.12
CSMT	215.0 (180.0 to 239.0)	223.5 (198.0 to 242.0)	.23
Inner macular ring AT	270.5 (257.0 to 282.7)	273.63 (254.5 to 293.0)	.59
Outer macular ring AT	241.0 (224.2 to 252.2)	238.12 (226.5 to 251.5)	.93
1 month			
TMV	7.31 (7.14 to 7.77)	7.05 (6.56 to 7.78)	.27
FT	218.0 (163.0 to 247.0)	210.0 (173.0 to 253.0)	.91
CSMT	244.0 (206.0 to 258.0)	221.0 (211.0 to 265.0)	.85
Inner macular ring AT	281.8 (275.0 to 317.5)	275.7 (261.0 to 297.7)	.45
Outer macular ring AT	253.6 (242.5 to 268.7)	238.2 (226.0 to 262.7)	.14

IQR = interquartile range, TMV = total macular volume, FT = foveal thickness, CSMT = central subfield macular thickness, AT = average retinal thickness

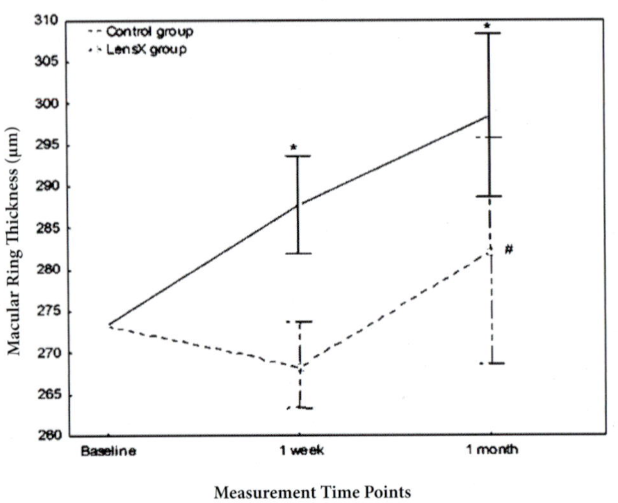

Figure 2. Mean values of inner macular ring thickness at baseline and 1 week and 1 month postoperatively in the study groups adjusted for age and preoperative inner macular ring thickness. *$P<.01$, #$P<.05$ compared to baseline. Whisker = 95% confidence limits of means. The dashed line represents the laser group and the continuous line represents the control group.

group (mean: 281.98 µm; 95% CL: 267.73-296.22; P=.02) and further increased in the control group (mean: 298.38 µm; 95% CL: 287.05-309.72; P=.003) compared to baseline.

DISCUSSION

The incidence of subclinical macular edema after uneventful cataract surgery has become a safety issue for this frequent operation, as studies have found angiographic leakage up to 19% postoperatively[11,12] and an increase of the perifoveal retinal thickness with OCT, which is detectable from the first week up to 6 months and peaks 4 to 6 weeks after surgery, in pseudophakic eyes.[14,16-18]

In our study, we detected the same subclinical parafoveal edema in the control group at 1 week and 1 month postoperatively with a continuous increase. However, in the laser group at 1 week, the thickness of the inner macular ring did not change; a slight increase was only detectable at 1 month. Based on our results, it is

TABLE 3

DIFFERENCE OF MACULAR THICKNESS MEASURED AT DIFFERENT AREAS IN EYES THAT UNDERWENT CONVENTIONAL AND FEMTOSECOND LASER–ASSISTED PHACOEMULSIFICATION*

Time/Macular Area	Difference (μm)	95% CL (μm)	P Value
1 week			
FT	−10.69	(−45.97-24.59)	.53
CSMT	0.86	(−16.42-18.14)	.92
Inner macular ring AT	21.68	(11.93-31.44)	<.001
Outer macular ring AT	11.67	(−9.21-32.55)	.26
1 month			
FT	41.19	(−29.40-111.79)	.24
CSMT	22.62	(−36.42-81.67)	.43
Inner macular ring AT	17.56	(−3.20-38.32)	.09
Outer macular ring AT	0.99	(−15.81-17.80)	.91

Difference = retinal thickness in control group–retinal thickness in laser group, CL = confidence limit, FT = foveal thickness, CSMT = central subfield macular thickness, AT = average retinal thickness
**Adjusted for age and preoperative thickness values.*

unlikely that the suction ring used during the positioning of the femtosecond laser had any harmful effect on macular structure, as macular thickening was not observed in the laser group 1 week after surgery. The substantially lower vacuum level (up to 40 mmHg) compared to LASIK (up to 90 mmHg) used during this procedure could explain this difference.

The delayed detection of macular thickening is probably due to the long-term subclinical inflammation triggered by intraocular tissue (iris) manipulation and mediated by prostaglandins in both groups.[19,20] In concordance with previous reports, we did not find any correlation between macular changes and ultrasound time,[21] suggesting that the blood–retinal barrier is more disrupted during the standard procedure than during femtosecond laser–assisted cataract surgery. The reduced manipulations of the anterior chamber during surgery may explain this phenomenon, which is our hypothesis for the difference found in postoperative macular edema.

Limitations of this study include a relatively small sample size and short follow-up period.

Our results suggest that both methods of cataract extraction are equally safe in terms of early macular thickness. Femtosecond laser–assisted cataract extraction resulted in significantly less early macular thickening compared to the standard procedure, although the differences beyond 1 month are unknown. This early difference may be particularly advantageous in patients who are at more risk for developing postoperative cystoid macular edema such as those with uveitis or diabetic retinopathy, although larger studies with longer follow-up will be necessary to make any substantive conclusions. Further randomized controlled studies with larger cohorts that evaluate exclusively diabetic patients or other patients particularly at risk for postoperative cystoid macular edema are necessary.

AUTHOR CONTRIBUTIONS

Study concept and design (M.E., K.M., Z.Z.N.); data collection (M.E., I.K., A.T., T.F., Z.Z.N.); analysis and interpretation of data (M.E., K.M., I.K.); drafting of the manuscript (M.E., I.K.); critical revision of the manuscript (K.M., I.K., A.T., T.F., Z.Z.N.); statistical expertise (K.M., I.K., A.T., T.F.); supervision (I.K., Z.Z.N.)

REFERENCES

1. Nagy Z, Takacs A, Filkorn T, Sarayba M. Initial clinical evaluation of an intraocular femtosecond laser in cataract surgery. *J Refract Surg.* 2009;25(12):1053-1060.
2. Vetter JM, Holzer MP, Teping C, et al. Intraocular pressure during corneal flap preparation: comparison among four femtosecond lasers in porcine eyes. *J Refract Surg.* 2011;27(6):427-433.
3. Davis RM, Evangelista JA. Ocular structure changes during vacuum by the Hansatome microkeratome suction ring. *J Cataract Refract Surg.* 2007;23(6):563-566.
4. Mirshahi A, Kohnen T. Effect of microkeratome suction during LASIK on ocular structures. *Ophthalmology.* 2005;112(4):645-649.
5. Luna JD, Artal MN, Reviglio VE, Pelizzari M, Diaz H, Juarez CP. Vitreoretinal alterations following laser in situ keratomileusis: clinical and experimental studies. *Graefes Arch Clin Exp Ophthalmol.* 2001;239(6):416-423.

6. Smith RJ, Yadarola MB, Pelizzari MF, Luna JD, Júarez CP, Reviglio VE. Complete bilateral vitreous detachment after LASIK retreatment. *J Cataract Refract Surg.* 2004;30(6):1382-1384.

7. Moshfeghi AA, Harrison SA, Reinstein DZ, Ferrone PJ. Valsalva-like retinopathy following hyperopic laser in situ keratomileusis. *Ophthalmic Surg Lasers Imaging.* 2006;37(6):486-488.

8. Conway ML, Wevill M, Benavente-Perez A, Hosking SL. Ocular blood-flow hemodynamics before and after application of a laser in situ keratomileusis ring. *J Cataract Refract Surg.* 2010;36(2):268-272.

9. Flach AJ. The incidence, pathogenesis and treatment of cystoid macular edema following cataract surgery. *Trans Am Ophthalmol Soc.* 1998;96:557-634.

10. Miyake K, Ibaraki N. Prostaglandins and cystoid macular edema. *Surv Ophthalmol.* 2002;47 Suppl 1:S203-S218.

11. Mentes J, Erakgun T, Afrashi F, Kerci G. Incidence of cystoid macular edema after uncomplicated phacoemulsification. *Ophthalmologica.* 2003;217(6):408-412.

12. Lobo CL, Faria PM, Soares MA, Bernardes RC, Cunha-Vaz JG. Macular alterations after small-incision cataract surgery. *J Cataract Refract Surg.* 2004;30(4):752-760.

13. Lederer DE, Schuman JS, Hertzmark E, et al. Analysis of macular volume in normal and glaucomatous eyes using optical coherence tomography. *Am J Ophthalmol.* 2003;135(6):838-843.

14. Biro Z, Balla Z, Kovacs B. Change of foveal and perifoveal thickness measured by OCT after phacoemulsification and IOL implantation. *Eye (Lond).* 2008;22(1):8-12.

15. Ghosh S, Roy I, Biscuvas PN, et al. Prospective randomized comparative study of macular thickness following phacoemulsification and manual small incision cataract surgery. *Acta Ophthalmol.* 2010;88(4):e102-106.

16. Jagow B, Ohrloff C, Kohnen T. Macular thickness after uneventful cataract surgery determined by optical coherence tomography. *Graefes Arch Clin Exp Ophthalmol.* 2007;245(12):1765-1771.

17. Hee MR, Izatt JA, Swanson EA, et al. Optical coherence tomography of the human retina. *Arch Ophthalmol.* 1995;113(3):325-332.

18. Perente I, Utine CA, Ozturker C, et al. Evaluation of macular changes after uncomplicated phacoemulsification surgery by optical coherence tomography. *Curr Eye Res.* 2007;32(3):241-247.

19. Frank RN, Schulz L, Abe K, Iezzi R. Temporal variation in diabetic macular edema measured by optical coherence tomography. *Ophthalmology.* 2004;111(2):211-217.

20. Lobo CL, Bernardes RC, de Abreu JR, Cunha-Vaz JG. One-year follow-up of blood–retinal barrier and retinal thickness alterations in patients with type 2 diabetes mellitus and mild non-proliferative retinopathy. *Arch Ophthalmol.* 2001;119(10):1469-1474.

21. Cagini CF, Iaccheri B, Piccinelli F, Ricci MA, Fruttini D. Macular thickness measured by optical coherence tomography in a healthy population before and after uncomplicated cataract phacoemulsification surgery. *Curr Eye Res.* 2009;34(12):1036-1041.

Central Corneal Volume and Endothelial Cell Count Following Femtosecond Laser–assisted Refractive Cataract Surgery Compared to Conventional Phacoemulsification

Ágnes I. Takács, MD; Illés Kovács, MD, PhD; Kata Miháltz, MD; Tamás Filkorn, MD; Michael C. Knorz, MD; Zoltán Z. Nagy, MD, DSC

ABSTRACT

PURPOSE: To compare the effect of conventional phacoemulsification and femtosecond laser–assisted cataract surgery on the cornea using Scheimpflug imaging and noncontact specular microscopy.

METHODS: In each group, 38 eyes (38 patients) underwent cataract surgery using either femtosecond laser–assisted (Alcon LenSx laser) (femtolaser group) or conventional phacoemulsification (phaco group). Central corneal thickness, 3-mm corneal volume, and Pentacam Nucleus Staging (PNS) were determined by a rotating Scheimpflug camera (Pentacam HR, Oculus Optikgeräte GmbH), and the volume stress index was calculated at 1 day and 1 month postoperatively. Endothelial cell count was measured by noncontact specular microscopy preoperatively, 1 day, 1 week, and 1 month postoperatively.

RESULTS: Central corneal thickness was significantly higher in the phaco group (607±91 μm) than in the femtolaser group (580±42 μm) on day 1, but did not differ significantly preoperatively and at 1 week and 1 month. Volume stress index at day 1 was significantly lower in the femtolaser group than in the phaco group ($P<.05$) but did not differ significantly at 1 month. Multivariate regression analysis showed that the type of surgery had a significant effect on central corneal thickness.

CONCLUSIONS: Femtosecond laser–assisted cataract surgery causes less corneal swelling in the early postoperative period and may cause less trauma to corneal endothelial cells than manual phacoemulsification. [*J Refract Surg.* 2012;28(6):387-391.]
doi:10.3928/1081597X-20120508-02

Originally published in Journal of Refractive Surgery, *June 2012.*

With the advent of femtosecond laser–assisted cataract surgery, a highly controlled and reproducible capsulotomy, efficient lens fragmentation or liquefaction, and precise and reproducible creation of a corneal incision became possible.[1-6]

Corneal edema is one of the most frequent early postoperative complications of phacoemulsification, which can sometimes lead to permanent and serious visual disturbances. Postoperative corneal swelling and endothelial cell loss are related to many factors, including phacoemulsification time and energy, cataract density, corneal pathology, anterior chamber depth, axial length, ocular trauma, free radical development, mechanical and heat injury, phacoemulsification technique, experience of the surgeon, and use of viscoelastic material.[7-13]

Corneal swelling can be determined by many techniques, including ultrasound or optical pachymetry, anterior segment optical coherence tomography (OCT), or Scheimpflug imaging.[14,15] Using the Pentacam HR (Oculus Optikgeräte GmbH, Wetzlar, Germany) as a three-dimensional method for evaluating the whole anterior segment adds the capability of measuring central corneal volume within a 3-mm area.[15]

Central corneal swelling must be discussed separately from peripheral corneal edema because of the difference in its origin and nature of its development. Pentacam analysis showed that although 3-mm corneal volume often returns to preoperative values by 1 month after phacoemulsification, 10-mm corneal volume remains high over 3 months, indicating that recovery from surgery takes longer near the incision site than at the central cornea.[15,16]

Suzuki et al[17] created a new formula that provides information about endothelial cell function, called volume stress index (VSI), a parameter that indicates the volume-homeostatic function for each corneal endothelial cell. This method is based

Nagy ZZ, ed. *Femtosecond Laser-Assisted Cataract Surgery: Facts and Results* (pp 135-139).

TABLE 1

DEMOGRAPHICS OF PATIENTS TREATED WITH AN INTRAOCULAR FEMTOSECOND LASER BEFORE PHACOEMULSIFICATION AND PHACOEMULSIFICATION ONLY

Demographic	Femtolaser Group	Phaco Group	P Value
Age (y)	65.81±12.42	66.93±10.99	>.05
Gender (M:F)	10:28	15:23	>.05
MRSE (D)	−1.00±4.70	−1.00±5.50	>.05

MRSE = manifest refraction spherical equivalent

on measuring the postoperative alteration of central corneal volume (in a 3-mm diameter area) and central endothelial cell density.

In our study, we aimed to analyze postoperative central corneal edema, endothelial cell count, and endothelial cell function, expressed by VSI, following femtosecond laser–assisted phacoemulsification compared to conventional phacoemulsification.

PATIENTS AND METHODS

Based on our preliminary data, at least 32 patients were required to achieve 90% power in statistical calculations. In this prospective study, femtosecond laser–assisted cataract surgery was performed in 38 eyes from 38 patients (femtolaser group) and conventional phacoemulsification in 38 eyes from 38 patients (phaco group) with various grades of cataract between February 2010 and February 2011. Patients were randomly assigned (using computer randomization) to either group by the surgeon (Z.Z.N.). Patients showing low cooperation, dense (grade 4+) or white cataract, corneal scars or opacities, anterior segment abnormalities, floppy iris syndrome, and poor pupillary dilation were not included in the study.

Demographics are shown in Table 1, and preoperative values in Table 2. No significant differences were present between groups.

The study was designed in accordance with the rules of the university's ethical committee. All study procedures followed the tenets of the Declaration of Helsinki. Informed consent was obtained.

All operations were performed under topical (proparacaine HCL 0.5%) anesthesia by the same surgeon (Z.Z.N.). Pupillary dilation was achieved with the instillation of one drop of tropicamide 0.5% every 15 minutes, three times before surgery.

In the phaco group, 2.8-mm clear corneal and side-port incisions were made with a disposable keratome (Alcon Laboratories Inc, Ft Worth, Texas). Continuous curvilinear capsulorrhexis was performed with a cystotome and a capsular forceps, and a divide-and-conquer phaco technique was used.

In the femtolaser group, the LenSx femtosecond laser system (Alcon LenSx Inc, Aliso Viejo, California) was used to generate a 4.75-mm capsulotomy, lens fragmentation in a cross pattern, and two corneal incisions

TABLE 2

ANTERIOR SEGMENT AND SURGICAL PARAMETERS OF EYES TREATED WITH AN INTRAOCULAR FEMTOSECOND LASER AND PHACOEMULSIFICATION AND PHACOEMULSIFICATION ONLY

Parameter	Femtolaser Group	Phaco Group	P Value
Preop CCT (μm)	545±32	550±39	>.05
Preop CV 3-mm (mm^3)	3.9±0.2	4.0±0.3	>.05
Corneal ECD (cells/mm^2)	2861±215	2841±215	>.05
ACD (mm)	2.57±0.39	2.62±0.45	>.05
Lens thickness (mm)	4.5±0.5	4.4±0.5	>.05
Axial length (mm)	24.1±3.0	23.9±2.9	>.05
Preop IOP (mmHg)	16.0±3.2	15.6±2.9	>.05
Scheimpflug-measured lens nuclear density	2.32±0.97	2.13±1.22	>.05
Phaco energy (%)	12.7±8.3	20.4±12.6	<.05
Phaco time (s)	0.56±0.6	0.67±0.75	>.05
Effective Phaco Time (s)	0.10±0.12	0.12±0.13	>.05

CCT = central corneal thickness, CV = corneal volume, ECD = endothelial cell density, ACD = anterior chamber depth, IOP = intraocular pressure

(a 2.8-mm two-plane main incision and a 1.0-mm single-plane side-port incision) as described previously.[3] Following femtosecond laser treatment, the corneal incisions were opened with a blunt spatula and the anterior chamber was filled with viscoelastic material (Provisc, Alcon Laboratories Inc). The edge of the laser-dissected anterior capsule was checked for complete separation with a cystotome, and the dissected capsule was pulled out of the eye with a forceps. Following hydrodissection, standard phacoemulsification was used to remove the four quadrants of the nucleus pre-chopped by the laser. In both groups, the Infinity phaco system was used (Alcon Laboratories Inc; vacuum 380 mmHg fixed, aspiration rate 35 cc/min fixed, bottle height 110 cm), and after cortex removal and implantation of the one-piece hydrophobic acrylic IOL (Alcon Laboratories Inc), the viscoelastic material was completely removed by irrigation-aspiration. Gentle hydration of the main corneal incision was performed in both groups.

Pre- and Postoperative Measurements

All patients underwent a complete ophthalmologic evaluation including corrected distance visual acuity, manifest refraction, slit-lamp examination, and intraocular pressure (IOP) measurement. Biometry was performed using a non-contact optical low-coherence reflectometer (Lenstar LS 900; Haag-Streit AG, Koeniz, Switzerland).

Pentacam HR Scheimflug imaging was used to measure 3-mm central corneal volume (3-mm CV) and thickness as well as nucleus density preoperatively (Pentacam Nucleus Staging [PNS]). Central endothelial cell count was measured with a Konan Noncon Robo Specular Microscope NSP-9900 (Konan Medical Inc, Hyogo, Japan). All measurements were repeated at 1 day, 1 week, and 1 month postoperatively. Examiners were not aware of which surgical procedure had been used when performing the postoperative examinations.

Volume stress index was calculated according to the formula described by Suzuki et al[15,17] as recommended: VSI = $\Delta V \div (CD \times 7.065)$ ($\Delta V = V2 - V1$). V2 is the 3-mm CV after phacoemulsification, V1 is the 3-mm CV before phacoemulsification, and $7.065 = 1.5 \times 1.5 \times 3.14$ (a 3-mm diameter area).

Statistical Analyses

Statistical analyses were performed with Statistica 8.0 (Statsoft Inc, Tulsa, Oklahoma). Departure from normal distribution assumption was tested by the Shapiro-Wilks W test. Due to normality of data, descriptive statistics show mean and standard deviation. For group comparisons of continuous variables, the independent-sample *t* test was used. To analyze changes in central corneal thickness over the time course, a repeated-measures analysis of variance was used. To test the effect of type of surgery on postoperative central corneal thickness, a multivariable regression analysis was performed. Preoperative central corneal thickness, central endothelial cell count, anterior chamber depth, PNS, and effective phacoemulsification time were incorporated as covariates in the multivariable regression model to adjust for their effects on postoperative central corneal thickness. Variables were kept in the model if they were associated with a *P* value <.05 and the overall fit of the model improved as indicated by the change of R^2, which was used to find the best fitting multivariable model. In all analyses, *P*<.05 was considered statistically significant.

TABLE 3

CENTRAL CORNEAL THICKNESS COMPARISON

Group	Central Corneal Thickness (µm) Preop	1 Day	1 Week	1 Month
Femtolaser	545±31	580±42*	554±36	545±31
Phaco	550±39	607±91*	559±52	557±42

*P<.05 compared to preoperative values using repeated measures analysis of variance.

RESULTS

Pentacam Nucleus Staging showed a statistically significant positive correlation with effective phacoemulsification time in both groups (r=0.35, *P*<.05, femtolaser group, and r=0.5, *P*<.05, phaco group). Central corneal thickness values in the two groups are shown in Table 3 and Figure A (on page 139). The final multivariable model, which included central endothelial cell count, PNS, preoperative central corneal thickness, and group as predictors, had the best-fit index with R^2=0.48. In this multivariable modeling, the type of surgery showed a significant effect on central corneal thickness at the first postoperative day whereas it was adjusted for the effect of the other factors.

In the femtolaser group, postoperative central corneal thickness on day 1 was significantly lower compared to the phaco group, with a mean difference of 29 µm (Table 3). Central endothelial cell count (*P*<.05), PNS (*P*<.05), and preoperative central corneal thickness (*P*<.001) had a significant effect on postoperative central corneal thickness. Anterior chamber depth and effective phacoemulsification time had no effect on

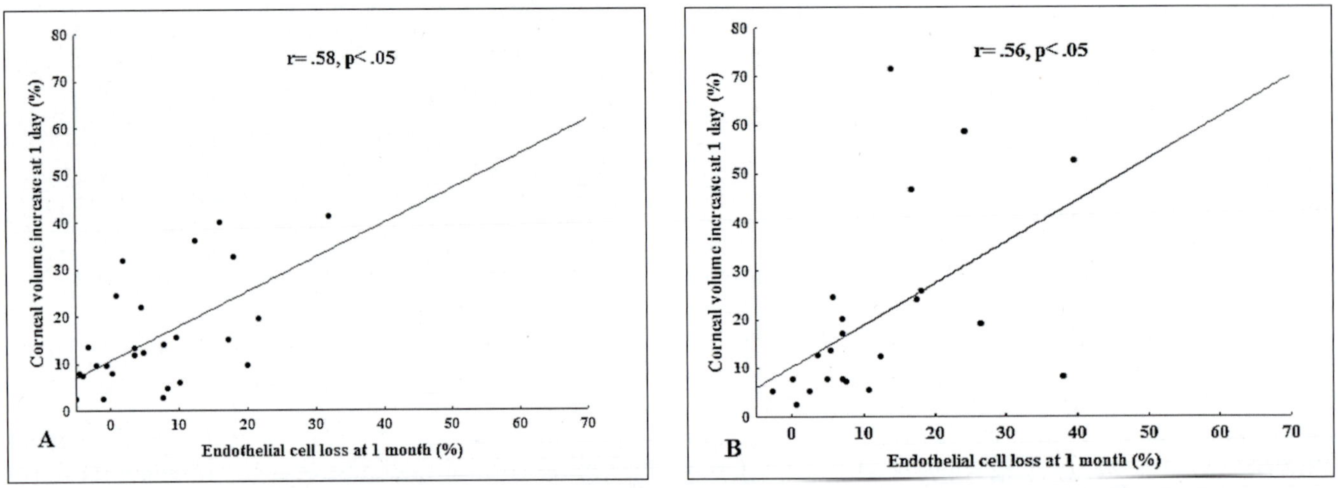

Figure 1. Correlation between corneal volume increase at 1 day (%) and endothelial cell loss at 1 month (%) in eyes treated with an intraocular femtosecond laser and phacoemulsification (femtolaser group) and with phacoemulsification only (phaco group). **A)** Femtolaser group, r=0.58, $P<.05$. **B)** Phaco group, r=0.56, $P<.05$.

Table 4
Corneal Endothelial Cell Count Comparison

Group	Endothelial Cell Count (cells/mm²)			
	Preop	1 Day	1 Week	1 Month
Femtolaser	2861±216	2860±217	2730±205	2738±245
Phaco	2841±215	2719±350	2669±377	2542±466

postoperative central corneal thickness ($P>.05$). Corneal endothelial cell counts were slightly lower in the phaco group at all postoperative follow-up examinations, but differences were not statistically significant, possibly due to the large standard deviation in the phaco group (Table 4).

Figure 1 shows a significant positive correlation between the 3-mm corneal volume increase at postoperative day 1 and endothelial cell loss at 1 month postoperative in both groups.

Volume stress index was $3.0 \pm 2.3 \times 10^{-5}$ in the femto-laser group and $5.3 \pm 6.0 \times 10^{-5}$ in the phaco group at postoperative day 1 and this difference proved to be statistically significant. The difference between the groups regarding VSI was not significant at 1 month, being $1.7 \pm 3.7 \times 10^{-6}$ and $1.7 \pm 3.5 \times 10^{-6}$, respectively (Fig 2).

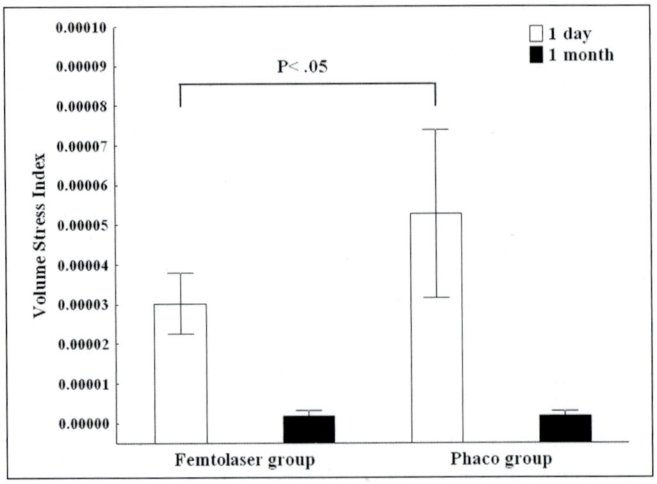

Figure 2. Volume Stress Index in eyes treated with an intraocular femtosecond laser and phacoemulsification (femtolaser group) and with phacoemulsification only (phaco group) ($P<.05$ at 1 day and $P>.05$ at 1 month).

Discussion

In our prospective study, we focused on the effect of femtosecond laser preoperative treatment of the nucleus on the postoperative central corneal thickness and central endothelial cell function, expressed by the VSI. We used Pentacam densitometry (PNS) to determine lens density, because it is an objective method and correlates strongly with the Lens Opacities Classification System (LOCS) III.[18] Cataract grades did not differ significantly between groups (Table 2).

Elnaby et al[19] described that mean effective ultrasound time intraoperatively and percentage of endothelial cell loss at 3 months postoperatively were significantly lower when the phaco prechop technique was used compared to the divide-and-conquer technique.

We also found that postoperative central corneal thickness was significantly lower in the femtolaser group compared to the phaco group on day 1, but not significantly different at 1 week and 1 month (Table 3). We also found a significantly lower VSI in the femtolaser group than in the phaco group 1 day postoperatively (see Fig 2). Phacoemulsification energy was also significantly higher in the phaco group than in the femtolaser group, and both phacoemulsification time and effective phacoemulsification time were higher in the phaco group, but differences were not statistically significant (Table 2). Corneal endothelial cell counts were lower in the phaco group at all postoperative follow-ups, but differences were not statistically significant, possibly due to the high standard deviation in the phaco group (Table 4).

Our study has a few limitations, eg, lack of an extended analysis of endothelial cell morphology (coefficient of variation, percentage of hexagonal cells). In addition, patients were not matched according to lens density, although mean values did not differ significantly between groups (Table 2), and randomization was done by the surgeon and not by randomization tables.

Despite these limitations, our findings indicate that pre-chopping the nucleus with a femtosecond laser reduces phacoemulsification power and endothelial cell trauma, as compared to standard phacoemulsification.

Author Contributions

Study concept and design (A.T., Z.Z.N.); data collection (A.T., I.K., K.M.); analysis and interpretation of data (A.T., I.K., K.M., T.F., M.C.K.); drafting of the manuscript (A.T., K.M.); critical revision of the manuscript (I.K., T.F., M.C.K., Z.Z.N.); statistical expertise (I.K., Z.Z.N.); administrative, technical, or material support (A.T.); supervision (K.M., Z.Z.N.)

References

1. Nagy Z, Takacs A, Filkorn T, Sarayba M. Initial clinical evaluation of an intraocular femtosecond laser in cataract surgery. *J Refract Surg*. 2009;25(12):1053-1060.
2. Nagy ZZ, Kránitz K, Takacs AI, Mihåltz K, Kovács I, Knorz MC. Comparison of intraocular lens decentration parameters after femtosecond and manual capsulotomies. *J Refract Surg*. 2011;27(8):564-569.
3. Kránitz K, Takacs A, Mihåltz K, Kovács I, Knorz MC, Nagy ZZ. Femtosecond laser capsulotomy and manual continuous curvilinear capsulorrhexis parameters and their effects on intraocular lens centration. *J Refract Surg*. 2011;27(8):558-563.
4. Mihåltz K, Knorz MC, Alió JL, et al. Internal aberrations and optical quality after femtosecond laser anterior capsulotomy in cataract surgery. *J Refract Surg*. 2011;27(10):711-716.
5. Nagy ZZ, Kránitz K, Takacs A, Filkorn T, Gergely R, Knorz MC. Intraocular femtosecond laser use in traumatic cataracts following penetrating and blunt trauma. *J Refract Surg*. 2012;28(2):151-153.
6. Ecsedy M, Mihåltz K, Kovács I, Takacs A, Filkorn T, Nagy ZZ. Effect of femtosecond laser cataract surgery on the macula. *J Refract Surg*. 2011;27(10):717-722.
7. Baradaran-Rafii A, Rahmati-Kamel M, Eslani M, Kiavash V, Karimian F. Effect of hydrodynamic parameters on corneal endothelial cell loss after phacoemulsification. *J Cataract Refract Surg*. 2009;35(4):732-737.
8. Takahashi H. Free radical development in phacoemulsification cataract surgery. *J Nihon Med Sch*. 2005;72(1):4-12.

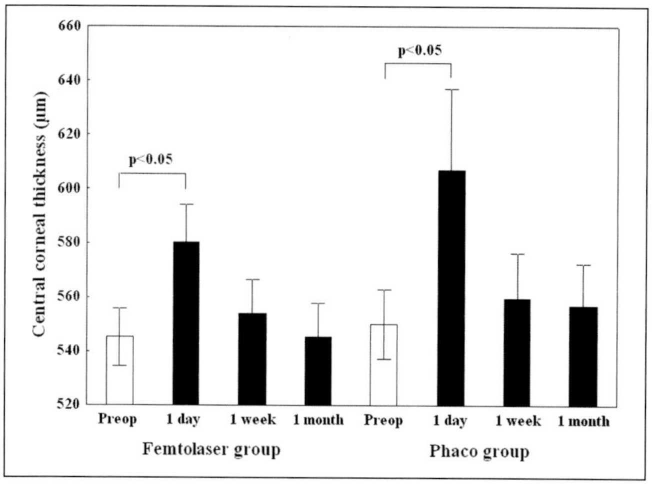

Figure A. Mean values of central corneal thickness in eyes treated with an intraocular femtosecond laser and phacoemulsification (femtolaser group) and with phacoemulsification only (phaco group) at different time points ($P<.05$ using repeated measures analysis of variance; whisker: 95% confidence limits of mean).

9. Yeniad B, Corum I, Ozgun C. The effects of blunt trauma and cataract surgery on corneal endothelial cell density. *Middle East Afr J Ophthalmol*. 2010;17(4):354-358.
10. Crema AS, Walsh A, Yamane Y, Nosé W. Comparative study of coaxial phacoemulsification and microincision cataract surgery. One-year follow-up. *J Cataract Refract Surg*. 2007;33(6):1014-1018.
11. Richard J, Hoffart L, Chavane F, Ridings B, Conrath J. Corneal endothelial cell loss after cataract extraction by using ultrasound phacoemulsification versus a fluid-based system. *Cornea*. 2008;27(1):17-21.
12. Storr-Paulsen A, Nørregaard JC, Farik G, Tårnhøj J. The influence of viscoelastic substances on the corneal endothelial cell population during cataract surgery: a prospective study of cohesive and dispersive viscoelastics. *Acta Ophthalmol Scand*. 2007;85(2):183-187.
13. Cho YK, Chang HS, Kim MS. Risk factors for endothelial cell loss after phacoemulsification: comparison in different anterior chamber depth groups. *Korean J Ophthalmol*. 2010;24(1):10-15.
14. Hutchings N, Simpson TL, Hyun C, et al. Swelling of the human cornea revealed by high-speed, ultrahigh-resolution optical coherence tomography. *Invest Ophthalmol Vis Sci*. 2010;51(9):4579-4584.
15. Suzuki H, Takahashi H, Hori J, Hiraoka M, Igarashi T, Shiwa T. Phacoemulsification associated corneal damage evaluated by corneal volume. *Am J Ophthalmol*. 2006;142(3):525-528.
16. Amann J, Holley GP, Lee SB, Edelhauser HF. Increased endothelial cell density in the paracentral and peripheral regions of the human cornea. *Am J Ophthalmol*. 2003;135(5):584-590.
17. Suzuki H, Oki K, Takahashi K, Shiwa T, Takahashi H. Functional evaluation of corneal endothelium by combined measurement of corneal volume alteration and cell density after phacoemulsification. *J Cataract Refract Surg*. 2007;33(12):2077-2082.
18. Grewal DS, Brar GS, Grewal SP. Correlation of nuclear cataract lens density using Scheimpflug images with Lens Opacities Classification System III and visual function. *Ophthalmology*. 2009;116(8):1436-1443.
19. Elnaby EA, El Zawahry OM, Abdelrahman AM, Ibrahim HE. Phaco prechop versus divide and conquer phacoemulsification: a prospective comparative interventional study. *Middle East Afr J Ophthalmol*. 2008;15(3):123-127.

Femtosecond Laser Cataract Incision Morphology and Corneal Higher-Order Aberration Analysis

Jorge L. Alió, MD, PhD; Ahmed A. Abdou, MD, PhD; Felipe Soria, MD; Jaime Javaloy, MD, PhD; Roberto Fernández-Buenaga, MD; Zoltán Z. Nagy, MD, DSC; Tamás Filkorn, MD

ABSTRACT

PURPOSE: Analysis of the femtosecond laser refractive lens surgery corneal incision configuration and corneal higher-order aberration (HOA) effect from the first postoperative day.

METHODS: High-resolution anterior segment optical coherence tomography was used to assess 20 eyes undergoing femtosecond laser refractive lens surgery with 2.2-mm minimal incision. The primary incision (tri-planar) actual length, cord length, surface angle, surface irregularity, and regional pachymetry values and the secondary incision (uni-planar) length, angle, surface irregularity, and pachymetry values were analyzed. Hartmann-Shack aberrometer was used to assess corneal HOAs to correlate the effect. Assessment was done preoperatively and 1 month postoperatively.

RESULTS: The actual length, cord length, and surface angle means for the primary incision in the first postoperative day and month were 1.50 ± 0.1 and 1.47 ± 0.2 mm ($P = .5$), 1.41 ± 0.1 and 1.42 ± 0.2 mm ($P = .8$), and 27° ± 4° and 23° ± 5° ($P = .07$), respectively. The length and surface angle for the secondary incision in the first postoperative day and month were 1.17 ± 0.01 and 1.04 ± 0.1 mm ($P = .05$) and 52° ± 3° and 42° ± 5° ($P = .007$). The regional pachymetry values for the primary and secondary incisions were significantly increased in the first postoperative day and then significantly decreased after 1 month. All irregularities occurred in the posterior surface (endothelium): 2 cases of posterior gap (first day) and 1 case of posterior retraction (first month). The HOAs had not significantly changed preoperatively and after 1 month.

CONCLUSIONS: The femtosecond laser refractive lens surgery incision is stable and does not significantly change the HOA.

[*J Refract Surg*. 2013;29(9):590-595.]

Originally published in Journal of Refractive Surgery, *September 2013.*

The wide range of applications of the femtosecond (10^{-15}) laser is due to its unique property to photodisrupt tissue with minimal collateral damage (1 μm).[1] This is attributed to the possibility to control many processes of the ultra-short femtosecond laser, such as cohort, electron direction of motion, breaking of chemical bonds, and absorption control.[2] The femtosecond laser can guarantee the stability, precision, length, shape, and width of the corneal incisions.[1] Another unique advantage is the possibility of imaging the cutting process, which can easily be done before, during, and after surgery. This is because the laser process is a three-dimensional scanning process and the essential three-dimensional beam delivery for acquiring three-dimensional image data is already part of the system. Thus, the target tissue can be scanned easily without making room for additional scanning mirrors and lenses for imaging using optical coherence tomography (OCT) imaging or other imaging technologies.[3]

Cataract surgeons are adopting femtosecond technology to perform laser capsulotomy, lens fragmentation, clear cornea incisions, and limbal relaxing incisions.[4] Studies have debated whether clear corneal incision (CCI)[5] is reliable or troublesome.[6-8] Anterior segment OCT (AS-OCT) has been used for analysis of CCI in phacoemulsification to evaluate the wound morphology, which is correlated to healing ability and adequacy.[9-14] Incision quality was also evaluated in many studies as corneal higher-order aberration (HOA) assessment.[15,16]

We aimed in this study to evaluate femtosecond laser refractive lens surgery incision by means of morphological AS-OCT analysis and corneal aberration effect. We also assessed the changes in both during the first postoperative month.

doi:10.3928/1081597X-20130819-01

Nagy ZZ, ed. *Femtosecond Laser-Assisted Cataract Surgery: Facts and Results* (pp 141-146).

Patients and Methods

Patients

A prospective, randomized, observational case series included 20 cataractous eyes undergoing femtosecond laser refractive lens surgery using 2.2-mm minimal incision. Patients were interviewed for demographic data and confirmation of ocular, systemic, and medical histories. All patients signed an informed consent. The study followed the tenets of the Declaration of Helsinki.[17] Ethical committee approval was obtained. Inclusion criteria were age between 50 and 90 years, a transparent central cornea, pupil dilation at the preoperative examination of at least 6.0 mm, grade II nuclear (or corticonuclear) cataract or higher (Lens Opacities Classification System III classification[18]), no glaucoma, normal fundus examination, no previous ocular surgery, and absence of any other ocular or neurological disease that could affect the visual acuity. Exclusion criteria were corticonuclear cataracts with grade less than or greater than II or other types of lens opacities, previous refractive corneal surgery, corneal pathology (eg, Fuchs' dystrophy), subluxated lens or weak zonules, failure of pupillary dilatation (< 6 mm), history of uveitis, history of retinal detachment surgery, and other ocular or neurological diseases that could affect visual acuity or the operation.

Patient Examination

Preoperative standard ophthalmic examination was performed. The examination included clinical data, refraction, uncorrected visual acuity and corrected distance visual acuity using Snellen charts (values expressed in decimal values), slit-lamp examination, intraocular pressure (IOP) measurement by Goldmann applanation tonometry, lenticular status with opacity grading, stereoscopic biomicroscopy of the macula, anterior corneal surface evaluation using the CSO topographer (Compagnia Strumenti Oftalmici, Florence, Italy), and corneal pachymetry with corneal AS-OCT Visante (Carl Zeiss Meditec, Jena, Germany) and KR1W Analyzer (Topcon Medical Systems, Santa Clara, CA) for aberration evaluation.

Postoperatively, we applied the following examination protocol: clinical slit-lamp examination with localization of the incision and confirmation that the incision was not leaking with Seidel test 30 minutes after surgery; visual acuity, refraction, IOP, slit-lamp examination, and analysis of the corneal incision using corneal AS-OCT Visante on the first postoperative day; and visual acuity, refraction, IOP, slit-lamp examination, and analysis of the corneal incision using corneal OCT and aberrometry at the first postoperative month.

Surgical Technique

Surgeries were done by multiple surgeons in Vissum Ophthalmology Corporation, Alicante, Spain, using LENSX (Alcon LenSx Inc., Aliso Viejo, CA) to perform a 2.2-mm clear corneal primary incision, anterior capsulotomy in the laser surgical operating room, and phacofragmentation followed by microcoaxial phacoemulsification, intraocular lens implantation, and completion of the surgery in the general operating room.

Topical anesthesia of preservative-free lidocaine 2% and adequate pupil dilatation (⩾ 6.0 mm) with cyclopentolate 1.0% were used in all patients before entering the laser surgical operating room.

After careful handling of the patient, femtosecond LENSX (Alcon Laboratories, Inc., Fort Worth, TX) docking was started, followed by precise adjustment of the lens capsule position, nucleus position, anterior capsulotomy site, and corneal incision configurations under three-dimensional OCT image guidance. Then nucleus fragmentation and anterior capsulotomy (5 mm) were followed by CCIs.

A tri-planar primary corneal incision (2.2 mm) was performed (first and third side cut angles 60° to 70° and second side cut angle 15° to 25°), which is used for microcoaxial phacoemulsification and intraocular lens implantation later on and a 90° apart uni-planar (1.0 mm) secondary corneal incision (side cut angle 30° to 45°) was performed for lens and intraocular lens manipulating instruments. The length of the incisions varies according to the corneal thickness and the side cut angles with average cord length 1 mm of the second plane "the longest" of the primary incision (**Figure 1**).

The patient was then transferred to the general operating room and placed under the usual operating microscope. The surgeon opened the incisions (2.2 and 1 mm) with a Sinskey hook and grasped the anterior capsule with Utrata forceps. Phacoemulsification and aspiration of the core previously fragmented with phacoemulsification with Stellaris (Bausch & Lomb, Rochester, NY) was performed.

The remaining steps, including the implantation of SA60 AcrySof intraocular lenses (Alcon Laboratories, Inc.), viscoelastic material aspiration, intraocular preservative-free cefuroxime 1.0% (0.1 cm^3), and testing of the sealing corneal wounds with or without hydration of the edges, were done as a conventional cataract procedure. No sutures were used in any eye. After surgery, patients were allowed to rest for 30 minutes and then examined at the slit lamp for the sealing of the corneal incision using a fluorescein Seidel test comprising 3.0 mL of 2.5 mg fluorescein sodium plus 4.0 mg oxybuprocaine chloride (Colircusi Fluotest; Alcon Cusí, El Masnou, Spain).

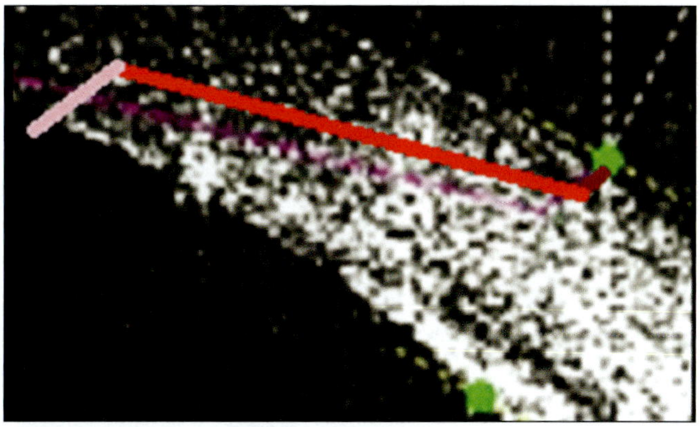

Figure 1. Tri-planar configuration of the primary incision.

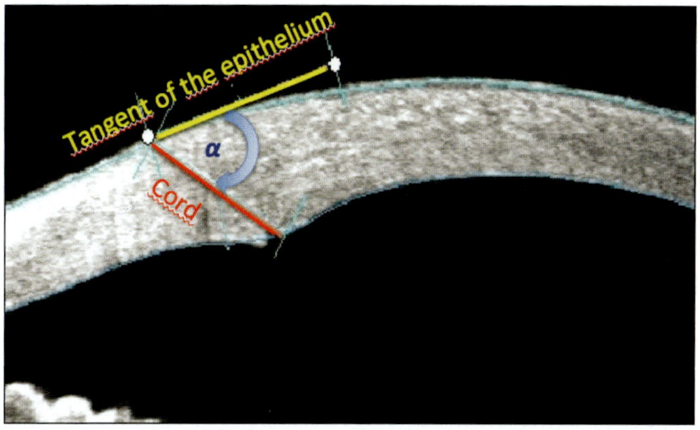

Figure 2. Uni-planar configuration of the secondary incision.

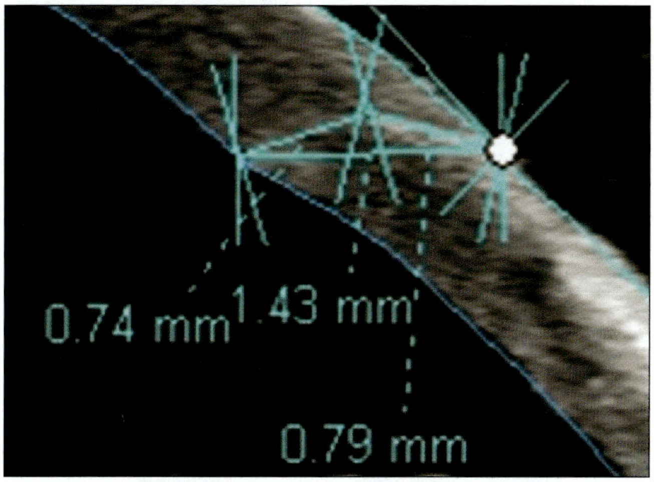

Figure 3. One-month postoperative length segments of tri-planar incision determined by anterior segment optical coherence tomography.

Postoperative topical therapy included topical ofloxacin 0.3%, dexamethasone alcohol 0.1%, and nonsteroidal anti-inflammatory drugs.

We evaluated the incision configuration with AS-OCT and then the corneal HOA effect with Hartmann-Shack aberrometer at 1 month postoperatively.

Corneal OCT was performed using the Visante system (Carl Zeiss Meditec, Jena, Germany), which uses an infrared light with a 1,310-nm wavelength to obtain interferometry scans of different anterior segment structures (high-resolution time-domain AS-OCT).[19] We used high-resolution corneal measurement to obtain accurate scans of the corneal structure. A linear scan with the same orientation of the incision was used, rotated 10 degrees clockwise and 10 degrees counterclockwise to find the image with the best resolution. Then the scanning was performed and an image acquired. We also performed an overall corneal pachymetry measurement to evaluate the regional corneal thickness of the primary and secondary incisions. The system is connected to a computer that has software with several options for image capturing and measurement.

We determined five variables for evaluation for the primary incision and four for the secondary incision. For the primary incision, we measured the actual length of the incision (segments x, y, and z); cord length (length between the epithelial and endothelial edges [**Figure 1**]); angle of the incision (the angle formed between the line of the second plane "the longest," which postoperatively appears to be extended to the surface as a straight line with the smallest first plane and the tangent line to the epithelial edge of the incision; surface irregularities (epithelial or endothelial gaps on the first postoperative day, retraction later on and bulge); and regional pachymetry of the area of incision. The same variables were measured for the secondary incision, with the exception of the cord length (because the incision is uni-planar and there was no difference between the actual length and the cord length) (**Figures 2-3**). The angle was measured for any configuration change of the incision.

Corneal Aberrometry

Corneal HOAs were measured using the KR-1W aberrometer (Topcon Medical Systems), an intraocular Hartman-Shack aberrometer that uses a rotational prism system that can give accurate data of HOAs in details (using Zernike polynomials) and is classified in ocular, internal, and corneal HOAs for 4- and 6-mm pupil diameter. We focused our analysis on the larger diameter (6 mm) and evaluated the root mean square (RMS) of the total HOAs coma Z (3, ± 1), and spherical aberration Z (4, 0).

Statistical Analysis

Data were recorded by Microsoft Excel 2010 (Microsoft Corporation, Redmond, WA) and the SPSS statistical software package for Windows (version 16; SPSS, Inc., Chicago, IL) was used for statistical analysis of the outcome means Wilcoxon test. A *P* value of less than .05 was considered significant.

Results

Patients

Twenty eyes of 20 patients (13 women, 65%; 7 men, 35%) were enrolled in the study. The mean age of the patients was 72.2 ± 6.9 years (range: 57 to 86 years).

AS-OCT Incision Analysis

Incision Length. There was minimal increase on the first day primary incision cord length mean after the first postoperative month (1.41 ± 0.1 and 1.42 ± 0.2 mm; $P = .8$) and an insignificant decrease in the actual length (1.50 ± 0.1 and 1.47 ± 0.2 mm; $P = .5$), whereas the decrease of the secondary incision length after the first month was 1.17 ± 0.01 and 1.04 ± 0.1 mm ($P = .05$) (**Figure 4A**).

Incision Angle. The primary incision angle decreased insignificantly after the first month (27° ± 4° day 1 postoperatively and 23° ± 5° month 1 postoperatively; $P = .07$), but the decrease of the secondary incision angle was significant (52° ± 3° day 1 postoperatively and 42° ± 5° month 1 postoperatively; $P = .007$) (**Figure 4B**).

Regional Pachymetry. Regarding the corneal thickness at the area of incisions, there was a significant increase in both primary (670 ± 41 µm preoperatively and 844 ± 94 µm day 1 postoperatively; $P < .001$) and secondary (664 ± 89 µm preoperatively and 779 ± 59 µm day 1 postoperatively; $P = .003$) incisions on the first postoperative day, which significantly decreased after the first month (731 ± 87 µm month 1 postoperatively for primary incision, $P = .02$; 673 ± 78 µm for day 1 postoperatively for secondary incision, $P = .008$) (**Figure 4C**).

Incision Quality. The high-resolution corneal scan revealed a high degree of wound integrity with straight line configuration. The second plane "the longest" appeared postoperatively as a single straight line with the first plane "the smallest." There were surface irregularities in three patients and all were posterior in the form of defects. One case had a posterior gap on the first postoperative day with Descemet membrane detachment in the primary incision and another case in the secondary incision, both of which completely resolved after the first month. The third case had posterior wound retraction of the primary incision after the first month.

Corneal Aberrometry. The HOAs increased after 1 month (0.69 ± 0.22 µm; $P = .10$) to almost the same preoperative mean value. The individual HOA (coma and spherical aberration) followed the same course as shown in **Table 1**.

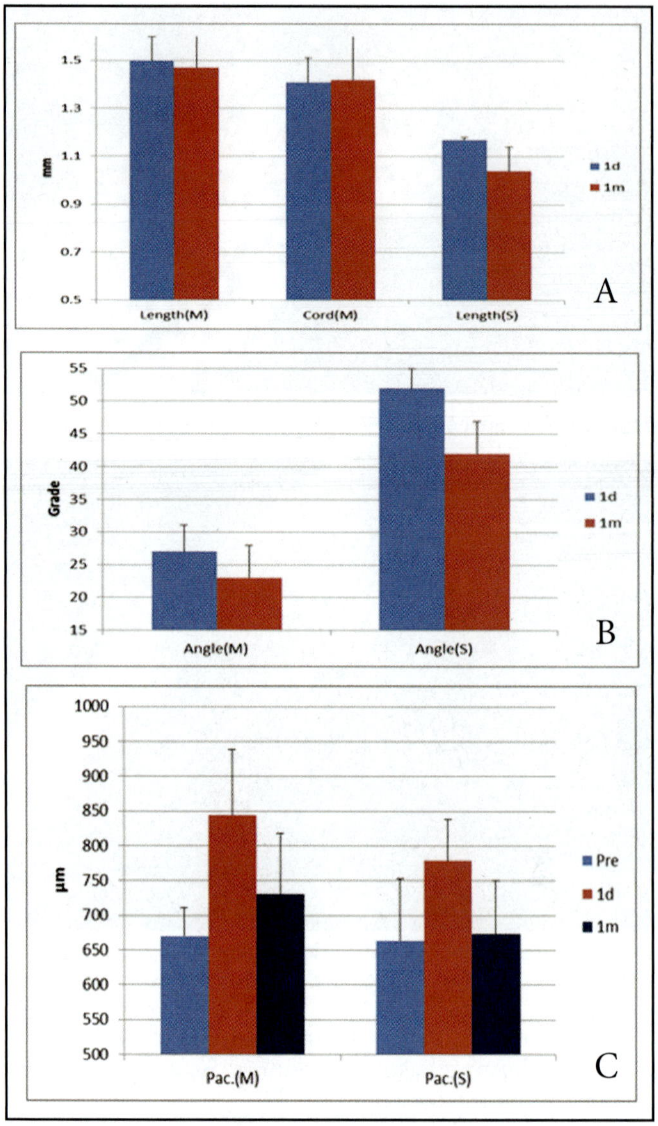

Figure 4. (A) Length, (B) angle, and (C) regional pachymetry of the primary (M) and secondary (S) incisions.

Discussion

Because the quality of the cataract incision has a great effect on the visual outcome, we tried to evaluate accurately the incision quality of femtosecond laser refractive lens surgery. We focused in our analysis on two methods (the wound configuration and integrity with high-resolution AS-OCT), which gives direct evaluation and analysis of the corneal HOA changes, which is the remote effect of the incision.

Our results revealed that the incision was precise even with different surgeons and both the length and angle changed minimally during the first postoperative month, achieving the desired preoperative parameters. The changes were less for the primary tri-planar incision with almost no change of the cord length, which reveals the stability of the tri-planar configuration. We agreed with other manual CCI studies about the insignificant decrease of the incision length during the postoperative first month, but this decrease was less with

Table 1
Mean ± SD (μM) Total and Individual HOAs

Visit	Total HOAs	Coma	Spherical Aberration	Trefoil
Preoperative	0.65 ± 0.45	0.27 ± 0.1	0.10 ± 0.3	0.37 ± 0.2
Postoperative 1 month	0.69 ± 0.22 (P = .330)	0.28 ± 0.1 (P = .649)	0.18 ± 0.2 (P = .041)	0.47 ± 0.2 (P = .075)

SD = standard deviation; HOA = higher-order aberration

the tri-planar femtosecond laser refractive lens surgery configuration.[13] The secondary incision angle mean value was similar to these studies[12,13] and the angles of all secondary incisions were in the range of what was described as critical angle, which provides a secure coapted ocular incision.[9,12] The tri-planar configuration angles provide the advantages of small secure angle entry and behave as if the larger angle (angle between the entry and exit) was the dominant one, adding more integrity with different levels of IOP.[9]

We agreed with other studies in finding a significant increase in the corneal thickness on the first postoperative day, which significantly decreased to almost the same preoperative level after the first month, whether with manual incision[12,20] or with femtosecond laser.[21] The increased thickness was more for the primary incision, which is attributed to the use of a phacoemulsification probe and the configuration of being larger and tri-planar.[22] We suggest that the greatest decrease in the incision length and the angle of the secondary incision despite a smaller diameter is related to a greater weakness of the biomechanics of the cornea with a loosening of its elasticity property. A larger incision with a tri-planar configuration of a greater diameter will create biomechanically a better conservation of the elasticity of the cornea. On the other hand, the Descemet membrane detachment that we encountered in one case may be related to a short "subendothelial" incision or inadvertent Sinskey hook manipulation.

Regarding the incision quality, it was obviously linear and distinct from the arcuate configuration of the manual one.[13,23] We did not find any epithelial defect at the site of incision and our reported endothelial gap, Descemet detachment, and retraction rates were much lower and healed faster than those reported in the literature.[12-14]

The insignificant change of the total HOAs and coma was similar to what was published by other studies on manual CCI after 1 month postoperatively and we reported from the first postoperative day.[12,15,16] The spherical aberration value is significant and slightly more positive due to the flattening of the cornea due to the incision. We reported an insignificant difference in postoperative trefoil after 1 month and this disagrees with other studies that found a significant increase of postoperative trefoil "surgically induced" with the manual CCI.[16,24] The slight increase of the total and individual HOAs after the first month could be related to restoration of the preoperative corneal thickness. Cataract surgery-related changes in corneal wavefront aberrations were dependent on incision size. It seems that 2 mm was the limit around which no optical changes are induced by cataract surgery in the human cornea.[15]

We believe that the tri-planar clear corneal incision is more stable due to its configuration[25] and long cord length that was approved to add stability and reproducibility in wound construction.[26] Moreover, our AS-OCT analysis reveals highly predictable incision angle and wound length even among different surgeons.

Femtosecond laser refractive lens surgery incision is stable and does not significantly affect the HOA with favorable results of the tri-planar configuration with highly predictable incision angle and wound length even among different surgeons.

Author Contributions

Study concept and design (AAA, JLA); data collection (AAA, JLA, FS); analysis and interpretation of data (AAA, JLA, RF-B, TF, JJ, ZZN); drafting of the manuscript (AAA, JLA, FS); critical revision of the manuscript (JLA, RF-B, TF, JJ, ZZN); statistical expertise (AAA, JLA); administrative, technical, or material support (JLA); supervision (JLA, RF-B, TF, JJ, ZZN)

References

1. Sugar A. Ultrafast (femtosecond) laser refractive surgery. *Curr Opin Ophthalmol.* 2002;13:246-2499.
2. Brumer PW, Shapiro M. *Principles of the Quantum Control of Molecular Processes.* Hoboken, NJ: John Wiley & Sons, Inc.; 2003.
3. Gibson EA, Masihzadeh O, Lei TC, Ammar DA, Kahook MY. Multiphoton microscopy for ophthalmic imaging. *J Ophthalmol.* 2011;2011:870879.
4. Uy HS, Edwards K, Curtis N. Femtosecond phacoemulsification: the business and the medicine. *Curr Opin Ophthalmol.* 2012;23:33-39.
5. Fine IH. Self-sealing corneal tunnel incision for small-incision cataract surgery. *Ocular Surgery News.* 1992;10:38-39.

6. Miller JJ, Scott IU, Flynn HW Jr, Smiddy WE, Newton J, Miller D. Acute-onset endophthalmitis after cataract surgery (2000-2004): incidence, clinical settings, and visual acuity outcomes after treatment. *Am J Ophthalmol.* 2005;139:983-987.
7. Monica ML, Long DA. Nine-year safety with self-sealing corneal tunnel incision in clear cornea cataract surgery. *Ophthalmology.* 2005;112:985-986.
8. Masket S. Is there a relationship between clear corneal cataract incisions and endophthalmitis? *J Cataract Refract Surg.* 2005;31:643-645.
9. Taban M, Rao B, Reznik J, Zhang J, Chen Z, McDonnell PJ. Dynamic morphology of sutureless cataract wounds -effect of incision angle and location. *Surv Ophthalmol.* 2004;49(suppl 2):S62-S72.
10. Schallhorn JM, Tang M, Li Y, Song JC, Huang D. Optical coherence tomography of clear corneal incisions for cataract surgery. *J Cataract Refract Surg.* 2008;34:1561-1565.
11. Dupont-Monod S, Labbé A, Fayol N, Chassignol A, Bourges JL, Baudouin C. In vivo architectural analysis of clear corneal incisions using anterior segment optical coherence tomography. *J Cataract Refract Surg.* 2009;35:444-450.
12. Elkady B, Piñero D, Alió JL. Corneal incision quality: microincision cataract surgery versus microcoaxial phacoemulsification. *J Cataract Refract Surg.* 2009;35:466-474.
13. Can I, Bayhan HA, Celik H, Bostanci Ceran B. Anterior segment optical coherence tomography evaluation and comparison of main clear corneal incisions in microcoaxial and biaxial cataract surgery. *J Cataract Refract Surg.* 2011;37:490-500.
14. Wang L, Dixit L, Weikert MP, Jenkins RB, Koch DD. Healing changes in clear corneal cataract incisions evaluated using Fourier-domain optical coherence tomography. *J Cataract Refract Surg.* 2012;38:660-665.
15. Alió JL, Elkady B, Ortiz D. Corneal optical quality following sub 1.8 mm micro-incision cataract surgery vs. 2.2 mm mini-incision coaxial phacoemulsification. *Middle East Afr J Ophthalmol.* 2010;17:94-99.
16. Tong N, He JC, Lu F, Wang Q, Qu J, Zhao YE. Changes in corneal wavefront aberrations in microincision and small-incision cataract surgery. *J Cataract Refract Surg.* 2008;34:2085-2090.
17. World Medical Association. *World Medical Association Declaration of Helsinki: Ethical Principles for Medical Research Involving Human Subjects.* Presented at the 52nd General Assembly; October 2000; Edinburgh, Scotland. Available at: http://www.wma.net/en/30publications/10policies/b3/. Accessed July 2012.
18. Chylack LT Jr, Wolfe JK, Singer DM, et al. The Lens Opacities Classification System III: the longitudinal study of cataract study group. *Arch Ophthalmol.*1993;111:831-836.
19. Radhakrishnan S, Rollins AM, Roth JE, et al. Real-time optical coherence tomography of the anterior segment at 1310 nm. *Arch Ophthalmol.* 2001;119:1179-1185.
20. Xia Y, Liu X, Luo L, et al. Early changes in clear cornea incision after phacoemulsification: an anterior segment optical coherence tomography study. *Acta Ophthalmol.* 2009;87:764-768.
21. Takács AI, Kovács I, Miháltz K, Filkorn T, Knorz MC, Nagy ZZ. Central corneal volume and endothelial cell count following femtosecond laser-assisted refractive cataract surgery compared to conventional phacoemulsification. *J Refract Surg.* 2012;28:387-391.
22. Vasavada AR, Dholakia SA. Corneal hydration intra-operatively during phacoemulsification. *Indian J Ophthalmol.* 2005;53:249-253.
23. Fine IH, Hoffman RS, Packer M. Profile of clear corneal cataract incisions demonstrated by ocular coherence tomography. *J Cataract Refract Surg.* 2007;33:94-97.
24. Can I, Bayhan HA, Çelik H, Ceran BB. Comparison of corneal aberrations after biaxial microincision and microcoaxial cataract surgeries: a prospective study. *Curr Eye Res.* 2012;37:18-24.
25. May WN, Castro-Combs J, Quinto GG, Kashiwabuchi R, Gower EW, Behrens A. Standardized Seidel test to evaluate different sutureless cataract incision configurations. *J Cataract Refract Surg.* 2010;36:1011-1017.
26. Masket S, Sarayba M, Ignacio T, Fram N. Femtosecond laser-assisted cataract incisions: architectural stability and reproducibility. *J Cataract Refract Surg.* 2010;36:1048-1049.

Intraocular Femtosecond Laser Use in Traumatic Cataracts Following Penetrating and Blunt Trauma

Zoltán Zsolt Nagy, MD, DSC; Kinga Kránitz, MD; Agnes Takacs, MD; Tamás Filkorn, MD; Róbert Gergely, MD; Michael C. Knorz, MD

ABSTRACT

PURPOSE: To investigate the use of femtosecond laser cataract surgery in traumatic cataracts of different origin.

METHODS: The first case developed acute traumatic cataract due to penetrating injury of the cornea and the anterior lens capsule; the second developed traumatic cataract 11 years after a penetrating corneal injury; and the third developed a "white" cataract 12 months after blunt ocular trauma. In all cases, 4.5-mm capsulorrhexis and corneal incisions were performed using a femtosecond laser system (Alcon LenSx Inc), and nucleus liquefaction with the laser was performed additionally in the second case.

RESULTS: In all patients, a capsulorrhexis could be created with the femtosecond laser. Preexisting radial tears were present in the first case, but the remaining anterior capsule could be cut with the laser. The second and third cases showed an intact 4.5-mm capsulorrhexis. Corneal incisions were stable in all cases, and nucleus liquefaction was possible in the second case (grade 1-2 nuclear density).

CONCLUSIONS: Results indicate that a femtosecond laser can be used successfully in certain instances of traumatic cataract after penetrating eye injury, even if an anterior capsule laceration is present, and also after blunt trauma resulting in "white" cataracts. [*J Refract Surg.* 2012;28(2):151-153.]
doi:10.3928/1081597X-20120120-01

Originally published in Journal of Refractive Surgery, *February 2012.*

Traumatic cataract is a frequent complication of eye injuries. Anterior lens capsule laceration occurs not only in penetrating injuries but also after blunt trauma rendering traumatic cataract surgery more difficult. Capsular complications (anterior and posterior capsular tear, vitreous loss, etc) during cataract extraction decrease the probability of achieving good long- and short-term postoperative results. Subjective complaints are more common in patients with capsular rupture and more myopic spherical equivalent and higher cylindrical refraction.[1-4] Until now, capsulorrhexis has been a manual multi-step procedure. With the aid of femtosecond lasers in ophthalmic surgery, a more precise and centred anterior capsulotomy became possible for routine cases.[5-8] This report presents the use of an intraocular femtosecond laser to perform capsulorrhexis, lens fragmentation, and corneal incisions in eyes with traumatic cataract either after penetrating globe injury, with or without anterior capsule laceration, or after blunt trauma.

CASE REPORTS

Case 1

A 28-year-old race car driver suffered a penetrating eye injury from a thread of wire that hit his left eye while working with a wire brush. He immediately removed the piece of wire from his eye and presented for treatment.

On admission, uncorrected distance visual acuity (UDVA) was 20/50. A 2-mm corneal laceration was visible mid-peripherally between 9 and 10 o'clock, and the iris had prolapsed. The corneal laceration was sutured (10-0 nylon interrupted sutures) and the iris was repositioned (Fig 1).

Nagy ZZ, ed. *Femtosecond Laser-Assisted Cataract Surgery: Facts and Results* (pp 147-150).

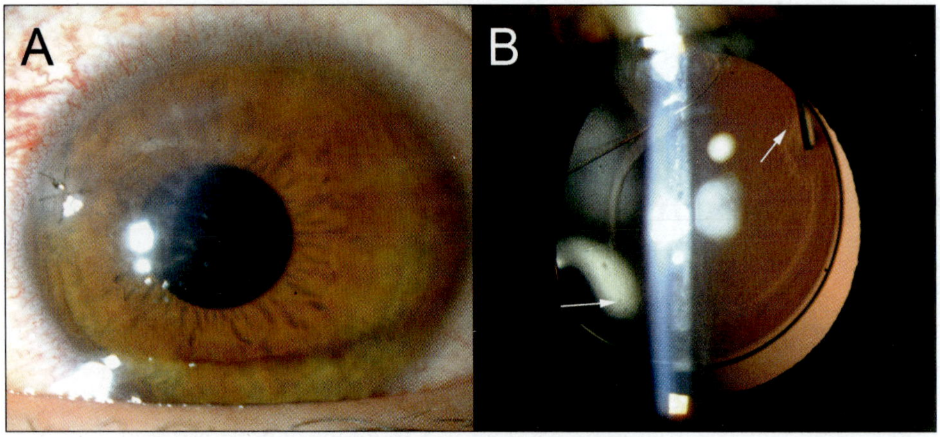

Figure 1. *Case 1.* Penetrating injury of the cornea and anterior lens capsule after cataract removal. **A)** Corneal sutures in place 1 day after cataract removal. **B)** Implanted IOL 1 week after surgery. Anterior capsule tears are visible at 2 and 8 o'clock.

After dilating the pupil, an oblique anterior capsule laceration from the center to the periphery between 8 and 2 o'clock became visible, but the lens was not removed at this stage. Two days later, cataract surgery was performed using an intraocular femtosecond laser (Alcon LenSx Inc, Aliso Viejo, California). As both eyes had no refractive error previously, data of the fellow eye were used to calculate intraocular lens (IOL) power.

After pupillary dilation (cyclopentolate 0.5%) and instillation of topical anesthetics (proparacaine 0.5%), the curved applanation lens was attached to the laser, docked to the eye, and suction was started. We did not anticipate a problem with wound leakage due to an increase in intraocular pressure caused by the suction because the wound was small and remained sealed as expected (see Fig 1). The laser has built-in optical coherence tomography and a scan was performed after suction was started. The start and endpoints of the circular cut of the 4.5-mm capsulorrhexis were placed 300 μm behind and 300 μm in front of the anterior capsule, respectively. The laser was also used to perform the main 3.2-mm corneal incision and a 0.9-mm side-port incision. No laser treatment of the nucleus was performed as it was assumed to be soft. Suction was released and the patient was transferred to the main operating room. After draping the eye, the incisions were opened with a blunt spatula and the anterior capsule was removed with capsulorrhexis forceps. Two radial tears of the anterior capsule at 8 and 2 o'clock, respectively, were noted. Between those tears, which we believe occurred during the initial trauma, the laser had cut a round capsulorrhexis. The soft nucleus and cortex were aspirated and a 3-piece acrylic IOL (+24.00 diopters [D], Acrysof MN60AC; Alcon Laboratories Inc, Ft Worth, Texas) was implanted into the capsular bag. The IOL haptics were oriented to 11 and 5 o'clock to minimize the likelihood of tear extension. The anterior tears did not extend into the posterior capsule.

Two weeks after surgery UDVA was 20/25 and corrected distance visual acuity (CDVA) was 20/20 (+0.50 +0.50 D × 40°). Intraocular lens tilt and decentration were measured using a Scheimpflug imaging system (Oculus Pentacam HR 70900; Oculus Optikgeräte GmbH, Wetzlar, Germany). The IOL was decentered 0.38 mm in the horizontal and 0.52 mm in the vertical direction, with a total decentration of 0.64 mm. Intraocular lens tilt was −8.09° around the vertical (y axis) and −1.74° around the horizontal axis (x axis). Slit-lamp examination showed a partial overlap of the anterior capsule over the IOL optic (overlap nasally and temporally), whereas the anterior capsule was peripheral to the IOL optic superiorly and inferiorly. One year later the result remained stable, UDVA was 20/20, and the patient continued as a successful race car driver.

Case 2

A 33-year-old woman, who presented in 2010, experienced a penetrating trauma in her left eye in 1999 caused by a pair of scissors. Slit-lamp examination showed a corneal scar starting paracentrally and extending to the periphery at 2 o'clock. Anterior synechiae were noted peripherally, causing slight pupil irregularity. The lens showed a cortical cataract anteriorly. Corrected distance visual acuity was 20/40. Cataract surgery was performed with the femtosecond laser. Pupil size was 8 mm after dilation. Nucleus liquefaction was performed using a pattern of stacked cylinders (largest diameter 4.5 mm, smallest 1 mm; starting 1.2 mm in front of the posterior capsule and ending 0.5 mm behind the anterior capsule). A 4.5-mm capsulorrhexis was created, and a 3.2-mm corneal incision and 0.9-mm side-port incision were performed with the laser. After transferring the patient to the main operating room, the surgery was uneventful; the capsulorrhexis was intact, the nucleus could be removed using aspiration only, and a 3-piece acrylic IOL (+22.00 D, Acrysof MN60AC) was implanted in the bag.

One month after surgery CDVA was 20/35 (+0.75 D cyl) (irregular astigmatism was due to a corneal scar between the paracentral and peripheral area from a childhood corneal injury). Intraocular lens decentration was 0.34 mm in the horizontal and 0.35 mm in the vertical direction, with a total decentration of 0.49 mm. The IOL tilt was −1.07° around the vertical (y axis) and 13.12° around the horizontal axis (x axis).

Case 3

A 48-year-old man suffered blunt trauma to his right eye from a piece of brick in December 2009 and presented in March 2010. Visual acuity was hand movements only. The cornea was clear, the anterior chamber was normal, pupil shape and response were normal, and the lens showed a complete "white" cataract. Cataract surgery was performed using the femtosecond laser to create a 4.5-mm capsulorrhexis, 3.2-mm corneal incision, and 0.9-mm side-port incision. No laser treatment of the nucleus was performed because of the lack of transparency. Intraoperativly, an intact 4.5-mm capsulorrhexis was found. Manual chopping of the nucleus and removal using standard phacomulsification were performed and a 3-piece acrylic IOL (+19.50 D, Acrysof MN60AC) was implanted in the capsular bag.

One week after surgery, CDVA was 20/20. Intraocular lens decentration was 0.07 mm in the horizontal and 0.48 mm in the vertical direction, with a total decentration of 0.49 mm. The IOL tilt was −9.84° around the vertical (y axis) and −2.64° around the horizontal axis (x axis) (Fig 2).

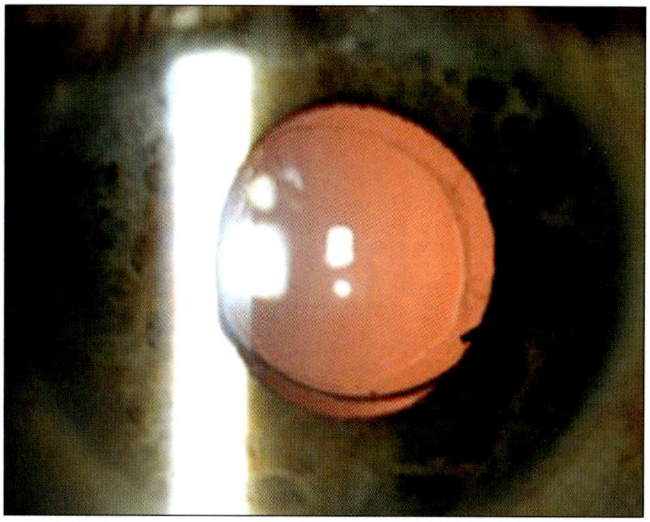

Figure 2. *Case 3.* Slit-lamp photograph 1 month after cataract surgery in an eye with "white" cataract following blunt trauma. The IOL optic is not symmetrically covered. Decentration was 0.07 mm in the horizontal direction and 0.48 mm in the vertical direction.

Discussion

Penetrating trauma often makes capsulorrhexis technically more difficult due to anterior capsule rupture. According to Marques et al,[9] in eyes with traumatic cataract the most common intraoperative complication is irregularity of the capsulorrhexis. A tear of the anterior capsule may extend to the posterior capsule, and into a radial anterior and posterior capsular tear that can complicate surgery at any stage. Capsule injuries have been reported to be not only the most frequent complications of traumatic cataract eyes but also prognostic factors for worse visual rehabilitation.[1-4] Anterior capsule tears as observed in case 1 may also affect IOL position. To minimize this, it is important to place the IOL haptics away from the anterior capsule tear, ideally 90° away.

We previously reported that reproducibility of the capsulorrhexis is significantly better with a femtosecond laser in non-traumatic cataract eyes.[5-8] A limitation of the femtosecond approach is the need for adequate pupil dilation. Pupil size must be 1- to 1.5-mm larger than the area treated with the laser (which means 0.5 to 0.75 mm on each side). We typically use a 4.5- to 5-mm capsulorrhexis and a 4.5-mm laser treatment diameter inside the nucleus; ie, the minimum pupil size must be 5.5 to 6 mm. The three cases reported herein indicate that a femtosecond laser–created capsulorrhexis is possible even if anterior capsule tears are present or in "white" cataracts. The laser-created capsulorrhexis may provide added safety in traumatic cataract cases.

Author Contributions

Study concept and design (Z.Z.N., R.G.); data collection (K.K., A.T., R.G.); analysis and interpretation of data (K.K., T.F., M.C.K.); drafting of the manuscript (Z.Z.N., R.G., M.C.K.); critical revision of the manuscript (K.K., A.T., T.F.); administrative, technical, or material support (Z.Z.N.); supervision (K.K., A.T.)

References

1. Lundström M, Behndig A, Montan P, et al. Capsule complication during cataract surgery: background, study design, and required additional care: Swedish Capsule Rupture Study Group report 1. *J Cataract Refract Surg.* 2009;35(10):1679-1687.
2. Artzén D, Lundström M, Behndig A, Stenevi U, Lydahl E, Montan P. Capsule complication during cataract surgery: case-control study of preoperative and intraoperative risk factors: Swedish Capsule Rupture Study Group report 2. *J Cataract Refract Surg.* 2009;35(10):1688-1693.
3. Johansson B, Lundström M, Montan P, Stenevi U, Behndig A. Capsule complication during cataract surgery: long-term outcomes: Swedish Capsule Rupture Study Group report 3. *J Cataract Refract Surg.* 2009;35(10):1694-1698.
4. Jakobsson G, Montan P, Zetterberg M, Stenevi U, Behndig A, Lundström M. Capsule complication during cataract surgery: retinal detachment after cataract surgery with capsule complication: Swedish Capsule Rupture Study Group report 4. *J Cataract Refract Surg.* 2009;35(10):1699-1705.

5. Nagy Z, Takacs A, Filkorn T, Sarayba M. Initial clinical evaluation of an intraocular femtosecond laser in cataract surgery. *J Refract Surg.* 2009;25(12):1053-1060.

6. Kránitz K, Takacs A, Miháltz K, Kovács I, Knorz MC, Nagy ZZ. Femtosecond laser capsulotomy and manual continuous curvilinear capsulorrhexis parameters and their effects on intraocular lens centration. *J Refract Surg.* 2011;27(8):558-563.

7. Nagy ZZ, Kránitz K, Takacs AI, Miháltz K, Kovács I, Knorz MC. Comparison of intraocular lens decentration parameters after femtosecond and manual capsulotomies. *J Refract Surg.* 2011;27(8):564-569.

8. Miháltz K, Knorz MC, Alió JL, et al. Internal aberrations and optical quality after femtosecond laser anterior capsulotomy in cataract surgery. *J Refract Surg.* 2011;27(10):711-716.

9. Marques FF, Marques DM, Osher RH, Osher JM. Fate of anterior capsule tears during cataract surgery. *J Cataract Refract Surg.* 2006;32(10):1638-1642.

Laser Refractive Cataract Surgery With a Femtosecond Laser After Penetrating Keratoplasty: Case Report

Zoltán Z. Nagy, MD, DSC; Ágnes I. Takács, MD; Tamás Filkorn, MD; Éva Juhász, MD; Gábor Sándor, MD; Andrea Szigeti, MD; Michael C. Knorz, MD

Cataract surgery after corneal transplant must minimize endothelial cell damage because postoperative transplant cell counts are lower than those of normal corneas. As the femtosecond laser was successfully introduced in cataract surgery,[1,2] we applied this technology in an eye that had a previous penetrating corneal transplant.

A 33-year-old man had a 7.0-mm diameter penetrating keratoplasty in his right eye 6 years prior to presentation. He later developed posterior polar cataract. The cornea was clear and corrected distance visual acuity (CDVA) was 20/40. Femtosecond laser–assisted cataract surgery (Alcon LenSx, Aliso Viejo, California) was performed as described previously.[1,2] The corneal scar was peripheral to the planned capsulotomy. Centration was assessed using the pupillary edge. A 4.8-mm capsulorrhexis was performed with the femtosecond laser and the nucleus was liquefied.

Corneal wounds were created with a 2.8-mm and 15° blade so as not to interfere with the transplant scar. The anterior chamber was filled with viscoelastic material, and the edge of the capsulorrhexis was identified with a cystotome and removed with a capsulorrhexis forceps. After hydrodissection, the lens nucleus and cortex were aspirated with the irrigation-aspiration handpiece. A +12.00-diopter (D) hydrophobic acrylic posterior chamber intraocular lens (Acrysof; Alcon Laboratories Inc, Ft Worth, Texas) was implanted in the capsular bag.

On postoperative day 1, CDVA was 20/200 because of slight corneal edema, which improved to 20/25 over the next 3 months. Subjective refraction was stable at +1.25 D sphere and −6.00 D cylinder at 1-year follow-up, with CDVA of 20/20. Corneal thickness measured with a Scheimpflug camera (Pentacam HR; Oculus Optikgeräte GmbH, Wetzlar, Germany) was 609 μm preoperatively and 598 μm 1 month postoperatively.

We report the first patient having successful laser refractive cataract surgery after penetrating keratoplasty. The curved interface aligned perfectly along the transplanted and donor cornea. Optical coherence tomography identified the scar line of the transplant and the scar did not interfere with the laser capsulotomy. The corneal incisions were created manually because of the peripheral localization of the transplant scar.

As reported previously,[1] the use of a femtosecond laser may minimize the ultrasound energy required to remove the nucleus, thereby preserving endothelial cells in postoperative transplant corneas. Graft failure following phacoemulsification and intraocular lens implantation is reported to be between 3% and 8%.[3,4] Endothelial cell loss related to ultrasound use is usually markedly higher in transplanted corneas than in normal, unoperated eyes.[5] In our case, most likely due to the use of the femtosecond laser to liquefy the nucleus, no ultrasound was required to remove the lens and endothelial cell count did not change up to 1 year after surgery.

References

1. Nagy Z, Takacs A, Filkorn T, Sarayba M. Initial clinical evaluation of an intraocular femtosecond laser in cataract surgery. *J Refract Surg*. 2009;25(12):1053-1060.
2. Nagy ZZ, Kranitz K, Takacs AI, Mihaltz K, Kovacs I, Knorz MC. Comparison of intraocular lens decentration parameters after femtosecond and manual capsulotomies. *J Refract Surg*. 2011;27(8):564-569.
3. Ohguro N, Matsuda M, Kinoshita S. Effects of posterior chamber lens implantation on the endothelium of transplanted corneas. *Br J Ophthalmol*. 1997;81(12):1056-1059.
4. Nagra PK, Rapuano CJ, Laibson PL, Kunimoto DY, Kay M, Cohen EJ. Cataract extraction following penetrating keratoplasty. *Cornea*. 2004;23(4):377-379.
5. Kim EC, Kim MS. A comparison of endothelial cell loss after phacoemulsification in penetrating keratoplasty patients and normal patients. *Cornea*. 2010;29(5):510-515.

doi: 10.3928/1081597x-20121228-01

Originally published in Journal of Refractive Surgery, *January 2013.*

Nagy ZZ, ed. *Femtosecond Laser-Assisted Cataract Surgery: Facts and Results* (p 151).

Femtosecond Laser-Assisted Cataract Surgery in Management of Phacomorphic Glaucoma

Kinga Kránitz, MD; Ágnes Ildikó Takács, MD; Andrea Gyenes, MD; Tamás Filkorn, MD; Róbert Gergely, MD; Illés Kovács, MD, PhD; Zoltán Zsolt Nagy, MD, DSC

Abstract

PURPOSE: To report the use of femtosecond laser-assisted cataract surgery in management of phacomorphic glaucoma.

METHODS: An 89-year-old patient developed acute phacomorphic glaucoma in her right eye with elevated intraocular pressure (62 mm Hg), shallow anterior chamber, and mature cataract. After conservative antiglaucoma therapy and Nd:YAG iridotomy, femtosecond laser-assisted cataract surgery was performed. A Malyugin ring was implanted for mechanical pupil dilatation and a 4.8-mm capsulorrhexis and lens fragmentation was performed using a femtosecond laser system (Alcon LenSx Inc., Aliso Viejo, CA) followed by in-the-bag intraocular lens implantation.

RESULTS: Intact 4.8-mm capsulorrhexis and successful lens fragmentation could be performed using femtosecond laser. After cataract surgery, the patient's visual acuity increased from hand motions to 0.4 (Snellen 4/10) and the intraocular pressure returned to normal range without antiglaucoma drop therapy.

CONCLUSIONS: The results indicate that femtosecond laser can be successfully used in certain cases of phacomorphic glaucoma, even if mechanical pupil dilatation is needed.

[*J Refract Surg.* 2013;29(9):645-648.]

Originally published in Journal of Refractive Surgery, *September 2013.*

Phacomorphic glaucoma can cause secondary angle-closure glaucoma due to increased lens thickness (advanced cataract, rapidly intumescent lens, or traumatic cataract) that narrows the iridoconeal angle via either a pupillary block or the forward displacement of the lens–iris diaphragm. Sudden rise in intraocular pressure can lead to irreversible visual loss in the affected eye.[1,2] Femtosecond laser-assisted cataract surgery has been used effectively for routine cases[3-5] and for traumatic cataracts.[6] Herein we report the effective use of this technology for managing phacomorphic glaucoma with a mature lens.

Surgical Technique

An 89-year-old woman was referred to the Ophthalmology Department of Semmelweis University, Budapest, Hungary, from a regional hospital due to acute angle-closure glaucoma with high intraocular pressure (62 mm Hg) in January 2013 after administration of conservative antiglaucoma therapy (pilocarpin, timolol, and dorzolamide eye drops supplemented with systemic carbonic anhydrase inhibitor acetazolamide). She had felt pain in her right eye for 3 days.

Slit-lamp biomicroscopy, applanation tonometry, gonioscopy, optical biometry, Scheimpflug imaging, and B-scan ultrasound examinations were performed on admission. Visual acuity was hand motions in the right eye and 0.2 (Snellen 4/20) in the left eye. Slit-lamp examination of the anterior segment showed significantly injected conjunctiva, mycrocystic and stromal corneal edema, and extremely shallow anterior chamber. The pupil was miotic due to previously applied parasympathomymetic eye drops. The intraocular pressure

doi:10.3928/1081597X-20130611-02

Nagy ZZ, ed. *Femtosecond Laser-Assisted Cataract Surgery: Facts and Results* (pp 153-156).

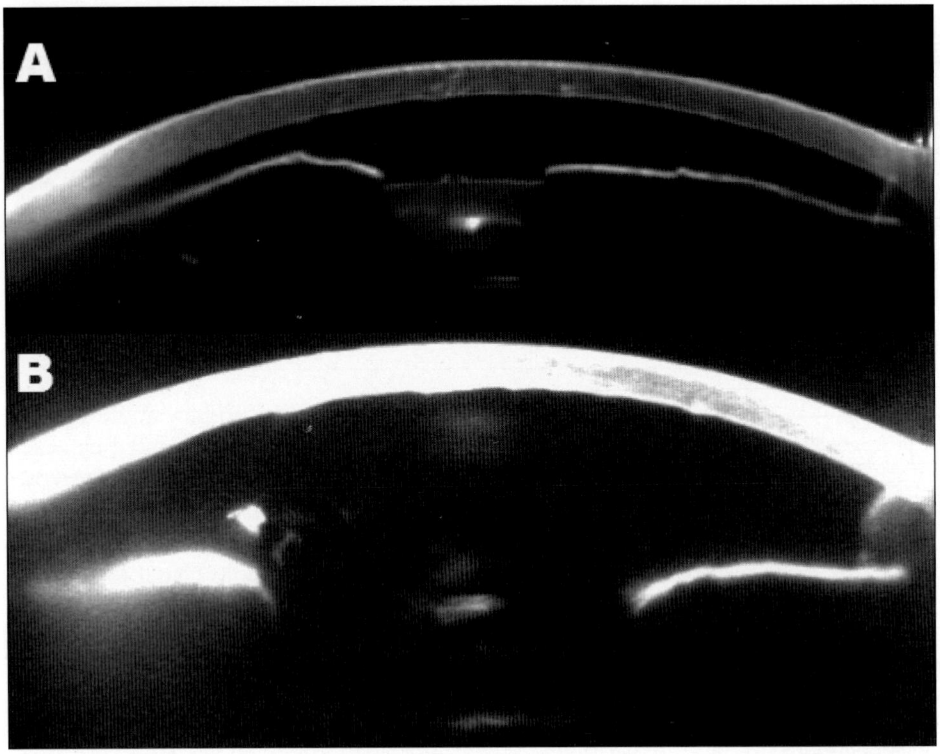

Figure 1. Scheimpflug-imaging. (A) Corneal edema, shallow anterior chamber, narrow chamber angle, and mature cataract preoperatively. (B) Deeper anterior chamber and wider chamber angle postoperatively.

was 40 mm Hg measured with Goldmann applanation tonometry. Closed anterior chamber angle was found in the superior and inferior quadrants with gonioscopy.

After Nd:YAG iridotomy and application of local antiglaucoma therapy, intraocular pressure decreased, ranging from 18 to 27 mm Hg, during the following days. The visual acuity increased to 0.4 (Snellen 4/10).

The extremely shallow anterior chamber and mature cataract supported the diagnosis of phacomorphic glaucoma previously suspected by Scheimpflug camera (Pentacam; Oculus Optikgeräte GmbH, Wetzlar, Germany) and optical biometry (Lenstar; Haag-Streit, Mason, OH) results (central corneal thickness: 703 μm, anterior chamber depth: 1.19 mm from endothelial layer to anterior lens surface) and lens thickness of 5.31 mm with an axial length of 20.33 mm (**Figure 1A**).

Considering the anterior chamber anatomical characteristics and lens thickness, femtosecond-laser assisted cataract surgery was performed to ensure the creation of intact capsulorrhexis on a tensioned lens capsule of a mature cataract.

Clear corneal incisions were created and a Malyugin ring was implanted for mechanical pupil dilation after lens capsule staining (methylene blue). After implantation of the Malyugin ring, the viscoelastic material was removed and the anterior chamber was filled with balanced salt solution. The corneal tunnel was sutured before docking the patient interface of the femtosecond laser system (**Figure 2A**).

The anterior crystalline lens surface was identified with an integrated optical coherence tomography imaging system. A 4.8-mm diameter capsulotomy was performed by scanning a cylindrical pattern starting 300 μm below the anterior capsule and ending at 300 μm above the capsule. Capsulotomy was followed by lens fragmentation (**Figure 2B**).

After femtosecond laser pretreatment, the corneal suture was removed. The anterior chamber was filled with viscoelastic material using a soft-shell technique applying Viscoat and Provisc (Alcon Laboratories, Inc., Fort Worth, TX). The free-floating stained capsulotomy was removed with a rhexis forceps while prefragmented lens quadrants were removed with phacoemulsification using the Infiniti Vision System (Alcon Laboratories, Inc.). Total phacoemulsification time was 67.2 seconds and phacoemulsification energy was 25%.

An Acrysof MA60AC (Alcon Laboratories, Inc.) hydrophobic intraocular lens was injected into the capsular bag and the Malyugin ring and viscoelastic material were removed from the anterior and posterior chambers after intraocular lens implantation. At the end of the procedure, 0.1 mL carbachol was injected intracamerally. All incisions were left sutureless (**Figure 2C**).

Within the first 10 days, the patient received a combination of antibiotic and steroid eye drops (dexamethasone and tobramycin). No postoperative complications occurred and no further antiglaucoma therapy was needed.

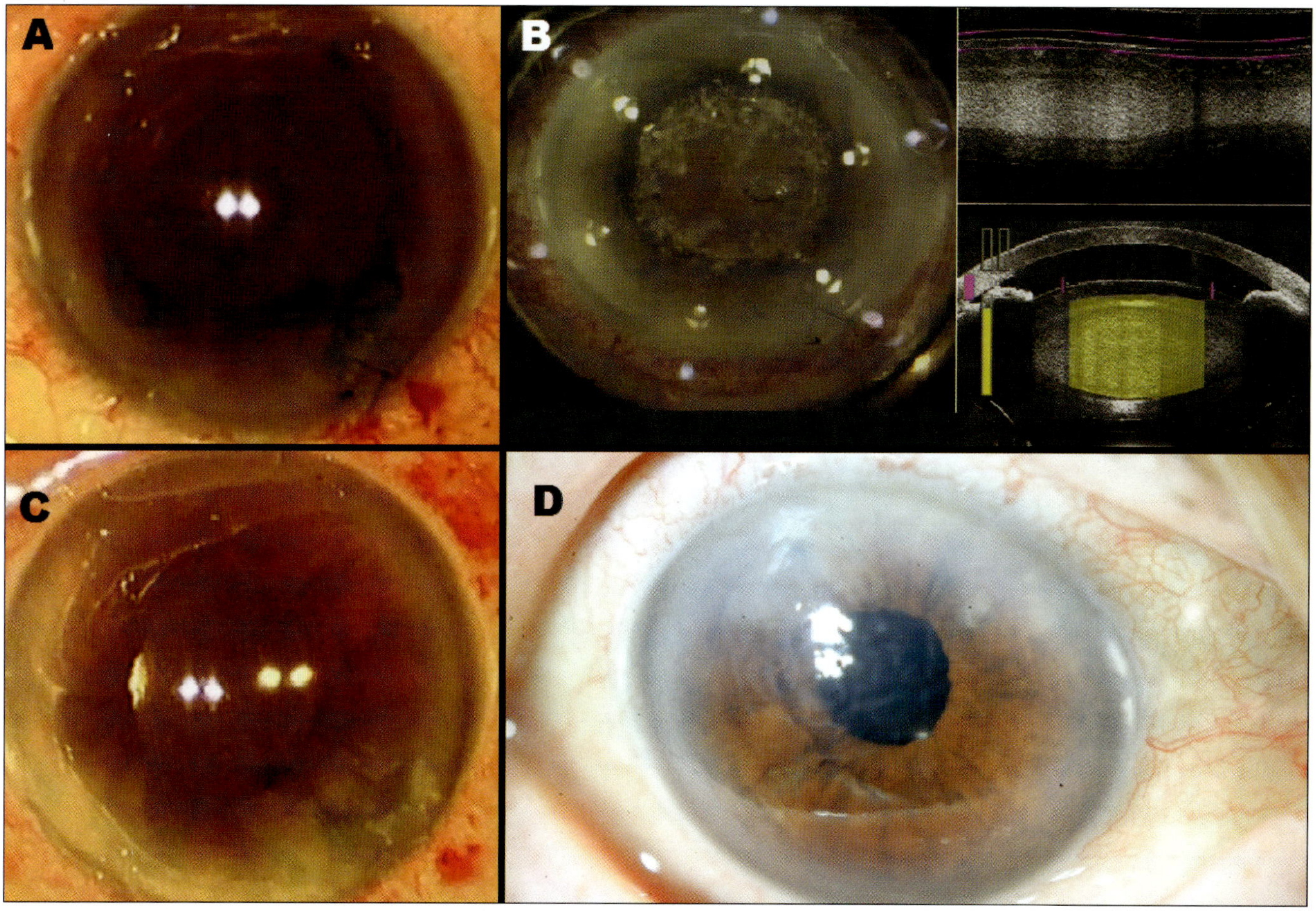

Figure 2. Intraoperative and postoperative state. (A) Clear corneal incisions, stained lens capsule, implanted Malyugin ring, and sutured corneal tunnel can be observed. (B) Femtosecond laser pretreatment: capsulorrhexis and lens fragmentation. (C) At the end of the surgery. (D) Digital photography of the anterior segment 1 week after cataract surgery.

One week after femtosecond laser-assisted cataract surgery, the corrected distance visual acuity was 0.4 (Snellen 4/10) as a result of postoperative corneal edema, which showed gradual improvement in the postoperative period. Intraocular pressure was 18 mm Hg without any concomitant antiglaucoma therapy. Deeper anterior chamber and wider chamber angle were measured using Scheimpflug imaging (**Figures 1B, 2C, and 2D**). The cornea was clear by 20 days postoperatively.

Discussion

Phacoemulsification is associated with smaller incision and less risk of suprachoroidal hemorrhage compared to extracapsular cataract extraction and thus was beneficial for management of phacomorphic glaucoma when possible. The shallow anterior chamber, intumescent cataract, and liquefied lens contents make the continuous curvilinear capsulorrhexis technically challenging and the presence of any corneal edema makes the whole surgical procedure more difficult.[1,2]

Femtosecond laser-assisted cataract surgery offers the possibility of a well-centered complete capsulotomy even in the case of an extremely shallow anterior chamber and intumescent cataract. Prefragmentation of the cataractous lens decreases the energy of the phacoemulsification procedure, reducing postoperative corneal edema.[3]

Proper pupil dilation is essential before femtosecond laser treatment to avoid iris cut. Therefore, the use of mechanical intraocular pupil dilators is recommended in the case of small pupils. According to our experience, implantation of a Malyugin ring is a safe method but the corneal wound needs to be sutured before docking the patient interface of the femtosecond laser.

Our results indicate that a femtosecond laser can be used successfully in certain instances of phacomorphic glaucoma, even if mechanical pupil dilatation is needed.

Author Contributions

Study concept and design (IK, KK, ZZN); data collection (AG, RG, IK, KK, ZZN, ÁIT); analysis and interpretation of data (TF, RG, IK, KK); drafting of the manuscript (IK, ZZN); critical revision of the manuscript (AG, TF, IK, KK, ZZN, ÁIT); statistical expertise (IK); administrative, technical, or material support (AG, KK, ZZN, ÁIT); supervision (RG, KK, ZZN)

References

1. Bhartiya S, Kumar MHM, Jain M. Phacomorphic glaucoma: evolving management strategies. *Journal of Current Glaucoma Practice.* 2009;3:39-46.
2. Lee JW, Lai JS, Yick DW, Tse RK. Retrospective case series on the long-term visual and intraocular pressure outcomes of phacomorphic glaucoma. *Eye (Lond).* 2010;24:1675-1680.
3. Nagy Z, Takacs A, Filkorn T, Sarayba M. Initial clinical evaluation of an intraocular femtosecond laser in cataract surgery. *J Refract Surg.* 2009;25:1053-1060.
4. Roberts TV, Lawless M, Bali SJ, Hodge C, Sutton G. Surgical outcomes and safety of femtosecond laser cataract surgery: a prospective study of 1500 consecutive cases. *Ophthalmology.* 2013;120:227-233.
5. Conrad-Hengerer I, Hengerer FH, Schultz T, Dick HB. Effect of femtosecond laser fragmentation on effective phacoemulsification time in cataract surgery. *J Refract Surg.* 2012;28:879-883.
6. Nagy ZZ, Kránitz K, Takacs A, Filkorn T, Gergely R, Knorz MC. Intraocular femtosecond laser use in traumatic cataracts following penetrating and blunt trauma. *J Refract Surg.* 2012;28:151-153.

Index